Program Evaluation
in the Health Fields

Social Problems Series

SHELDON R. ROEN, Columbia University, *Editor*

Program Evaluation in the Health Fields:
A Book of Selected Readings

Edited by HERBERT C. SCHULBERG, Ph.D.,
ALAN SHELDON, M.D., and FRANK BAKER, Ph.D.

Psychiatric Disorder and the Urban Environment:
A Cornell Social Science Seminar Book

Edited by BERTON H. KAPLAN, Ph.D., in collaboration with ALEXANDER H.
LEIGHTON, M.D., JANE MURPHY, Ph.D., and NICHOLAS FREYBERG, Ph.D.

Research, Planning, and Action for the Elderly:
The Power and Potential of Social Science

DONALD KENT, Ph.D., ROBERT KASTENBAUM, Ph.D., and SILVIA SHERWOOD, Ph.D.

Crisis of Family Disorganization
Edited by ELEANOR PAVENSTEDT, M.D. and VIOLA W. BERNARD, M.D.

Program Evaluation in the Health Fields

edited by

HERBERT C. SCHULBERG, Ph.D.
ALAN SHELDON, M.D.
FRANK BAKER, Ph.D.

Harvard Medical School
Boston, Massachusetts

Behavioral Publications
New York, N.Y.

Contents

Contributors

STIG ANDERSEN, M.A. Resident Representative, United Nations Development Programme, Algiers, Algeria. Formerly Senior WHO Officer, National Tuberculosis Institute, Bangalore, India.

ANITA K. BAHN, Sc.D. Associate Professor of Biostatistics, Department of Preventive Medicine, Women's Medical College, Philadelphia, Formerly Chief, Outpatient Studies Section, Biometrics Branch, National Institute of Mental Health, Chevy Chase, Md.

MAUDE BAILEY, R.N., M.A. Director, Public Health Nursing, South Carolina State Board of Health, Columbia, S. C.

FRANK BAKER, Ph.D. Lecturer in Psychology, Department of Psychiatry, Harvard Medical School, Boston, Mass.

BERNARD J. BERGEN, Ph.D. Associate Professor, Department of Psychiatry, Dartmouth Medical School, Hanover, N. H.

DAVID G. BERGER, Ph.D. Research Director, Community Mental Health Center, Temple University, Philadelphia, Pa. Formerly Research Coordinator, State of Oregon Department of Mental Health, Salem, Oregon.

DONALD T. CAMPBELL, Ph.D. Professor, Department of Psychology, Northwestern University, Evanston, Ill.

ANTONIO CIOCCO, Sc.D. Professor, Department of Biostatistics, Graduate School of Public Health, University of Pittsburgh, Pittsburgh, Pa.

EDWARD COHART, M.D. Professor of Public Health, School of Public Health, Yale University, New Haven, Conn.

O. LYNN DENISTON, M.P.H. Research Associate and Lecturer in Public Health Administration, Department of Community Health Services, University of Michigan School of Public Health, Ann Arbor, Mich.

PAUL M. DENSEN, Sc.D. Professor of Community Health, Harvard School of Public Health, Boston, Mass. Formerly Deputy Commissioner and Director, Office of Program Planning, Research, and Evaluation, New York City Department of Health.

AVEDIS DONABEDIAN, M.D. Professor of Medical Care Organization, University of Michigan School of Public Health, Ann Arbor, Mich.

JOSEPH W. EATON, Ph.D. Professor of Social Work Research, Sociology and Economic and Social Development, University of Pittsburgh, Pa.

H. S. ELWOOD, Research Assistant, Boston Poison Information Center, Boston, Mass.

AMITAI ETZIONI, Ph.D. Professor, Department of Sociology, Columbia University, New York, N. Y.

ANDREW C. FLECK, M.D. First Deputy Commissioner, New York State Department of Health, Albany, N. Y.

HOWARD E. FREEMAN, Ph.D. Professor of Social Research, Florence Heller Graduate School for Advanced Studies in Social Welfare, Brandeis University, Waltham, Mass.

ELMER A. GARDNER, M.D. Professor of Psychiatry, Temple University Health Sciences Center, and Director, Community Mental Health Center, Philadelphia, Pa.

VLADO A. GETTING, M.D., Dr. P.H. Professor of Public Health Administration, Department of Community Health Services, University of Michigan School of Public Health, Ann Arbor, Mich.

JOSEPH GORDON, B.S. Director, Bureau of Health Information, City Department of Health, Baltimore, Md.

JOANNA F. GORMAN, M.S.S.W. Lecturer in Public Health and Social Welfare, School of Social Welfare, University of California, Berkeley, Calif.

LEE GUREL, Ph.D. Director, Program Evaluation Staff, Department of Medicine and Surgery, Veterans Administration, Washington, D. C.

ROBERT J. HAGGERTY, M.D. Professor, Department of Pediatrics, University of Rochester School of Medicine and Dentistry, Rochester, N. Y. Formerly Executive Secretary, Boston Poison Information Center and Associate in Pediatrics, Harvard Medical School, Boston, Mass.

HAROLD P. HALPERT, Dr. P.H. Chief, Systems Research Section, Applied Research Branch, National Institute of Mental Health, Chevy Chase, Md.

G. HALSEY HUNT, M.D. Executive Director, Educational Council for Foreign Medical Graduates, Philadelphia, Pa. Formerly Chief, Division of General Medical Sciences, National Institutes of Health, Bethesda, Md.

GEORGE B. HUTCHISON, M.D., M.P.H. Staff Member, Michael Reese Hospital and Research Institute, Chicago, Ill. Formerly of the Division of Research and Statistics, Health Insurance Plan of Greater New York and Harvard School of Public Health.

HOWARD P. IKER, Ph.D. Research Assistant Professor in Psychology, Department of Psychiatry, University of Rochester School of Medicine and Dentistry, Rochester, N. Y.

GEORGE JAMES, M.D., M.P.H. Dean, Mount Sinai School of Medicine, New York, N. Y. Formerly Commissioner, New York City Department of Health.

ANDIE L. KNUTSON, Ph.D. Professor, School of Public Health, University of California, Berkeley, Calif.

THEODORE LANDSMAN, Ph.D. Professor of Education, College of Education, University of Florida, Gainesville, Fla.

PAUL V. LEMKAU, M.D. Professor of Mental Hygiene, School of Hygiene and Public Health, Johns Hopkins University, Baltimore, Md.

BRIAN MACMAHON, M.D., Ph.D. Professor, Department of Epidemiology, Harvard School of Public Health, Boston, Mass.

KENNETH M. McCAFFREE, Ph.D. Professor, Department of Economics, University of Washington, Seattle, Wash.

JOSEPH E. McGRATH, Ph.D. Professor, Psychology Department, University of Illinois, Urbana, Ill.

HERBERT MENZEL, Ph.D. Professor, Department of Sociology, New York University, New York, N. Y.

HAROLD C. MILES, M.D., M.P.H. Clinical Assistant Professor of Psychiatry, School of Medicine and Dentistry, University of Rochester, Rochester, N. Y.

MARY MONK, Ph.D. Associate Professor, Department of Environmental Medicine and Community Health, Downstate Medical Center, State University of New York, Brooklyn, N. Y.

JOHN S. NEILL, M.D., M.P.H. Director, Hillsborough County Health Department, Tampa, Fla.

TRAVIS J. NORTHCUTT, Ph.D., M.P.H. Associate Professor of Sociology and Research Associate in the Institute for Social Research, Florida State University, Tallahassee, Fla. Formerly Social Scientist, Bureau of Mental Health, Florida State Board of Health, Jacksonville, Fla.

MAURICE E. ODOROFF, M.A. Assistant Professor, Community Medicine and International Health, Georgetown University School of Medicine, and Associate Coordinator, Metropolitan Washington Regional Medical Program, Georgetown University Medical Center, Washington, D. C.

THOMAS F. PUGH, M.D., M.P.H. Associate Professor, Department of Epidemiology, Harvard School of Public Health, Boston, Mass.

CHARLES E. RICE, Ph.D. Associate Professor, Department of Psychology, George Washington University, Washington, D. C. Formerly Research Psychologist, Veterans Administration Hospital, Perry Point, Md.

GEORGE L. ROBB, M.D. Assistant in Medicine, Children's Hospital Medical Center, Boston, Mass.

DANIEL D. ROMAN, Ph.D. Professor of Management, School of Government and Business Administration, George Washington University, Washington, D. C.

JOHN ROMANO, M.D. Distinguished University Professor of Psychiatry, and Chairman of the Department, University of Rochester School of Medicine and Dentistry, Rochester, N. Y.

IRWIN M. ROSENSTOCK, Ph.D. Professor of Public Health Administration, Department of Community Health Services, University of Michigan School of Public Health, Ann Arbor, Mich.

HERBERT C. SCHULBERG, Ph.D., S.M. in Hyg. Assistant Clinical Professor of Psychology, Department of Psychiatry, Harvard Medical School,. Boston, Mass., and Associate Executive Director of United Community Services of Metropolitan Boston.

ROBERT E. SERFLING, Ph.D. Chairman, Department of Biostatistics, Tulane University Medical School, New Orleans, La. Formerly Chief, Statistics Section, Epidemiology Branch, Communicable Disease Center, Public Health Service, Atlanta, Ga.

LEE G. SEWALL, M.D. Clinical Professor of Psychiatry, University of Arkansas Medical Center, and Director. Arkansas State Community Mental Health Services, Little Rock, Arkansas.

ALAN SHELDON, M.A., M.B.B., D.P.M., S.M. in Hyg. Assistant Professor, Department of Psychiatry, Harvard Medical School, Boston, Mass.

MINDEL C. SHEPS, M.D., M.P.H. Professor of Biostatistics, School of Public Health, University of North Carolina, Chapel Hill, N. C. Formerly at Department of Preventive Medicine, Harvard Medical School, Boston, Mass.

IDA L. SHERMAN, M.S. Acting Chief, Statistics Section, Epidemiology Branch, Communicable Disease Center, Public Health Service, Atlanta, Ga.

CLARENCE C. SHERWOOD, Ph.D. Professor, John Jay College, City College of New York, N. Y. Formerly Research Director, Action for Boston Community Development, Boston, Mass.

MATTHEW TAYBACK, Sc.D. Assistant Secretary of Health and Mental Hygiene and Scientific Affairs, Baltimore City Health Department, Baltimore, Md.

LEONARD P. ULLMANN, Ph.D. Associate Professor, Department of Psychology, University of Illinois, Urbana, Ill.

CHARLES M. WYLIE, M.D., Dr. P.H. Professor of Public Health Administration, Department of Community Health Service, University of Michigan School of Public Health, Ann Arbor, Mich. Formerly Assistant Professor of Public Health Administration, School of Hygiene and Public Health, Johns Hopkins University, Baltimore, Md.

Acknowledgments

Section I

James, George. Evaluation in Public Health Practice.
  Reprinted by permission of the author and the American Public Health Association from Am. J. Publ. Hlth. 52: 1145-1154, 1962.

Knutson, A. L. Evaluation for What?
  Reprinted by permission of the author from the Proceedings of the Regional Institute on Neurologically Handicapping Conditions in Children held at the University of California, Berkeley, June 18-23, 1961.

MacMahon, Brian; Pugh, Thomas F.; and Hutchison, George B. Principles in the Evaluation of Community Mental Health Programs.
  Reprinted by permission of the authors and the American Public Health Association from Am. J. Publ. Hlth. 51: 963-968, 1961.

Hutchison, G. B. Evaluation of Preventive Services.
  Reprinted by permission of the author and the publisher from J. Chronic Dis. 11: 497-508, 1960.

Freeman, Howard E., and Sherwood, Clarence C. Research in Large-Scale Intervention Programs.
  Reprinted by permission of the authors and the Society for the Psychological Study of Social Issues from J. Soc. Issues, 21 (1): 11-28, 1965.

Fleck, Andrew C. Evaluation Research Programs in Public Health Practice.
  Reprinted by permission of the author and the publisher from Ann. N. Y. Academy of Sciences, 107: 717-724, 1963.

Etzioni, Amitai. Two Approaches to Organizational Analysis: A Critique and a Suggestion.
  Reprinted by permission of the author and the publisher from Admin. Sci. Quart. 5: 257-278, 1960.

Bergen, B. J. Professional Communities and the Evaluation of Demonstration Projects in Community Mental Health.
  Reprinted by permission of the author and the American Public Health Association from Am. J. Publ. Hlth. 55: 1057-1066, 1965.

Section II

McGrath, Joseph E. Toward a "Theory of Method" for Research on Organizations.
  Reprinted by permission of the author and the publisher from W. W. Cooper; H. J. Leavitt; and M. W. Shelly II (Eds.), New Perspectives in Organizational Research. New York: John Wiley, 1964, pp. 533-556.

Campbell, Donald T. Factors Relevant to the Validity of Experiments in Social
    Settings.
    Reprinted by permission of the author and the American Psychological Association
from Psych. Bull. 54: 297-312, 1957.

Donabedian, Avedis. Evaluating the Quality of Medical Care
    Reprinted by permission of the author and the publisher from the Milbank Memor-
ial Fund Quarterly, 44: 166-203, 1966.

Deniston, O. L.; Rosenstock, I. M.; and Getting, V. A. Evaluation of Program Effec-
    tiveness.
    Reprinted by permission of the authors and the publisher from Publ. Hlth. Rep.
83: 323-335, 1968.

Section III

Roman, Daniel D. The PERT System: An Appraisal of Program Evaluation Re-
    view Technique.
    Reprinted by permission of the author and the publisher from J. Acad. Man. 5:
57-65, 1962.

Andersen, Stig. Operations Research in Public Health.
    Reprinted by permission of the author and the publisher from Publ. Hlth. Rep.
79: 297-305, 1964.

Ciocco, Antonio. On Indices for the Appraisal of Health Department Activities.
    Reprinted by permission of the author and the publisher from J. Chronic Dis.
11: 509-522. 1960.

Rice, Charles E.; Berger, David G.; Sewall, Lee G.; and Lemkau, Paul V. Measuring
    Social Restoration Performance of Public Psychiatric Hospitals.
    Reprinted by permission of the authors and the publisher from Publ. Hlth. Rep.
76: 437-446, 1961.

Gardner, Elmer A.; Miles, Harold C.; Iker, Howard P.; and Romano, John. A Cum-
    ulative Register of Psychiatric Services in a Community.
    Reprinted by permission of the authors and the American Public Health Associa-
tion from Am. J. Publ. Hlth. 53: 1269-1277, 1963.

Section IV

Bailey, Maude Conway. Evaluation of Public Health Nursing Services Through a
    Study of Patient Progress.
    Reprinted by permission of the author and the American Public Health Association
from Am. J. Publ. Hlth. 55: 892-900, 1965.

Monk, Mary; Tayback, Matthew; and Gordon, Joseph. Evaluation of an Antismoking
    Program among High School Students.
    Reprinted by permission of the authors and the American Public Health Associa-
tion from Am. J. Publ. Hlth. 55: 994-1004, 1965.

Serfling, Robert E., and Sherman, Ida L. Survey Evaluation of Three Poliomyelitis Immunization Campaigns.
Reprinted by permission of the authors and the publisher from Publ. Hlth. Rep. 78: 413-418, 1963.

Robb, G. L.; Elwood, H. S.; and Haggerty, R. J. Evaluation of a Poison Center.
Reprinted by permission of the authors and the American Public Health Association from Am. J. Publ. Hlth. 53: 1751-1760, 1963.

Wylie, Charles M. Use of Death Rates in Evaluating Multiple Screening.
Reprinted by permission of the author and the publisher from Publ. Hlth. Rep. 76: 1111-1116, 1961.

Hunt, G. Halsey, and Odoroff, Maurice E. Followup Study of Narcotic Drug Addicts After Hospitalization.
Reprinted by permission of the authors and the publisher from Publ. Hlth. Rep. 77: 41-54, 1962.

Gardner, Elmer A.; Bahn, Anita K.; and Miles, Harold C. Patient Experience in Psychiatric Units of General and State Mental Hospitals.
Reprinted by permission of the author and the publisher from Publ. Hlth. Rep. 79: 755-767, 1964.

Ullmann, Leonard P., and Gurel, Lee. Size, Staffing, and Psychiatric Hospital Effectiveness.
Reprinted by permission of the author and the American Medical Association from Arch. Gen. Psychiat. 11: 360-367, 1964.

McCaffree, Kenneth M. The Cost of Mental Health Care Under Changing Treatment Methods.
Reprinted by permission of the author and the American Public Health Association from Am. J. Publ. Hlth. 56: 1013-1025, 1966.

Northcutt, Travis J.; Landsman, Theodore; Neill, John S.; and Gorman, Joanna F. Rehabilitation of Former Mental Patients: An Evaluation of a Coordinated Community Aftercare Program.
Reprinted by permission of the authors and the American Public Health Association from Am. J. Publ. Hlth. 55: 570-577, 1965.

Section V

Menzel, Herbert. Scientific Communication: Five Themes From Social Science Research.
Reprinted by permission of the author and the American Psyhological Association from Am. Psychol. 21: 999-1004, 1966.

Halpert, Harold P. Communications as a Basic Tool in Promoting Utilization of Research Findings.
Reprinted by permission of the author and the publisher from Com. Ment. Hlth. J. 2: 231-236, 1966.

Eaton, Joseph W. Symbolic and Substantive Evaluative Research.
Reprinted by permission of the author and the publisher from Admin. Sci. Quart. 6: 421-442, 1962.

Densen, Paul M.; James, George; and Cohart, Edward. Research, Program Planning, and Evaluation.
  Reprinted by permission of the author and the publisher from Publ. Hlth. Rep. 81: 49-56, 1966.

Gardner, Elmer A. The Use of a Psychiatric Case Register in the Planning and Evaluation of a Mental Health Program.
  Reprinted by permission of the author and the publisher from R. Monroe, G. Klee, and E. Brody (Eds.), Psychiatric Epidemiology and Mental Health Planning. Washington: American Psychiatric Association, 1967, pp. 259-281.

Schulberg, Herbert C., and Baker, Frank. Program Evaluation Models and the Implementation of Research Findings.
  Reprinted by permission of the authors and the American Public Health Association from Am. J. Publ. Hlth. 58: 1248-1255, 1968.

Preface

THE need for a single volume bringing together materials relevant to the evaluation of health programs has long been evident. In spite of the burgeoning interest in this field, no comprehensive reference has yet been assembled for the researcher or administrator concerned with the numerous issues raised in the evaluation of existing or new programs. This work grew from the Editors' experiences in trying to evaluate the changing nature of health programs and in teaching this topic to students. While attempting to teach program evaluation, we have been impressed by the need to first gently disillusion the naive student who expects to have a magically succinct evaluation technique presented to him, before proceeding with a careful elaboration of what current conceptions of evaluation can and cannot accomplish. It is unclear how much of the current emphasis upon evaluation stems from the practical needs of legislators and granting agencies and how much emerges from the implicit promises of researchers. What is clear, though, is that this emphasis will quickly subside and join a long list of previous false panaceas unless some clear, realistic concepts and methodologies for evaluation are developed.

In assembling almost three dozen papers which bear upon the evaluation of health programs, we have tried to select those materials which could meet the needs of both researchers and program directors. It is our firm conviction that in spite of the well-known differences in orientation and priorities which these two groups frequently exhibit, nevertheless there exists a wide span of common concern which needs only to be properly plumbed. To capitalize upon the mutual interests of researchers and practitioners and to demonstrate opportunities for fruitful collaboration, we have emphasized papers of potential interest to both groups and avoided selections which were overly skewed toward the needs of only one of them. Many other sources are available for the study of program development or research methodology but this volume differs in its attempt to integrate what generally have been dichotomous fields of interest.

In addition to informing the administrator about some of the complexities and difficulties in program evaluation, and hopefully helping him to make realistic judgments about his own needs, the selected readings also are intended to raise questions for the researcher by indicating gaps in our concepts and techniques so that he may strive to develop appropriate solutions. The book should have an academic use as well, and prove to be particularly valuable as a source of reading for courses offered in schools of public health or social welfare on social-research techniques applied to problems of health program planning and evaluation.

The preparation of this book was supported by NIMH Research Grant MH-09214 to the Laboratory of Community Psychiatry, Harvard Medical School, and we would like to thank Dr. Gerald Caplan for his encouragement and assistance. Particular appreciation is due our research assistants, Mrs. Tema Halpern and Miss Rachel Glass, for their conscientious efforts in performing necessary editorial tasks, and our secretary, Mrs. Rose Marie Toon, for her typing of the manuscript.

HERBERT C. SCHULBERG, Ph.D.
ALAN SHELDON, M.D.
FRANK BAKER, Ph.D.

Section I

Concepts and General Issues

1

Introduction

HERBERT C. SCHULBERG, ALAN SHELDON, and FRANK BAKER

INTEREST in program evaluation is a relatively recent development and, although various efforts date back many decades, widespread concern for information about health program effectiveness can be considered essentially a post-World War II phenomenon. The literature in this field continues to grow and increasingly sophisticated overviews have been prepared by the US Public Health Service,[1] Herzog,[2] Bloom,[3] and Suchman.[4] Concern with evaluation has been building to a rapid crescendo and has even evolved to a point where serious Congressional attention is being given to the formulation of national social indicators for assessing the status of Great Society programs.[5]

There are numerous reasons for this recent surge of interest and they include pressures from within the health field, as well as forces at play on the greater social scene. The health professional's quest for data about program effectiveness is part of a widespread effort to impose internal quality controls. As a result, we have moved from narrow inquiries about the success or failure of given procedures with individual patients to broader concern for the efficacy of programs with large population groups.

The most significant feature of the recent interest in program evaluation, however, is the fact that it is no longer professionals alone who are asking what hitherto had been academic questions about the outcome of their efforts. Equal, if not greater, interest in program effectiveness is being displayed by legislators and executives preoccupied with expanded demands upon limited tax funds and it is from this quarter that the most pertinent and difficult questions are being posed. The exponential growth of Federal funding and participation in social action programs, particularly for health services, certainly has been a major stimulus for greater governmental concern but there are other bases for this as well. The long-standing American belief that any program can be successful if its budget is expanded is being questioned more and more, while disillusionment is being

3

expressed with the competing technologies and programs proposed by professionals. Greenberg and Mattison[6] have noted that a tone of skepticism, characterized by an attitude of healthy questioning, pervades many traditional activities. The motives and ideologies of such long-standing institutions as the clergy, business, education, and government have all been subjected to close scrutiny in recent years.

We will soon be at the point of finally having to indicate whether inquiries about health program effectiveness can be answered with a minimum of obfuscation, or whether program evaluation is so complex that assessment attempts only produce overly simplistic formulations. If health professionals decide that the latter response is most appropriate, we must be prepared to accept as a consequence the fact that nonprofessional observers will determine program effectiveness and set priorities. Although this option has certain genuine merits, we would contend that it has an equal number of drawbacks, since the abandonment of professional responsibility for program evaluation can ultimately be profoundly harmful. We cannot legitimately expect legislators and administrators to fully appreciate the complexities of our endeavors. Their assessment criteria perforce must be different from our own, and their decisions are often based upon pragmatic as well as scientific factors. Accepting the professional's responsibility for actively participating in the assessment of his efforts, let us proceed to consider some of the variables implicit in the concept of evaluation. What questions should the health professional pose, what methodological procedures should he undertake, and how can he use his findings most effectively?

In reviewing the variety of papers which could have been selected to answer these questions, we have been impressed by several striking paradoxes which can be taken as a direct reflection of the current status of program evaluation in the health fields. First, program evaluation has by now assumed a secure position in the ranks of those deities to whom we pay homage and obeisance, and yet we blithely ignore its teachings and injunctions. Second, the administrator's desire to have his program evaluated has a potent initial quality and yet research efforts frequently limp to a sterile halt. Third, the methodological procedures for evaluating a health program are in many ways similar to those of any other research effort, and yet it is often impossible to develop a practical design for this type of study. Fourth, the potential programmatic implications of evaluative findings can be much more direct and specific than those from other types of research, and yet the results of these studies generally remain shrouded in confusion and mystery.

The reasons for these paradoxes are diverse but interrelated, and carry many implications for the future of this field. This introductory chapter, following the outline of the book, reviews the major outstanding issues and points to the manner in which the papers included in each section reflect upon them.

Concept of Program Evaluation

It has been wryly observed that the popularity of program evaluation stems from its ambiguity, and it is not surprising that this term has come to have diverse implications among researchers and administrators in view of its numerous connotations and the wide-ranging motivation of participants in such studies. Some of the differences in regard to the meaning of "evaluation" are conceptually significant while others simply produce unnecessary confusion. Before proceeding, however, with an analysis of how we view evaluation, it is equally necessary to comment on the diversity of opinions regarding the nature of a health "program." In the field of organizational study, programs generally are defined as a set of activities occuring within a social enterprise which have specific inputs of resources and conditions, certain ways of organizing and processing these resources and conditions, techniques for establishing relations among them, and certain outputs which can be evaluated against given standards. Additionally, aspects of the organization's patterned activities occur not only within its own structure but also in relation to other organizations as well.

While difficulties certainly arise in applying this definition of "program" to industrial activities, they are of a relatively minor nature when compared to the complexities encountered in the health field. It is the unusual health activity which has clearly delineated its scope of concern and effort along the parameters of this straight-forward definition of "program" and the researcher frequently is required to clarify, or even impute, the nature of the program's characteristics. This problem becomes particularly evident in attempts to define a program's goals and objectives. For the purposes of this book we are subscribing to the foregoing definition of a "program," and our thoughts about program evaluation, including the examples of program evaluation selected for inclusion in Section IV, reflect this approach.

Returning to the issue of how to define evaluation, a frequent starting point for differing conceptions of this term is the relationship between evaluation studies and other types of research. James (Chapter 2) considers program evaluation distinct from other research, since it does not seek new knowledge but attempts instead to mark progress toward prestated objectives. Hutchison (Chapter 5), on the other hand, has noted that evaluative efforts nevertheless require more rigorous methodology than program demonstrations or reviews. While we agree with these general characterizations of evaluation, we must also point to their arbitrariness. The information obtained by assessing a program's ability, or inability, to meet prestated objectives can be useful not only for pragmatic reasons but also for generating new knowledge about the disease entity being treated.

Despite current ambiguity, the most common usage of the term "program evaluation" is thought to be consistent with the American Public Health Association's[7] statement that evaluation is the process of determining the value or amount of success in achieving a predetermined objective. The following four steps are inherent in such a process: formulating the objective; identifying proper criteria to be used in measuring success; determining and explaining the program's degree of success; and recommending further program activity. A most crucial implication emerging from this conception of evaluation is that the researcher's prime focus should be on whether or not the program under study attains a prespecified objective. The point is emphasized because this conception of evaluation presents the researcher with a specific set of hypotheses and suggests the methodology to be employed in studying their validity. Although in reality ample latitude and discretion are actually available to the researcher, evaluation studies stemming from this "goal-attainment" model are necessarily of a different and more restricted nature than those conducted by a researcher on the basis of a "systems model" of evaluation. This latter approach contends that organizations constantly pursue multiple objectives and the effectiveness with which any one goal is attained must be studied in the context of its influence upon the attainment of other goals. Since these two differing conceptions of evaluation are the major ones being utilized at this time, their salient features warrant further consideration in this introduction.

Goal-Attainment Model

Most researchers concerned with program evaluation agree that, although clarification of a program's objectives is one of the most difficult phases in this process, it is also one of the most critical. The emphasis stems from a conception of evaluation as measurement of the degree of success or failure encountered by the program in reaching predetermined objectives. Health programs generally can be viewed as having the ultimate objective of improving health and reducing morbidity and mortality. Such global objectives are too distant and abstract, however, to be used as operational indexes in evaluating a program and so the researcher must seek to evaluate program objectives at a level which is both measurable and relevant. A common alternative, therefore, is to measure a program's success in reaching practical objectives rather than ideal ones. This takes the form of substituting for study a variety of initial and intermediate goals, with the assumption that ultimate ones will be affected if a series of prior accomplishments are fulfilled. The distinctions between varying levels for studying goals are illustrated in MacMahon, Pugh, and Hutchison's (Chapter 4) description of ways for evaluating accomplishment, an ultimate objective, in contrast to procedures for evaluating technique, and intermediate objective. The evaluation of accomplishment is intended to test the hypothesis that a certain practice has a beneficial outcome. The evaluation of technique is concerned with determining whether a specific technique has been performed within specified limits and cause and effect are not directly at issue.

Studies of intermediate objectives are generally easier to carry out but the information thus derived must necessarily be more limited. This evaluation strategy can be justified only when the relationship between intermediate and ultimate objectives already has been demonstrated or will be tested in subsequent studies. Even when the relationship between the different levels of program objectives has been demonstrated, however, Hutchison (Chapter 5) warns that changes may occur over time as a result of technological modifications or changes in the natural course of the disease. Evaluating the extent to which an intermediate objective, such as an immunization program, has been successfully achieved is meaningless if the vaccination no longer provides immunity. In reality, most health programs could never be undertaken if assumptions were not made about the validity of intermediate objectives and James (Chapter 2) emphasizes that, in the absence of facts, the public expects health professionals to use expert opinion.

Accepting the legitimacy and significance of evaluating many objectives other than the ultimate one, the researcher is still confronted with the practical problem of how to select appropriate objectives for study. As a starting point it is essential that he clarify the program director's motivation for seeking an evaluation, since this will affect many aspects of his work. The variety of reasons for undertaking an evaluation have been categorized by Knutson (Chapter 3) as those which are organization oriented and those which are personally oriented. It well behooves the researcher to determine which is paramount in his particular instance so that he may select the relevant sections of the program for study, formulate appropriate validity assumptions, design an adequate methodology and, perhaps most important, gain cooperation from those participating in the program.

Assuming that this condition has been met, evaluation can then be performed at one of a variety of levels which James (Chapter 2) has classified in the following way:

1. Evaluation of effort: how do the practices of the program under study compare with local or national standards? The use of such yardsticks as patient-staff ratios provides a simple but limited assessment of the program's functioning.

2. Evaluation of performance: what outcomes have the program's efforts produced? This approach assumes that services were provided correctly to those individuals helped.

3. Adequacy of performance: to what extent has the community's total problem been solved by this program? Services directed to a minority of individuals are less adequate than those focused upon the total population.

4. Evaluation of efficiency: can the same end result be achieved at lower cost? Screening programs frequently are evaluated in this manner by considering the number of false positives and false negatives produced by them.

In assessing the significance of an evaluation study, considerable difficulty arises from the confusion about different levels of objectives so that the researcher is faced with the dilemma of whether or not to actively participate with the program developer from the very outset in clearly specifying goals. Differences of opinion about this matter exist among researchers and administrators, sometimes depending upon whether the evaluation is to be conducted by an internal or external group, but perhaps the most determined stand is that taken by Freeman and Sherwood (Chapter 6). They contend that if the researcher is going to act responsibly as an agent of social change through his evaluation, then it is mandatory that he personally become involved in the program's development. Freeman and Sherwood argue that the researcher must participate with the administrator in identifying the program's goals, describing its input and output variables, and specifying the relationship between input variables and goals. Once an impact model has been formulated, the researcher should oppose modifications in the program and any of its procedures which potentially could render his evaluation efforts useless.

This conception of evaluation, and the researcher's role in it, exemplifies the goal-attainment model and simultaneously points to many of its problems. While lucidly elaborating the rationale of certain programmatic efforts and ultimate goals, this model, when carefully adhered to, also restricts the program director's flexibility in periodically modifying his services. The well-known frictions between researchers and clinicians described by Andrew[8] and by Bergen in Chapter 9 arise from the differing interests and goals of these two groups, and a program evaluation study is a vehicle par excellence for exacerbating these differences. It should be noted that not all researchers take as firm a position as do Freeman and Sherwood in opposing program modifications during the period of data collection, and some research methodologies actually allow for these changes.

In spite of its limitations, the goal-attainment model of evaluation is the one most commonly used at the present time and almost all of the evaluation examples presented later in this book are based upon this approach. The model presents an easily conceived relationship between a specific service and an ultimate effect, while the methodology to be used in assessing outcome generally is drawn from the well-established designs of researchers.

The Systems Model

An alternative conception of program evaluation can be found in the systems model. This approach warrants considerably more attention from researchers and program administrators than it has obtained thus far, and it is striking that Suchman's[9] otherwise fine overview of program evaluation completely omits any consideration of the systems model. In contrast to the goal-attainment approach which directs evaluation efforts at measuring how well a specific organizational goal was achieved, the systems model contends that such an approach is unproductive and even misleading, since an organization constantly functions at a variety of levels. Even though directing part of its means directly to the goal activities, an organization must simultaneously devote segments of its resources to such other vital functions as maintenance and recruitment.

Etzioni (Chapter 8), who is the foremost proponent of this approach, argues that the starting point for a study of program effectiveness should not be the specific goal or objective but rather a working model of the social unit which is capable of achieving a goal. The systems approach assumes that certain resources must be devoted to vital nongoal activities such as those mentioned previously, and the central question in a study of effectiveness should be: How close does the organization's allocation of resources approach an optimum distribution? What counts, Etzioni emphasizes, is a balanced distribution of resources among all organizational needs and not the maximal satisfaction of any one. Overattention to a specific goal will lead to underconcern for other activities. In terms of the goal-attainment model, the fact that an organization can become less effective by allocating more means to achieve a goal is a paradox, but the systems model recognizes that organizational ineffectiveness may arise by allocating a surfeit of resources as well as by withholding them.

The relevance to the health field of the systems model, and its conception of multipurpose organizations, can be illustrated in a number of ways. First, in addition to improving the health of a target population, the personnel of a health facility generally are also concerned with their own personal growth and the organization's continued development and expansion. Second, the motivation for developing and evaluating an innovative treatment program usually stems from factors related to the needs of a patient population but it also includes the personnel's desire for control of organizational resources and the maintenance of personal influence and status. Third, the teaching hospital's goal of excellent patient care to a total population must compete with its other goal of providing interns and residents with a requisite range of experiences and responsibilities.

The systems model's significance in the evaluation of health programs is also evident in its stress on the fact that evaluation studies themselves necessarily occur within an organizational context. Organizations vary in their degree of receptivity to such research and more serious constraints may be imposed upon study design and data collection by administrative resistance than by the complexities of the clinical program under study. Fleck (Chapter 7) has noted that any formal organization is influenced by two antithetical needs. The first is stability, which requires regular routines, and the second is survival, which necessitates change. The organization primarily emphasizing stability will only tolerate "ritualistic" or "operational" evaluations of its programs. Both of these approaches involve the collection of routine data about technical efficiency but give no insight into the conditions under which operational patterns should be modified. The organization primarily concerned with its other need of survival and interested in modifying routines at all levels, by contrast, requires a "behavioral" evaluation which includes the previous indexes but which also assesses such covert organizational variables as points of resistance and privately held goals. The organizational context of the program is also relevant to the generalization of evaluation findings. For example, a program may be evaluated as effective when operated by the highly motivated and well-trained staff of a teaching hospital but prove to be ineffective under the aegis of less motivated or less trained personnel in a small community hospital.

Having discussed the relevance of the systems model, it is necessary also to point out the drawbacks of this approach to evaluating health programs. The model's major liability is the increased expense and complexity which it imposes upon the researcher and this probably is the major reason why it is not utilized more frequently. In contrast to the goal-attainment model which simply requires that the researcher specify the particular organizational goal which he wishes to study, the systems model requires the evaluator to determine what he considers a highly effective allocation of means and then to study the organization's degree of success in achieving this optimal distribution. To undertake a systems study, the researcher must have considerable knowledge about the varied purposes and operating routines of the organization and the acquisition of such information is often a demanding, tedious process. A larger research staff usually is needed to complete such a study and the research director must be capable of simultaneously overseeing the development and conducting of numerous data collection procedures. The information to be gathered about the program's functioning may be of a qualitative as well as a quantitative nature, and adroit conceptual skills are required in ultimately integrating these diverse assessments.

As we have already indicated, the health field is notably lacking in evaluations which have incorporated the complex concepts and strategies of the systems model. Although industry and business have long been comfortable about engaging in such studies (e.g., Georgopoulos and Tannenbaum[10]), it is only in the past few years that sporadic systems assessments have begun to appear in the health field. The papers by Gardner and his colleagues (Chapters 19, 26, and 34) illustrate the range of uses to which systems data gathered by a psychiatric case register can be applied in the evaluation and planning of community mental health programs, while recent papers by Baker[11] and Schulberg and Baker[12] describe the application of systems concepts to the evaluation of a mental hospital in transition.

Research Designs and Evaluation Indexes

The formulation of a research design and the selection of evaluation indexes should occur within the framework of how one conceptualizes the process of evaluation. The previous discussion has described the different perspectives on this process and we will now proceed to consider the alternative methodological designs which stem from use of either the goal-attainment or the systems model of evaluation. Before proceeding to do so, it would be helpful to consider the variety of general methodological issues pertinent to both approaches.

Research Designs

One of the first questions to confront the program evaluator is that of research design. How loose or how rigorous should it be? Although papers like those by Borgatta,[13] Freeman and Sherwood (Chapter 6), and Deniston, Rosenstock, and Getting (Chapter 13), imply that a rigorous experimental design is the most appropriate one for program evaluation, the variety of legitimate alternatives is actually broader. We would contend that design selection should be related to the degree of knowledge currently available about the program under study. Less rigorous designs can be appropriately employed when ambiguity is great, while more rigorous designs should be utilized as knowledge about relevant variables increases. Many administrators have been reluctant to permit the requirements of rigorous methodology to be imposed upon their fledgling efforts in fear of being overly constrained, and such hesitation is thought to be justified. On the other hand, a well-developed service has far less basis for resisting the imposition of rigorous research procedures and a looser methodological approach for evaluating such a program might indeed be a wasteful effort.

The variety of methodological designs appropriate for program evaluation range from those involving highly realistic field studies to artificial computer simulations based upon mathematical models. An overview of these different approaches is presented by McGrath (Chapter 10) and they can be categorized in the following manner:

1. *Field study investigations* obtain data directly from existing organizations of the kind to which the results will apply and the subjects being studied are operating under usual motivational forces. The field study's rigor varies, since procedures for conducting such an evaluation range from observational, subjective data collection to the systematic objective methods.

2. *Experimental studies* incorporate the classical features of research design, including appropriate subject sampling, the assignment of subjects to experimental and control groups, and control over exposure to the treatment variable. Many general discussions of field experimentation can be found in the program evaluation literature[14-16] and its use is particularly advocated in the goal-attainment model of evaluation. The experimental study theoretically can provide specific evidence that an objective has been achieved and delineations can be made in the measurement of intermediate and ultimate goals.

In reality, however, one is hard pressed to uncover any successfully completed studies of this type in the health field. An obvious reason for this void is the tremendous difficulty encountered in fulfilling the requirements of true experimentation in natural social settings. Certain modifications can be applied, however, and McGrath suggests the use of experimental simulation techniques through which a relatively faithful representation of the program can be created under quasi-laboratory conditions. The simulated program can be set in motion and its operations can be studied as they are expressed in the behavior of humans who are assigned roles within the program.

A more common alternative to the experimental evaluation of real-life programs are the quasi-experimental designs refined by Campbell. These designs permit the researcher to capitalize upon the idiosyncratic aspects of any particular situation in constructing unique tests of causal hypotheses while still considering factors of validity. In Chapter 11, Campbell presents a variety of preexperimental and experimental designs with an indication of how each deals with problems of internal validity, i.e., did in fact the experimental stimulus make a significant difference in this specific instance, and the problem of external validity, i.e., to what populations, settings, and variables can this effect be generalized? The relative strengths and weaknesses of ten quasi-experimental designs are also considered by Campbell,[17] and he comments on the manner in which each handles the challenges of internal and external validity.

3. *Laboratory experiments* constitute refined attempts to abstract appropriate variables from real-life situations by representing them in a more fundamental form. No attempt is made in this methodological approach to recreate reality and instead the emphasis is placed upon analysis of the basic processes which presumably underlie human functioning in a broad range of programmatic settings. In spite of the rigor of this method, its artificial nature has led to little application in the health field.

4. *Computer simulations* are based upon mathematical models and are distinguished from experimental simulations because they are closed or complete models of the program being simulated. All variables, including the dependent or output variables which result from the system's operation, are built into a simulation model and thus it does not involve actual performance by human participants. The increasing availability of large electronic computers has given impetus to the use of simulation models in public health problems and they are particularly applicable to the systems approach.

Each of these four different research designs contains many advantages and disadvantages and the choice of any one for evaluating a health program will depend upon the relative importance of realism, precision of measurement, opportunities for manipulating variables, and other relevant features of the research situation. McGrath considers the different designs to be complementary rather than interchangeable and he presents a series of guidelines in Chapter 10 through which the researcher can make an appropriate rational choice.

Evaluation Indexes

Just as the researcher is confronted with the necessity of choosing an appropriate research design, so must he deliberately select relevant evaluation indexes from the great variety of data potentially available to him. An example of the questions which he must resolve is whether it is valid to use indexes reflecting assumed change rather than direct measures of the desired change. This problem is particularly acute when scores on attitude scales are substituted for measures of overt behavior and it leads to the dilemma of deciding whether a program has achieved its ultimate goal or only an intermediate one. The study by Monk, Tayback, and Gordon (Chapter 21) of attitudes toward smoking and smoking behavior provides a case in point. Despite many complexities, choices must be made and Jackson[18] urges that the researcher not await that millenium when agreement can be obtained from all parties concerned. It is necessary, as well as sufficient, that the criterion measures reflect an intensive and extensive knowledge of the program being evaluated.

The requirements for an appraisal index are thought by Ciocco (Chapter 16) to be the following:

1. The count or measurement of the phenomena being studied should be objective, reliable, accurate, and easily obtainable.

2. Knowledge should be available about the properties of the average or ratio being employed, and of factors related to variations in its numerical value.

3. It should be possible to establish a link between the index and the objective of the activity which it is supposed to measure.

In describing the evolution of health indexes, Ciocco laments the fact that the increased complexity of public health activities has resulted in the introduction of many indexes which measure the operation of the program itself (evaluation of effort) rather than the bearing of these operations on the health of the community (evaluation of accomplishment). This situation is particularly true in the field of chronic disease where such indexes as staff-patient ratios, per diem expenditures, and so on, are commonly cited as indications of a program's effectiveness.

Along with the thought which is devoted to selecting a valid evaluation index, the researcher must also consider the ease or difficulty of collecting data to derive it. The many evaluation studies which develop unique indexes and data collection procedures will not be considered further here but we would like to dwell upon one alternative, which is that of utilizing the data routinely and systematically collected by the organization itself.

Existing clinical and administrative records contain a veritable gold mine of information which can be modified for use as assessment indexes and, as a result, this resource has become the basis for the common medical audit. Despite the reservations which Donabedian (Chapter 12) notes about the completeness and validity of clinical records, culling them has become a refined procedure and many studies of the quality of medical care are based upon a professional's review of routine patient records. The evaluation of programs through medical audit could advance to the point where the overall effectiveness of a given facility could be represented by a single total score but Sheps (Chapter 17) thinks that such a composite index would obscure important differences. She suggests that a number of measurements about each facility continue to be made and that each be allowed to stand for itself as part of a total profile. More detailed consideration of the varied indexes which can be used for evaluating the effort or performance of public health and general hospital programs is found in the papers by Donabedian (Chapter 12), Ciocco (Chapter 16), and Sheps (Chapter 17).

The medical audit has also been utilized in the evaluation of psychiatric programs. The degree to which the various subobjectives of a mental hospital are attained can be studied through use of routinely collected data such as those suggested by Heymann and Downing,[19] the American Public Health Association,[20] and Rice, Berger, Sewall, and Lemkau (Chapter 18). Indexes such as discharge rates can be utilized as a measure of the extent to which a facility is discharging its patients back to the community (an initial subobjective) while readmission rates can shed light on the hospital's effectiveness in maintaining patients in the community (a later subobjective). A variety of evaluation indexes based upon regular hospital records are suggested by Rice, et al; and an instance of their application is seen in the study of Veterans Administration Hospital effectiveness by Ullmann and Gurel (Chapter 27).

An expanded variation of the medical audit for use in monitoring the effectiveness of several community programs is evident in the recently developed psychiatric case register which is composed of centrally assembled cumulative patient records updated periodically. The detailed procedures needed to maintain such a register are described by Gardner, Miles, Iker, and Romano (Chapter 19) and they suggest that it can be used, for example, to evaluate the impact of new services upon the caseloads of individual agencies which participate in the total community network. The uses of a psychiatric case register are further explicated by Bahn,[21] and there is little doubt that this technique constitutes an excellent mechanism for assembling the basic, routine data needed for program evaluation. Unfortunately, the expense of maintaining a community-wide case register is still quite high so that its applications thus far have been limited.

In addition to the relevant data available through standard archival records, many other forms of data are readily accessible and they can be appropriately used for program evaluation. The variety of assessments which can be accomplished through analysis of the physical condition of structures, simple observations, the unobtrusive use of hidden hardware, etc., are detailed by Webb, Campbell, Schwartz, and Sechrest.[22] They particularly stress the advantages of nonreactive measures for minimizing the possibility that data collection will alter the very nature of the service being evaluated.

Goal-Attainment Model Studies

Having considered the issues of methodology relevant to assessment efforts in general, the discussion turns to how they specifically apply to the goal-attainment model. In terms of research design, the predominant emphasis has been upon experimental approaches because of this model's central concern with measuring the degree of success in achieving specified objectives.

Many fine descriptions exist of ways to apply experimental design to goal-attainment program evaluation. Greenberg and Mattison[23] provide a flow chart indicating the optimal procedures to be followed in measuring criteria of success, starting with a clarification of the target population to whom the program is being directed and concluding with a comparison of the impact of the experimental service upon this group in contrast to a control group. The manner in which objectives and subobjectives are defined and measured carries specific implications for the design of a goal-attainment evaluation because of the relationship between the assumptions which are made initially and the interpretations which can be applied later. Deniston, Rosenstock, and Getting (Chapter 13) present very precise definitions of relevant terms so that each of the steps in the goal-attainment approach can be conducted uniformly by researchers. A particularly elegant formulation of an experimental design for evaluating the objectives of a school mental health program was offered by Glidewell, Mensh, Domke, Gildea, and Buchmueller,[24] through which it would be possible to test a program's success independent of (a) the conditions under which the program functions and (b) the effects of other influences operating simultaneously in the community.

Even when an experimental design is utilized, some ambiguity still remains about the time at which measurements are to be made. Knutson (Chapter 3) asserts that the purposes of evaluation require that two types of complementary assessment be made, i.e., measuring both program achievement (the ultimate objective) and program progress (the intermediate objectives). Limiting assessment to that of achievement can be wasteful since, if errors occur early in the program, the opportunity for correction will be lost if measurements are not obtained until the end. The measurement of a program's progress helps identify the processes affecting it so that ultimate success or failure can be explained more intelligently.

A special administrative tool of considerable value in the Knutson approach to assessment is the Program Evaluation and Review Technique (PERT). It is essentially a planning and control concept to focus the administrator's attention on key program parts, to point up potential problem areas which could disrupt program goals, to evaluate progress toward the attainment of program objectives, and to give management a prompt mechanical reporting device (Roman, Chapter 14). The fundamental information used in the PERT approach emerges from a quantified description of the program's flow plan which is composed of a series of related events and activities. The more complex the program is, the greater the number of events included in the flow plan. Merten[25] suggests that the most effective use of PERT occurs after the selection of specific objectives and during the implementation and evaluation phases. The application of the PERT approach to a multiple-screening program is illustrated by Merten and he indicates that it has its greatest value when applied to programs with simultaneous activities and time limitations. The growing PERT literature was reviewed in the past by Dooley[26] and he has categorized it according to the uses to which one might wish to put this technique.

The methodological rigor of experimental designs confronts the evaluator with a host of complex demands but it also makes it possible for him to determine whether specific objectives have been attained. Deniston, et al. suggest a series of ratios which can be computed to determine effectiveness, the most complex of which recognizes that a program's actual attainment must be examined relative to its planned attainment and the attainments which have resulted from nonprogrammatic efforts. In this regard, it is important to heed Hutchison's (Chapter 5) cautionary note that in evaluating a preventive service, the researcher should not confuse the additional time of observation with an added life increment due to improved treatment.

Systems Model Studies

In contrast to the goal-attainment model's clear-cut emphasis upon experimental designs, the systems model utilizes a variety of non-experimental approaches for dealing with the fact that it minimizes sharp differentiations between independent and dependent variables. The ideal laboratory paradigm, with well-defined inputs and outputs, the varying of an experimental condition while everything else is held constant, etc., is considered unrealistic and inapplicable to health programs by the systems model. It emphasizes that programs are complex social situations in which numerous events and conditions occur simultaneously and the researcher, therefore, is confronted with the problem of determining which aspects of the total situation are related to outcome measures. It should be noted that the selection of criterion variables can also be conducted differently in a systems evaluation. Yuchtman and Seashore[27] and Bennis[28] have pointed to the inadequacies of the traditional measures of organizational effectiveness, i.e., indexes of performance and human resources, and Bennis has suggested alternatives extracted from the normative and value processes of science.

Since the systems model indicates that all variables are dependent or reciprocal in nature, appropriate methodological techniques include multivariate analysis and path analysis. Randell[29] has addressed himself to the problem of applying appropriate multivariate techniques to the study of systems and suggests that canonical analysis is of value in apportioning the causal contribution of inputs, constraints, and treatments to outcomes. Canonical methods give the maximum correlation between two sets of variables and thus indicate the degree of association that could be obtained between systems variables and outcome measures, if the set of criteria were optimally weighted.

In developing an understanding of the statistical relationships between variables in a systems model, recent discussions of linear causal models offer further intriguing possibilities. Blalock[30] was one of the first to advocate the use of path analysis in clarifying complex causal arguments of the type encountered in the systems model. Diagrammatic representations of the system are constructed and the numerical values of path coefficients are inserted to indicate the nature of the relationship between each determining variable and the variable dependent on it. Werts[31] has described the advantages of a path diagram in bringing to light previously overlooked relationships that might well be brought into the theoretical analysis. As a technique for developing heuristic and evaluation models of complicated systems, path analysis offers great promise since it allows the researcher to deal with the reciprocal causality which is basic to the systems model.

We indicated earlier that computer simulations represented an increasingly appropriate methodological approach to evaluation and these techniques have been particularly relevant to systems models. The most common application of computer simulations to evaluation is seen in the field of operations research which Andersen (Chapter 15) describes as an attempt to study the system as a living organism in its proper environment without the artificial qualities of laboratory research. Andersen explored the types of problems which an operations research team would encounter when dealing with public health problems and illustrated the manner in which formal models derived from previously collected data can be refined to produce optimal solutions whose efficacy can subsequently be evaluated.

The general feeling has arisen that operations researchers pay a great deal of attention to model construction, some to model validation, but very little to the tactical problems posed in the use of such models for generating evaluation data of value to decision-makers. In an effort to shift this balance of emphasis, Fetter and Thompson[32] have constructed a set of simulation models describing the essential features of general hospital subsystems and they hope to extend their models further so that they can be used to predict and evaluate the consequences of various alternatives pertaining to patient and staff organization. A similar application of operations research to environmental health programs is found in a paper by Harrington.[33]

Examples of Program Evaluation

Having analyzed the conceptual and methodological principles relevant to the design of an evaluation study, consideration turns to how well the principles have been applied in the actual evaluation of programs. It is quickly evident that there is a striking difference between the high quality and sophistication of the theoretical papers in this field and the lower quality research emerging from actual studies of programs. Many of the evaluations reported in the literature suffer, unfortunately, from a variety of shortcomings which reflect either lack of awareness of relevant conceptual and methodological principles or an inability to apply them properly.

The reason for the discrepancy between theory and practice may be attributed to the fact that evaluation studies belong to the category of enterprises that are easy to formulate and criticize but exceedingly difficult to carry out. Another reason may be the difference in the type of individual who writes and reads about the theory and method of evaluation as contrasted with the one who is concerned about the actual findings of evaluation research. This contention is supported by an inspection of the original publication outlets for the papers included in this volume. In contrast to the wide range of journals from which the papers for Sections I-III could be drawn, the case examples of program evaluation had to be culled almost entirely from the *American Journal of Public Health* and *Public Health Reports*. It has been primarily the public health practitioner who has subscribed to the theoretician's preachings about the imperative nature of evaluation but has found that, unfortunately, it is easier to agree with the sermon than to apply it.

In selecting examples of program evaluation, we have tried to focus upon research assessing the effectiveness of a specific set of activities which in their totality constitute an organizationally based program. The papers presented in Section IV illustrate program evaluation approaches at the levels of primary, secondary, and tertiary prevention and also indicate the wide variety of health programs amenable to studies of effectiveness. A recent paper by Collins[34] reviews further ongoing evaluation research in the field of community psychiatry.

We have noted earlier that case examples which stem from the goal-attainment model of evaluation are more common than studies based upon the systems model. The only systems-oriented study included in Section IV is the one by Gardner, Bahn, and Miles (Chapter 26). They considered the question of how existing mental health services contribute to a community's caregiving network by conducting input-output analyses of a local mental hospital and the psychiatric unit of a general hospital. Rigorous experimental methodology would require greater comparability between the organizational structure, the personnel, the inputs, etc., of the two programs. However, these differences are grist for the mill in a systems analysis, and one product of this type of study could be a series of recommendations regarding the optimal functions of each facility.

Even though most evaluation studies are based upon the classical goal-attainment model, many of them implicitly recognize that the ultimate decision about a program's effectiveness cannot be reached solely within the study's precise frame of reference. For example, in assessing the effectiveness with which a Poison Information Center was attaining its primary objectives, Robb, Elwood, and Haggerty (Chapter 23) found that the Center was saving few lives but that related educational activities had gained sufficient professional and lay approval to warrant the program's continuation. Hunt and Odoroff's (Chapter 25) methodologically excellent follow-up of drug addicts demonstrates the limited utility of evaluating a program's impact upon the basis of a single criterion, such as rate of readdiction. A broader-ranging analysis of other objectives relevant to the addict's rehabilitation is also needed when evaluating the effectiveness of programs directed at such a group.

Space does not permit a detailed analysis of the specific conceptual and methodological concerns raised by each case example and such a critique is left as a learning exercise for the reader. We will comment here only on one major problem which pervades most reports of evaluation research. A common significant shortcoming is the researcher's failure to specify whether his study is that of a program's progress, i.e., whether it has attained initial and intermediate subobjectives, or that of a program's achievement, i.e., whether it has attained ultimate goals. This confuses the reader interested in the validity of the criterion being measured by the researcher and the appropriateness of its linkage to the program's objective. Much of the criticism directed at the studies conducted by Ullmann and Gurel (Chapter 27) and Ullmann[35] of Veterans Administration Hospital effectiveness stems from the heavy emphasis which these researchers placed upon speed of discharge as the primary criterion of effectiveness. Although this measure is an appropriate index of a psychiatric program's ability to attain its initial subobjective, as suggested in Chapter 18 by Rice, et al., the question of whether further subobjectives, like patient adjustment in the community, have been attained is of equal or greater concern to most readers.

The problem of understanding the link between a program's objective and the criterion being used to measure its attainment is further compounded by the failure of most researchers to include in their reports a description of the process through which a program's objectives were to be achieved. The report, for example, by Northcutt, Landsman, Neill, and Gorman (Chapter 29) that a coordinated rehabilitation program failed to attain better success in meeting certain objectives than an uncoordinated program has limited generalization value because little indication was given by the authors as to how coordination was intended to produce more effective results.

Although James (Chapter 2) has suggested that the evaluation of a program's efficiency in achieving a specific objective per unit of expenditure is a highly valuable type of assessment, few instances of this approach can be found in the health literature. A conceptual assumption for the evaluation of efficiency is that two alternative programs demonstrate equally good success on a series of criteria measures and that relative cost is their major differentiating feature. The more efficient program would be that with the lower cost. In reality, however, it has been quite difficult to find similar health programs to which such an assumption could be applied and tested. The rare studies of efficiency that have been conducted have examined the relationship between varying rates of effectiveness and differential levels of financial support. The papers by Ullmann and Gurel (Chapter 27) and McCaffree (Chapter 28) represent rare attempts to analyze the impact of higher per diem expenditures in psychiatric hospitals upon their efficiency in discharging patients. The McCaffree study utilized cost accounting procedures which have seldom been applied in the psychiatric field and it thus makes a particularly valuable contribution.

Implementing Research Findings

Fundamental to any comprehensive conception of program evaluation is the notion that findings emerging from research endeavors should be employed subsequently in the modification of existing programs and the planning of new ones. Unfortunately, this final step in the evaluation model has received little attention and even less use. Despite the careful concern which has been directed toward the formulation of rigorous research designs employing valid criterion measures, little concern has been exhibited by program evaluators and administrators for the factors crucial to the implementation of evaluation findings.

The reasons for this state of affairs are numerous and bear a similarity to the factors producing the previously noted gap between the theory and practice of program evaluation. Once again it is relevant to point to the differences in goals and operating procedures of those individuals conducting research studies and those who are responsible for program development. As a result, many of the same issues which affected the original initiation of the evaluation effort (Bergen, Chapter 9) again arise to plague attempts at program modification. It is generally acknowledged that individual behavior in accepting or rejecting change takes place in the context of an organization or social system and that the ideology of science, which supports the interpretation and communication of research results, now conflicts with certain organizational values. The latter frequently

favor symbolic or ritualistic evaluation of the type described by
Fleck (Chapter 7) so that even though homage is regularly paid by
the organization to the theoretical value of assessment there is also
routine avoidance of the substantive data emerging from such studies.

Sarason[36] has contended that any attempt to implement research
findings which does not come to grips with man-systems relationships
is incomplete and potentially misleading. Rodman and Kolodny[37]
have similarly stressed the significance of the social organization
within which evaluation occurs and that such research usually is
undertaken because of the administrator's needs rather than those of
practitioners. Because of the researcher's initial link to the administrator, the practitioner may feel that his work is being assessed by
someone with a vested interest in discerning and reporting errors
and he therefore employs a variety of psychological defense mechanisms for ignoring the researcher's findings. A study by Eaton (Chapter 32) of the professional personnel at Veterans Administration
clinics and Department of Correction institutions revealed a con-
tradiction between an individual's subscribing to the avowed objectives of research and his acceptance of research findings. The majority of personnel expressed reluctance to interpret evaluative data,
although there was greater readiness to interpret encouraging findings than discouraging ones. Only a minority of individuals are willing to risk the criticism which would be created by widely dissemi-
nating information with evaluative implications.

Given the likelihood that evaluation findings will encounter widespread avoidance, denial, or apathy, what steps can be taken to minimize such an eventuality? It appears appropriate to refer once
again to the features of the two program evaluation models considered
throughout this introduction, since the characteristics and limitations of each directly affect the implementation of research findings.
After analyzing the goal-attainment and systems models, Schulberg
and Baker (Chapter 35) concluded that the major conceptual and
methodological strengths of the former are often irrelevant at the
point of implementation. Since the goal-attainment model assumes
that specific goals can be assessed in isolation from the other goals
being sought by the organization, it is relatively insensitive to the
systemic forces affecting the implementation of findings.

In this approach to evaluation, the researcher runs the additional risk of selecting for study publicly stated organizational goals
which were never meant to be achieved. When this is the case, the
administrator will feel little need to alter his program to accommo-

date the researcher's findings. Schulberg and Baker contend that the systems model, on the other hand, by focusing upon the various factors determining research design and data interpretation offers more promise for programmatic utilization of evaluation findings. The systems model also suggests a variety of linkages and feedback mechanisms which can be used to bridge the gap between research data and program modification.

To assist in the feedback of research findings to the program administrator, increasing attention is being given to the field of scientific communication, with particular interest being displayed in the relationship between the systems supplying specialized information and the publics which are consumers of it. Studies of scientists' information-gathering behavior have become progressively more sophisticated and outstanding work is evident in the American Psychological Association's Project on Scientific Information in Psychology,[38, 39] which refined innovative research techniques for studying communication networks. The subtler aspects of communication are analyzed by Menzel in Chapter 30 and he describes five themes which he considers central to scientific communication. Of particular interest is the finding that just as health organizations must simultaneously pursue multiple goals so too must scientific information systems do so, even though the achievement of some goals may be antithetical to the satisfaction of others. For example, many journals attempt on the one hand to present the scientist with highly concise direct messages and, on the other hand, to bring to his attention information which he may not have appreciated as being relevant to his own interests. A variety of different communication methods for promoting the utilization of research findings are suggested by Halpert (Chapter 31). They range from the routine distribution of key documents summarizing research data to the novel notion of backstopping familiar communication techniques with consulting "detail men" who follow up on plans and help the agency put them into effect.

As an illustration of specific ways in which research findings are directly utilized for program modification and planning, we have included in Section V reports by Densen, James, and Cohart (Chapter 33) and Gardner (Chapter 34) of procedures through which they bridged the gap between research and service programs. The New York City Health Department established an Office of Program Planning, Research, and Evaluation through which it was possible to translate gains achieved through laboratory and epidemiologic investigation into programs of potential benefit to the population. Densen, et al., reported that of particular value to the Office's effectiveness in evaluating and modifying programs was the fact that its director was a deputy commissioner with clear access to the commissioner and all program directors.

Psychiatric case registers (development and uses for program evaluation are described by Gardner and his colleagues in Chapters 19 and 26) can be of particular value in modifying existing programs and planning new ones. The registers provide data about a wide variety of factors relevant to a program's operation and include additional information about other facets of the total system. Gardner (Chapter 34) describes the utilization of case register data in the planning of a new psychiatric unit for a general hospital by estimating utilization patterns from the previous experiences of an existing unit.

Summary

In this introductory chapter we have sought to familiarize the reader with what we consider to be the major issues confronting the researcher or administrator attempting to evaluate a health program. The goal-attainment model and the systems model were identified as the two major approaches to evaluation and we have described the implications of each for conceptualizing the process of evaluation, selecting an appropriate research design and valid indexes, and finally for implementing research findings. The papers which follow were selected for their relevance to these issues and because of their explication of the topics introduced in this chapter. In certain ways, many of these papers will be more effective at raising further questions than in providing irrefutable answers. This is entirely appropriate, since the evaluation of health programs still requires considerable thought and effort if the paradoxes described early in this chapter are to be more fully resolved.

REFERENCES

1. U. S. Public Health Service. Evaluation in Mental Health. Washington: PHS Publication No. 413.
2. Herzog, E. Some Guide Lines for Evaluative Research. Washington: Children's Bureau, Publication No. 375-1959.
3. Bloom, B. Mental Health Program Evaluation: 1955-1964. Denver: National Institute of Mental Health, 1965.
4. Suchman, E. Evaluative Research: Principles and Practice in Public Service and Social Action Programs. New York: Russell Sage Foundation, 1967.

5. Bauer, R. (Ed.) Social Indicators. Cambridge, Mass.: M.I.T. Press, 1966.
6. Greenberg, B., and Mattison, B. The Whys and Wherefores of Program Evaluation. Can. J. Publ. Hlth. 46: 293-299, 1955.
7. American Public Health Association. Glossary of Administrative Terms in Public Health. Am. J. Publ. Hlth. 50: 225-226, 1960.
8. Andrew, G. Some Observations on Management Problems in Applied Social Research. Am. Sociol. 2: 84-90, 1967.
9. Suchman, op. cit.
10. Georgopoulos, B., and Tannenbaum, A. A Study of Organizational Effectiveness. Am. Soc. Rev. 22: 534-540, 1957.
11. Baker, F. An Open-Systems Approach to the Study of Mental Hospitals in Transition. Comm. Ment. Hlth. J. 5, 4: 403, 1969.
12. Schulberg, H., and Baker, F. The Changing Mental Hospital: A Progress Report. Hosp. Comm. Psychiat. 20: 159-165, 1969.
13. Borgatta, E. Research Problems in Evaluation of Health Service Demonstrations. Milbank Mem. Fund Quart. 44: 182-201, 1966.
14. Herzog, op. cit.
15. Suchman, op. cit.
16. Greenberg, and Mattison, op. cit.
17. Campbell, D. T. Experimental and Quasi-Experimental Designs for Research on Teaching. In Gage, N. L. (Ed.) Handbook of Research on Teaching. Chicago: Rand McNally, 1963.
18. Jackson, D. Some Issues in Evaluating Programs. Hosp. Comm. Psychiat. 18: 161-170, 1967.
19. Heymann, G., and Downing, J. Some Initial Approaches to Continuous Evaluation of a County Mental Health Program. Am. J. Publ. Hlth. 51: 980-989, 1961.
20. American Public Health Association. Data Collection and Analysis for Program Planning and Evaluation. In Mental Disorders: A Guide to Control Methods. New York: American Public Health Association, 1962.
21. Bahn, Anita. Research Tools for Planning and Evaluation. In Williams, R. and Ozarin, Lucy (Eds.). Community Mental Health: An International Perspective. San Francisco: Jossey-Bass, 1968, pp. 292-304.
22. Webb, E., Campbell, D., Schwartz, R., and Sechrest, L. Unobtrusive Measures: Nonreactive Research in the Social Sciences. Chicago: Rand McNally, 1966.
23. Greenberg and Mattison, op. cit.
24. Glidewell, J., Mensh, I., Domke, H., Gildea, M., and Buchmueller, A. Methods for Community Mental Health Research. Am. J. Orthopsychiat. 27: 38-51, 1957.
25. Merten, W. PERT and Planning for Health Programs. Publ. Hlth. Rep. 81: 449-454, 1966.
26. Dooley, A. Interpretations of PERT. Harvard Bus. Rev. 42: 160-167, 1964.
27. Yuchtman, E., and Seashore, S. A System Resource Approach To Organizational Effectiveness. Am. Soc. Rev. 32: 891-903, 1967.
28. Bennis, W. Towards a 'Truly' Scientific Management: The Concept of Organizational Health. General Systems, 18: 269-282, 1962.
29. Randell, G. A Systems Approach to Industrial Behavior. Occup. Psychol. 40: 115-127, 1966.
30. Blalock, H. Causal Inferences in Non-Experimental Research. Chapel Hill: University of North Carolina, 1964.
31. Werts, C. Path Analysis: Testimonial of a Proselyte. Am. J. Soc. 73: 509-512, 1968.

32. Fetter, R., and Thompson, J. The Simulation of Hospital Systems. Operations Res. 13: 689-711, 1965.
33. Harrington, J. Environmental Hazards: Operations Research—A Relatively New Approach to Managing Man's Environment. New Engl. J. Med. 275: 1341-1350, 1966.
34. Collins, J. Evaluative Research in Community Psychiatry. Hosp. Comm. Psychiat. 19: 97-102, 1968.
35. Ullmann, L. Institution and Outcome: A Comparative Study of Psychiatric Hospitals. New York: Pergamon Press, 1967.
36. Sarason, S. Towards a Psychology of Change and Innovation. Amer. Psychol. 22: 227-233, 1967.
37. Rodman, H., and Kolodny, R. Organizational Strains in the Researcher-Practitioner Relationship. Hum. Org. 23: 171-182, 1964.
38. American Psychological Association. Reports of the American Psychological Association's Project on Scientific Information Exchange in Psychology. Vol. 1. Washington: APA, 1963.
39. American Psychological Association. Reports of the American Psychological Association's Project on Scientific Information Exchange in Psychology. Vol. 2. Washington: APA, 1965.

2

Evaluation in Public Health Practice

GEORGE JAMES

ACCORDING to the American Public Health Association's definition, evaluation is the "process of determining the value or amount of success in achieving a predetermined objective. It includes at least the following steps: Formulation of the objective, identification of the proper criteria to be used in measuring success, determination and explanation of the degree of success, recommendations for further program activity."[1]

It differs from research primarily in that it does not seek new knowledge, but attempts to mark progress toward a prestated objective. While research can end with the presentation of results, evaluation is viewed as part of a circular process. Its findings are reincorporated into the specific program from which they came. Evaluation utilizes the same general statistical, epidemiological, and technical methods as research.

Although evaluation has always been an important concern of health workers, it is no secret that its priority ran well behind that given to the administration of the program itself. So great was our faith in service technics that we begrudged any diversion of effort from them. During the 1930's, when handicapped children's programs achieved nation-wide scope, the cry was for more clinics, more children brought to care, more programs offering corrective services. Not one carefully planned, controlled, prospective evaluation study of the long-range restorative power of the program was begun. Tuberculosis case-finding efforts, child health clinics, and child guidance clinics have increased to meet "obvious" demands for such services without the development of methodical attempts to evaluate how well the underlying health needs were being met.

Recently, it began to appear that public health workers intend to pay much more serious attention to evaluation. They are becoming increasingly concerned because their best efforts are not effective against the major health problems of the present era. Of the 20 leading causes of death, only two are now capable of being controlled. We

are fighting current health problems fully equipped to win the struggle against those of 1920. The hope for solution must rest in a greater
emphasis upon research and demonstration.[2,3] This costs money,
money which must come at least partially from the budgets of some
of the traditional but no longer essential programs. It is not easy to
convince both the public and many public health workers that certain
services long provided are no longer required.

The evaluation process is a circular one, stemming from and returning to our value system. The steps in the process are outlined below.[4]

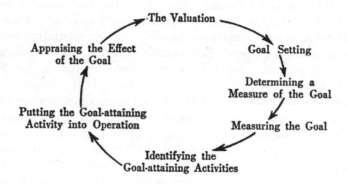

A discussion of the practical application of this evaluative process to
public health services must begin with a brief comment about the
three keystones of program planning: needs, resources, attitudes. A
public health need is the lack of a service or program required to
protect the public health. To be directly useful as a goal of public
health effort it must be rendered in practical terms.

It is not very productive for the health officer to dwell upon the fact
that coronary disease is the leading cause of death among males in the
United States. Not until he can find a facet of the problem that can be
solved by the application of specific resources can he hope to have
an impact upon it. In tuberculosis control, for example, the over-all
need to reduce morbidity and mortality from the disease must be expressed by certain practical objectives such as (a) the examination of
all familial contacts of a case of tuberculosis; (b) the routine x-ray
examination of admissions to general hospitals as a good source of new
cases of tuberculosis. These are practical expressions of a need for
tuberculosis control in the community, and can lead directly to the
formulation of specific objectives and action programs aimed at meeting these practical needs.

In order to describe a need in practical terms we must possess an available and useful resource. Until such a resource has been developed and its effectiveness proved, research and demonstration constitute our most useful program, unless we wish to proceed by faith alone.

Concern for community attitudes is equally important. In setting objectives we are quite dependent upon our cultural value systems. Often we are forced to yield to pressures exerted by a vocal but uninformed minority, illogical or unscientific as it may be.

We may find ourselves deeply involved in programs of minor value to disease control or prevented from performing an effective health service control because of forceful community attitudes.

Utilizing our knowledge of needs, resources, and attitudes, we then proceed to establish program objectives. The first and most all-embracing of these is the ideal objective or statement of purpose. This defines our ultimate goal in disease control such as "the elimination of all tuberculosis cases and deaths." Although such a formulation suggests neither a specific set of activities nor a timetable for effort, it does provide us with (a) a reason for our program, (b) a specific end point which defines what we consider to be ultimate success, and (c) a set of mortality and morbidity rate yardsticks against which all other measures of success must some day be validated.

Nevertheless, despite the above defense of the ideal objectives, it is the practical objectives which are the translation from purpose to program, and which make health services possible. Program evaluation consists essentially of the measurement of our success in reaching the practical objectives.

Some students of administration speak of "objectives," "steps," and "activities" as a descending order, with each of the latter terms used to denote action taken to implement a former one. Others, including myself, prefer to use the single term "objective." These objectives are then considered as making up an ordered series, each of which is dependent for its existence upon an objective at the next higher level, and each in turn is implemented by means of lower level objectives. In this framework there is a descending order of objectives beginning at the ideal objective and ending at the lowest level at which the task is to be subdivided. One can consider that, in general, the line officer of highest rank in a health department is responsible for the highest order objective, with each of the succession of lower ranked workers charged with one of the objectives of the descending scale.

Let us use a county dental health program as an illustration. The ideal objective is complete dental care for all children in the county.

A high order practical objective for the health officer might be the complete dental care of school children through a combination of private dental care, school dental corrections, and topical fluoride. His dental director may adopt as his 1961 practical objective the complete dental care of all first-grade children. The school dentist implements this, and his practical objective might be to achieve complete dental care for all first-grade children at the Central Avenue school. His dental hygienist has the task of applying topical fluoride to the first-grade children's teeth after the dentist completes the operative work. Her assistant is responsible for the objective of obtaining parental consent to all dental procedures.

Some may feel that the lower levels in this example should not be dignified by the term "objective." Significant evaluations have been performed at lower levels than these, i.e., how to write letters that bring consent, or how to educate the parent so that he demands dental care for his child.

Program evaluation should be applied to the lowest levels first and then successively to each objective up the scale. After we know the degree to which we have met an objective, this finding then becomes a step toward the next highest objective. If each of the dental hygienists in our illustration does her task satisfactorily, the resulting progress then becomes a part of the program for each school dentist. If each dentist carries out his full responsibility (part direct service and part administration) the combined result satisfies the dental director's objective for the year.

Most of the difficulty in communication about evaluation has occurred because of the confusion between these levels of objectives. Some have felt it sufficient to evaluate a training program by noting that the student has learned his lesson well. Others insist we must first prove that his learning has actually resulted in his doing better work, before we can state the program has been a success. According to the framework described here, they are both right—they are merely talking about objectives at different levels.

The cement which holds our hierarchy of objectives together, and which is the cause of so much poor communication and argument in the entire field of evaluation, rests on the assumptions we must make whenever we create a new objective. These assumptions are of two essential types, value assumptions and validity assumptions. We will say little here about the value assumptions, although they are a rich field for discussion,[5] particularly, but by no means exclusively, as we deal with foreign lands and subcultures within our own. Such value assumptions are: the value of saving a human life, our complete lack of interest in the survival of such species as the rat or M. tuberculosis compared to our great cultural concern for the dog. They include the value people put on health in relation to other human needs. They are highly significant, but not as treacherous to our practical understanding of evaluation as are the validity assumptions.

An assumption of validity must be made whenever we move from a higher order objective to a lower one. Hence, every lower level objective must assume all of the assumptions we have made for all of the objectives above it in the scale. Any program which is based upon a set of false major assumptions cannot be rescued by its lower level objectives, although quite valid evaluations might still be made for each of them individually. It is possible to evaluate the ways of making a pamphlet more readable, even if the public health facts in the reading matter are false. It was quite feasible to show that mothers could be motivated to feed their babies on a rigid time schedule, even though today we believe that this principle is wrong.

There are only two ways one can move up the scale of objectives in an evaluation: (a) by proving the intervening assumptions through research effort, i.e., changing an assumption to a fact, or (b) by assuming their validity without full research proof. When the former is possible, we can then interpret our success in meeting a lower level objective as automatic progress toward a higher one. Knowing the high potency of tetanus toxoid, we can equate a certain program of immunization to a given level of community immunity. Similarly, we can feel fairly sure that a 1 ppm sodium fluoride concentration in our water supply is a valid expression for a 60 per cent caries reduction among the children drinking it since birth.

When an assumption cannot be proved, we still must attempt to progress upward in interpreting an evaluation, since, as program administrators, none of us wishes to defend low order objectives for their own sake. But we go upward at our peril.

Public health as well as all other community services would be impossible unless validity assumptions were made. It is part of our value system that the population will not forgive our failure to make validity assumptions—in the absence of fact they expect us to use our expert opinion. During the polio outbreak 15 years ago some health officers were severely criticized for not closing schools and swimming pools while others who took these epidemiologically unproved steps received high praise. Perhaps the real objective involved was to allay fear and insecurity which is satisfied by forthright expert action no matter how unproved its effectiveness. Our task today, however, is not to examine the reasons why validity assumptions are made but to emphasize that they are made liberally in every one of our health programs.

Despite such apologies for freely made validity assumptions, it has become apparent that their cost can come too high. Newer health programs, particularly those in the chronic disease field, could bankrupt any community which wished to proceed too vigorously along the path of current assumptions. Could we afford the cost of all-out obesity control, a continuous program to promote the unsaturated-fat diet, a public program of annual physical examinations? The health officer's answer to this general problem is the demonstration. He tries out such programs on a small scale while awaiting and hopefully contributing to the research solutions required to prove validity.

The only sure answer to this dilemma for the evaluation is to identify each validity-assumption clearly and meticulously both at the time it is made and again at the time of evaluation. Only in this way can we keep clear the lines of communication between the professionals in our field and openly invite research investigation.

A group of people belonging to the same profession tend to make the same assumptions. This situation generally relegates evaluation to a low priority, since a low level evaluation may be too readily accepted as proof of attainment of a higher level objective. Charles Ascher compares this to the story of the emperor's new clothes. Not until a stranger from a far away empire remarked out loud about the emperor's robeless costume did the natives dare believe what their eyes revealed. Public health workers need consultants from fields such as social science to help them become alert to the many assumptions implied in health programs. We must learn other ways of building more dissatisfaction into our programs, to keep us alert, critical, and flexible instead of smug, self-satisfied, and rigid. One such way is to provide for a periodic review by a critical advisory committee with a changing membership.

The establishment of evaluation standards is a task familiar to health workers. A standard is a practical objective, and once established serves as a measure of progress. There is much which is dangerous in this practice. It is difficult to find the source for the fact that 2,400 Escherichia coli per ml is the upper limit of safety for beach water, let alone the proof we have of its validity. We must expect that every standard has in it a number of validity assumptions which should be methodically identified, listed, and described at the time the standard is established. Each of the assumptions of the objectives must be identified at each step in ascending order up to and including the ideal objectives dealing with the elimination of disease and the development of optimal health. If we do this we need not argue too vehemently over exactly what the standard should be. We will have provided the challenge for its own eventual refinement. If we do this we will avoid being classified with the members of those learned boards of expert nutritionists during the 1930's who, as McCollum once remarked, spent so much of their time "solemnly passing biologic laws."

Let us use the familiar program of tuberculosis control as an example of how to handle assumptions. The ideal objective is "the elimination of all morbidity and mortality from tuberculosis." Its chief assumptions are as follows:

a. Man's life is worth prolonging. His productivity should be kept high as long as possible, and disease and suffering are to be avoided. This is a value assumption which requires no further justification in our culture.

b. The continued biologic existence of the tubercle bacillus is unnecessary and undesirable. Although partly a value assumption, this is also partly a validity assumption. It is possible that the eradication of tuberculosis could lead to circumstances which would be even more unfavorable for mankind. However, in the absence of such evidence, we must make the assumption.

c. The total physical, social, and emotional cost of tuberculosis control will be less than that of the disease. This is another part value, part validity assumption, which we can restudy from time to time as our program proceeds.

The next lower level of objectives would include: "The earliest possible detection and isolation of all cases of reinfection tuberculosis." Let us examine the assumptions associated with this objective:

a. The disease spreads from infectious persons to others, hence prompt detection and isolation of these cases will reduce tuberculosis incidence. This is a validity assumption which we will probably never test under controlled-study conditions. We must confess that tuberculosis case and death rates have fallen as rapidly in many areas which have not had specific case finding and case control programs. Moreover, despite all of the years of intensive community x-ray effort aimed at early detection, we still seem unable to increase appreciably the proportion of early stage cases among the total cases reported.

b. Infectious cases may be discovered by modern technics. This validity assumption has been proved as essentially correct as long as one is willing to note the problems of reliability which exist to a predictable degree if only one person reads the chest x-ray.

c. A chest x-ray is a relatively harmless procedure.

A next lower order of objectives of the objective discussed above would be: "The examination by x-ray of all contacts to known cases of tuberculosis." The chief assumption implied here is that this group not only has a higher incidence of infection than average but one sufficiently higher to justify its being singled out for special follow-up. The truth of this assumption may vary from area to area and from time to time. The problem becomes more complicated if we try to compute the changing relative priority of contact examinations as a method of case finding with, for example, the examination of old cured cases, inmates of nursing homes, jails, or general hospitals.

The next level of case-finding objectives brings us finally to practical goals: "At least one x-ray examination on all (or 80 per cent if one wishes to be even more practical) of the contacts to cases of reportable tuberculosis, and one such examination per year thereafter for those remaining in contact with active cases." Now we have finally arrived at what we commonly recognize as a "standard of recommended practice." If we wish this standard to be considered as a true expression of the ideal objective "the elimination of tuberculosis" we must remember the crucial effect of each of the assumptions we have made so far. In addition, we have made a new assumption in establishing the present objective or standard; namely, that this specific procedure is the most valid, reliable, efficient, and adequate method for detecting these particular tuberculosis cases.[6]

When one considers all of the assumptions which have been made, it is not surprising that we feel dissatisfied with our final standard. This is all very well, and it is far better that we, as professionals, should be the first and not the last to experience these doubts! Such insecurities lead to a frequent restudy of the problem, a healthy sharing of experience with our colleagues and further refinements of the standard. The alternatives are dogmatism, lack of flexibility and an outdated concern with an armamentarium incapable of solving the health problems of our times.

Let us here emphasize again that if one of the key assumptions of our higher objectives is proved wrong, the standard must inevitably collapse. If, for example, the chest x-ray were found to be a significantly harmful procedure, or if tuberculous disease in a future era became largely endobronchial in site and could not be detected by x-ray, then our illustrative standard would be meaningless. These are not all far-fetched possibilities. Concern with ionizing radiation has already had an impact upon the frequency of the chest x-ray examination of certain groups in the community.

Evaluation in public health can be performed under several categories: effort, performance, adequacy of performance, and efficiency. Effort evaluations are those whose yardsticks and objectives are based either upon the capacity for effort or on the actual effort itself. It is obvious that such objectives and evaluations assume that the specific effort involved is a valid means of attaining a higher order objective of health accomplishment. Effort evaluation is the easiest to perform in public health. As a matter of fact, the best currently available measure of the adequacy of local health services in this country is a very general capacity-to-serve measure: the presence of a sufficient number of specific kinds of qualified health personnel.

The next category of evaluation is performance, which is an end result of effort. Performance occurs at several levels. It could be, for example, the number of cases of tuberculosis found after x-ray, the number of these cases hospitalized or the number cured after hospitalization. It is not generally recognized, but there are a number of key validity assumptions involved in many evaluations of performance. The fact that a number of children are reported as having received complete dental care does not insure that all of this care was done properly and was truly completed. Problems of reliability are common in performance standards, and must be taken into consideration whenever they might be of major significance. For example, the proportion of diabetics diagnosed in a case-finding program will vary with the blood sugar test used, the age groups tested, the time elapsed after the last meal and the follow-up procedures used. Hence every evaluation standard devised must specify all modifying conditions of significance.

An evaluation of a community health program can be made more meaningful if, in addition to performance, it is able to give some measure of the extent of the total problem solved. Such an evaluation tells us how adequate the program has been in terms of the denominator of total need. Although accurate data describing the unmet need are not generally available, some estimates have been made which are useful. The National Tuberculosis Association has estimated the total unknown cases of tuberculosis in the United States, and the American

Diabetes Association the number of those with unrecognized diabetes. The National Health Survey is expected to supply much valuable data on unmet needs for various disabling illnesses. It can be recognized that the ideal objective always includes an adequacy concept.

It might be useful to present an actual example of a state-wide evaluation utilizing the concept of adequacy of performance. The New York State Health Department knew that fluoridation of the public water supply could reduce dental caries among children by 60 per cent and that topical fluoride applied to the teeth of children who were not served by public water supplies could reduce dental caries by 40 per cent.

At the time the evaluation was made, 20 per cent of the upstate New York population had fluoridated water supplies and 30 per cent of the preschool population were receiving topical applications of fluoride. The effectiveness of these methods of preventing dental caries in children can be seen in Table 1.

TABLE 1. CARIES PREVENTION IN CHILDREN IN
UPSTATE NEW YORK, 1954

	A	B	C
Method of Fluoridation	Per cent Children Affected	Per cent Effectiveness of Procedure	Per cent Caries Prevented (AXB)
Water supply	20.0	60.0	12.0
Topical application	30.0	40.0	12.0
Total	50.0		24.0

Thus it is seen that 24 per cent of dental caries in children were prevented by the state's program at the time of the evaluation.

The study then considered the potential possibility for the prevention of caries. If all communal water supplies in upstate New York were fluoridated, 80 per cent of the population would be affected. Children in the remaining 20 per cent of the area could be given topical fluoride. Table 2 shows how effective such a program would be in caries prevention.

Potentially 56 per cent of the dental caries in children in upstate New York could be prevented. It is known from local studies that the practicing dentists in New York State are able to take care of almost

TABLE 2. POTENTIAL CARIES PREVENTION IN
CHILDREN IN UPSTATE NEW YORK

Method of Fluoridation	A Per cent Children Affected	B Per cent Effectiveness of Procedure	C Per cent Caries Prevented (AXB)
Water supply	80.0	60.0	48.0
Topical application	20.0	40.0	8.0
Total	100.0		56.0

40 per cent of the caries load and that after fluoridation they appear to continue to fill the same number of dental caries. Hence, the full application of fluoridation in this state plus the regular dental correction program would meet 56 per cent plus 40 per cent of the prefluoridation unmet need and hence would be 96 per cent adequate. The present program is meeting only 24 per cent plus 40 per cent of the total dental caries need among children and hence has an adequacy rating of 64 per cent.

Despite the great value of the evaluation by adequacy of performance, it is not sufficient for the practitioner of public health. Few programs can be justified at all cost and a measure of efficiency should be included whenever possible. The emphasis on efficiency is closely related to the health officer's attempt to streamline traditional programs. Can the same end result be achieved at lower cost? Can less skilled personnel substitute adequately for physicians, nurses, and engineers? Can self-inspection programs achieve an effective degree of restaurant sanitation control? Such questions point out that standards of performance will be improved if they can consider the effort-costs involved and arrive at a comparative efficiency rating.

Efficiency concepts do dominate many of the public health decisions made in chronic disease programs. When any new test is considered as a possible addition to the armamentarium for mass screening, careful attention must be paid to the number of false-positives which will occur. The individuals who are screened as positive must be followed by more elaborate and costly examination procedures. A screening program which results in a large number of false-positives could rapidly overwhelm the follow-up mechanisms of a community. Hence, any technic which gives a high proportion of false-positives will be discarded for practical use. A history of chest pain as an indication of coronary heart disease, the measurement of obesity as an index of suspicion of hypertension, the presence of low gastric acidity as a warning sign for incipient cancer of the stomach are all screening tests which have not been widely accepted as practical for health department detection programs because of their high number of false-positives.

In addition to the four categories, every evaluation exercise should also analyze the processes involved in the program. What is it that has made the program succeed or fail? What changes in technics or methods could have improved program effectiveness? Which recipient of the program benefited the most and which the least? What did the program accomplish in terms of originally unforeseen objectives? Each program is a potential target for numerous research questions. The findings of the evaluation study, aimed though they may be at determining progress toward a specific objective, should be analyzed closely to see which additional questions might also be answered.

A few words should be included here on the desirability of building evaluation into the health program. The health officer sets up controls to keep him posted on results as the program proceeds. This feedback information is another means of stimulating dissatisfaction and allows him the opportunity to institute prompt corrective measures when necessary. This same information can offer valuable data for the performance of evaluation studies. Recently in New York City the early feed-back data on the cancer detection clinic program indicated that the particularly susceptible population was not well represented in the patient load. Even after the clinic had been moved to an area of the city where these persons resided, they still did not make use of the clinic. Further study revealed that large numbers of women of the high risk group were patients at the department's social hygiene clinics as well as certain hospitals, and the detection program was instituted there. The first year of operation of this changed program found six times as many patients with cancer of the cervix than had been found previously.

Building evaluation into the program permits data collection to proceed at the time the events occur, a far better method than later retrospective search for data of possible significance. In establishing health programs, the general rules for the development of a longitudinal study should be followed, and the evaluation of the results is similar to the hypothesis-proving analysis of longitudinal data in an experimental design.

In conclusion, the following major rules of evaluation should be observed by the modern public health worker:

1. The practical objectives of each program to be evaluated should be clearly stated.

2. The underlying assumptions of validity associated with each objective should be meticulously identified.

3. Evaluations by effort should always be done. Evaluations by performance, adequacy of performance, and efficiency should be done whenever possible.

4. The entire program should be reexamined in the light of the findings arising from the evaluation exercise.

5. To insure the reliability of any standards developed as aids to evaluation, the status of all significant conditions associated with the use of the standard must be specified.

6. The ultimate value of evaluation to public health programs will depend to a great extent upon research proof of the validity of the assumptions involved in the establishment of key objectives.

7. As in every new field there is a period of time set aside for clarification of terms and construction of conceptual frameworks. Further progress will then occur only from the performance of actual evaluation projects, carefully designed and analyzed. Public health practitioners today need the stimulation which can be achieved only through the critical appraisal of a large number of such studies. The time for such work is now!

NOTES AND REFERENCES

1. Glossary of Administrative Terms in Public Health. A.J.P.H. 50: 225-226, 1960.
2. James, G. Research by Local Health Department: Problems, Methods, Results. Ibid. 48: 353-361, 1958.
3. James, G. Public Health Program Planning in Our Present Era. Nursing Outlook, 8: 334-337, 1960.
4. Elinson, J. Lecture at Columbia University School of Public Health and Administrative Medicine—Course Title: Evaluation in Public Health—1959.
5. Vickers, G. What Sets the Goals of Public Health? Lancet, 1958, pp. 599-604.
6. There is also a special assumption involved whenever we pick a practical goal which is less than 100 per cent of approved practice. We, of course, are implying that the group not reached is substantially similar to the group reached.

3

Evaluation for What?

ANDIE L. KNUTSON

ONE might define evaluation as the process of determining the value or worth of something relative to a given purpose or standard. It is the process of making decisions, drawing together evidence, weighing the pros and cons of various suggestions, and selecting courses of action.

Each of us is constantly making evaluations in his daily life, judging the worth of alternatives against his own background of knowledge and experience. We judge ideas or actions as right or wrong, good or bad, honest or dishonest, practical or impractical so frequently that we are often unaware of doing so. When the weighing process is subconscious or intuitive, major decisions may be made without considering pertinent evidence at hand. Motives underlying evaluations are seldom pinpointed and discussed.

Most of our evaluations in daily life are made without help from specialists. From time to time, however, we do seek out persons who are trained to serve in some evaluative role. We may turn to the physician or nurse, the psychiatrist or psychologist, the judge or lawyer, the consulting engineer, the real estate appraiser or any one of a wide range of experts.

The first questions such an expert is likely to ask are, "Why have you come to me? What is your problem? Why do you need help?"—questions which are concerned with the reasons for the evaluation.

"Why do you want to evaluate?" "Evaluation for what?"—deserves the most critical attention of those concerned with evaluation. Most of the major decisions that need to be made in planning and conducting an evaluation hinge on the answer to this question.

Program evaluation, like all research, tends to start with some concern, curiosity, uncertainty or what Whitehead has called "a ferment already stirring in the mind." Some element of desire or need to know seems necessary if any steps toward evaluation are to be taken at all. Whoever wants to evaluate wants to evaluate for some reason, in order to make some kind of decision or to serve some personal or group purpose.

It is essential to know why a person wants to evaluate in order to help him identify the kind of evidence he will need in making his decision. His reasons for evaluating ought to determine not only the kind of evidence, but also the amount and quality of evidence required and, accordingly, the methods of measurement to be used.

The evaluation of a particular program or program activity may be undertaken for any number of explicit or covert reasons. In general, these reasons fall into two groups: (a) those that are organization-oriented, and (b) those that are personally-oriented.

From the point of view of the organization, a program evaluation may be undertaken:

1. to demonstrate to others that the program is worthwhile;
2. to determine whether or not a program is moving in the right direction;
3. to determine whether the needs for which the program is designed are being satisfied;
4. to justify past or projected expenditures;
5. to determine the costs of a program in terms of money or human effort;
6. to obtain evidence that may be helpful in demonstrating to others what is already believed to be true regarding the effectiveness of a program;
7. to gain support for program expansion;
8. to compare different types of programs in terms of their relative effect;
9. to compare different program methods or approaches in terms of effect;
10. to satisfy someone who has demanded evidence of effect.

Even in stating some of these organization reasons for evaluating, we reveal the influence of personal values. When we say, for example, that we wish to "justify our efforts" or "to demonstrate effect" these statements suggest a certain degree of effectiveness has been assumed even before the evaluation is initiated.

An individual may have many personal reasons for wanting to evaluate:

1. he may see evaluation as "the thing to do" if one wants to belong;
2. he may wish to make an evaluative study as a means of bringing favorable attention, better budgets, and better staff to his unit;
3. he may see it as a means of gaining status and acceptance of peers and superiors;

4. he may see it as a way of making his job easier and more interesting;

5. he may see it as a step toward promotion;

6. he may simply have a vague but urgent need to know if he is progressing.

It is easy to see that a wide range of personal as well as group reasons may underlie the desire to seek evidence of program success or failure. The individual may never realize these personal values are influencing his decisions, for values are slithery things and creep in to influence many areas of decision in ways that those involved may never recognize.

An expert drawn in to assist in planning or carrying out an evaluation also has personal and group interests in the activity. Sometimes satisfaction of these specialists' interests may take precedence in his mind over achievement of the purposes of the program being evaluated. The expert may be more interested in research papers than in program improvement. These motives of the evaluator also need to be identified and understood.

The mere fact that we want to evaluate a program assumes that evaluation is good, but is this assumption always sound? Is evaluation always good? Do the reasons leading to evaluation justify the effort in each instance? Over-evaluation may be as serious a program weakness as under-evaluation.

Someone has suggested that evaluation is like salt—nearly all foods taste better with some salt. Some foods need more salt than others, but too much salt can ruin the meal.

It is impossible to identify all the reasons involved in the decision to evaluate any particular activity; yet it is important to identify these reasons with as much precision as possible, for many aspects of the evaluation hinge upon the individual and group motivations for undertaking evaluation. For example:

1. The reasons for evaluation may govern the kind of program selected for evaluation and the part of the program to be evaluated. If the underlying purpose of the evaluation is to demonstrate to others, to bring attention to the department, or to achieve status for evaluation it may be important to focus attention upon some program that has status within the eyes of one's peers. At the present time, for example, programs like cancer, heart disease or mental health are likely to be more attractive as areas in which to carry out evaluative research than are programs which have their setting in the laboratory or in

the activities of administration. As a result it may be much easier to employ good people to carry out evaluations in the former areas.

2. The reasons for evaluation will tend to govern the kinds of assumptions the evaluator is willing to accept or reject. They will help to identify the action level at which evaluation is desired. It may be necessary in one situation to assume that an urgent need for the program exists; whereas, the need itself may be the focus of critical review at another time. It may be appropriate in one instance to assume certain case finding methods are valid and reliable so that the evaluation can be focused on ways of applying these methods. Or it may be necessary to assume that the diagnosis is adequate and valid if the primary purpose of the evaluation concerns comparative treatment. At times it may be assumed that the number of qualified professional persons on the staff yields an index of effectiveness so that programs in various areas can be compared for budgetary or planning purposes. Under other circumstances evaluation might focus attention on the effectiveness of these specific professional services.

3. The reasons for evaluation tend to govern the type of program methods to be compared and the standards of judgment or value against which effectiveness will be measured. If the program decision to be made concerns a choice between alternatives, then it is important that the data obtained permit a valid choice between the alternatives suggested.

4. The reasons for evaluation likewise govern the intensity of the investigation to be undertaken and the level of critical analysis to be completed. They suggest the criteria to be used in determining whether or not the effort is successful, and accordingly the types of evidence to select or collect in order to measure satisfaction of the criteria. If we accept the general idea that the criterion of success equals yield divided by effort, then we need to know the reason for evaluation to determine what data to include in judging the yield. This may depend in part on who is making the final judgment; that is, whose reasons are governing the evaluation. What one group or individual holds as valid evidence may not be so perceived by a member of another group. For example, a person who is looking critically in terms of dollars and cents spent may not be impressed with data concerning public acceptance or even with data related to human suffering. On the other hand, if his interest is strongly focused toward the saving of lives, cost figures may not impress him.

5. Above all, a frank answer to the question "Why do you want to evaluate?" will help to set the general orientation of staff and consul-

tants to the process of evaluation. On this answer rest the decisions regarding who should be involved in planning and conducting the evaluation; the type and manner of controls; the nature and frequency of feedback or reporting; and the extent to which provision will be made to incorporate findings into program change.

One must know as early as possible whether a "tender-minded" approach or a "tough-minded" approach will best serve the purposes defined. The action research which contributes so much to program progress cannot substitute for the tightly controlled studies necessary for measuring program achievement. Long-range controlled studies cannot yield early feedback.

The primary purposes of evaluation are to provide objective estimates of achievement and to provide guidance for the conduct of program activities. Achieving these purposes requires two types of evaluation, namely: (a) the evaluation of program achievement, and (b) the evaluation of program progress.

Public health programs are not like laboratory experiments. They seldom start and end at specific predetermined points. Baselines and final measurements cannot be clear-cut; nor can measurements be completely independent of the educational process. We know for example, that the likelihood of success is increased if leaders in the community have a part in setting objectives and policies. Yet this very process of jointly establishing objectives and program plans, which must be completed before baselines are obtained, is itself educational. Interviewing to obtain baseline measurements may also influence behavior.

It may be helpful to think of a new program as a growing type of operation as illustrated in the diagram.

A program may be initiated by one person or a small group of persons who have identified a problem and are seeking a solution. They will first attempt to define the problem specifically, to identify the primary needs or wants, and to determine the nature of the situation about which something must be done. Decisions made during this exploratory phase of the program are often key to the success of the program.

We next move into that phase of the program in which specific objectives become crystallized. Agreements are reached on the philosophy and policies to be followed, the kinds of persons needed to work on the program, the resources to be made available, the methods or techniques and procedures to be used.

At this time a baseline may be drawn to obtain data on the existing status relative to the specific program objectives. Then after the pro-

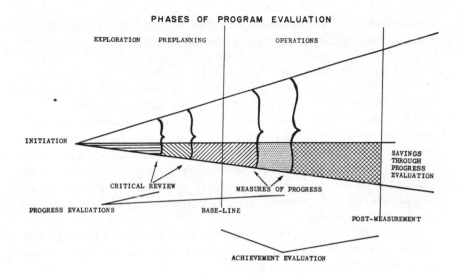

gram has been in operation for a long enough time to expect results, a post-measurement may be taken to determine whether the program is achieving its long-range objectives. This process might be called evaluating program achievement.

Limiting evaluation to the evaluation of achievement is wasteful. Suppose, for example, an error occurs in the beginning of the program. If we do not evaluate until the program is completed, we may not identify that error, and the opportunity to correct it will be lost.

Progress evaluation helps us to identify these errors when they occur. Its purpose is to provide guidelines for the conduct of program activities. The principles and techniques of progress evaluation can be applied during this process of program planning and development to improve the quality of decisions made.

Progress evaluation requires an attitude of critical self-appraisal. It involves the systematic application of the best available techniques and approaches for the purpose of ferreting out program weaknesses and detecting ways of reorienting efforts along more profitable lines. It is a means of identifying barriers that lie ahead and of finding ways of removing them before they disrupt the program. Discussions, interviews, questionnaires, statistical data, or almost any other technique of evaluation available may be applied for this purpose. The critical factor is not the evaluation technique to use but the kinds of questions to explore.

This approach to evaluation has special values that recommend it for those responsible for on-going public health programs. It can be applied to any aspect or part of the program with little loss of time and without excessive controls. It can be applied by every member of the staff. Usable results can be obtained and used while the program is in action and before the program money and efforts are spent.

A variety of means can be employed during the planning, development and operation of a program to identify possible weaknesses or fruitful alternative methods before great expenditures have been made. Improvements can then be initiated quickly and at minimum cost. In general, however, this positive approach to evaluation involves two types of approach: critical reviews, and objective tests and measures of progress.

The critical review, a familiar public health tool, yields the greater returns during the early steps in planning. Some of the issues to consider in this type of review include:

1. Have the needs, wants or concerns the program is intended to serve been adequately identified? Has the public to be served been represented in defining the needs? Is it possible that one of our difficulties in public health is that we are attempting to teach people to become concerned about what *we believe* to be important? Would we be more successful if we try to find out what *they* consider to be important and develop ways of fitting our efforts into their patterns of interest and concern?

2. Have the objectives of the program been specifically defined and written down? Are they tied in with the over-all objectives and philosophy of the program? Have lay, as well as professional people, had a share in setting the objectives to assure that they are directly related to existing concerns and are understood and accepted? Are these objectives based on scientifically valid and adequate evidence? Are they stated in terms of the specific changes in behavior to be achieved? Is it physically, socially and psychologically possible for the individual concerned to carry out the action recommended? Are the objectives sufficiently limited so that one can reasonably hope to achieve them?

3. Have the criteria to be used in measuring achievement been clearly stated and agreed upon so that baselines can be established and measurement of achievement is possible?

4. Have steps been taken to obtain a baseline from which progress can be measured? Are the baseline measures *directly* related to specific program objectives? Have other possibilities for comparison been considered?

5. Have the objectives been broken down into intermediate steps or sub-goals so that it is possible to plan the program more pointedly, and to measure progress while the program is in operation?

As the program moves into the operational phase, the questions of evaluation include: Are the methods and approaches employed in the program adequate for the purposes of the program? Are significant barriers to success identified and corrective actions taken?

Answers to questions such as these may be obtained by various types of objective measures while the program is in progress. Program methods may be pretested in pilot situations. Materials may be tested for their understanding and usefulness. Observational studies or surveys may yield information useful in guiding the program. Many ways may be found to obtain public interpretations while the program is in progress.

For example, through such means it may be possible to determine whether the community opinion leaders most closely related to the program feel that their views are being considered as the program develops. Have efforts been made to assure that they are prepared and eager to support the program, and to help interpret it to those with whom they relate?

To the extent that valid and reliable answers are obtained to the questions of progress evaluation and the results of these evaluations are applied, the likelihood of program success will be increased. The data obtained in evaluating program progress are not valid, however, for determining whether or not the objectives of the program have been achieved. For this purpose, sound studies of program achievement are essential.

Concrete evidence that an objective has been achieved is the only realistic criterion for measuring achievement. Such evidence should be clearly distinguished from evidence that intermediate goals have been achieved.

Three steps must be taken in order to evaluate the achievement of a public health program. If the principles of progress evaluation have been applied, the first two steps will have been taken and the third already planned.

First, it is essential to have a precise statement of the program objectives and the specific, agreed-upon criteria that will be used to determine whether or not these objectives have been achieved.

Secondly, it is essential to have a baseline measurement of the status of the situation at the time the objectives are established; or if that should be impossible, some other agreed-upon and appropriate programs for comparison. Data obtained concerning the status of the program should relate directly to these specific objectives.

Having such a baseline measurement is essential because public health programs seldom, if ever, start from absolute zero. The group concerned is likely to have some knowledge, some attitudes and some practices relating to public health before the program starts. Having incorrect information is not the same thing as having no information at all. Unlearning may be more difficult than learning anew.

Thirdly, it is essential to know the status of the program relative to objectives at some point sufficiently advanced in time so that changes as a result of the program effort can reasonably be expected. Usually the methods of measurement employed to obtain baseline data may also be used to obtain follow-up data. We need to be aware, however, that the process of interviewing or collecting data is in itself an educational process. In evaluating programs, therefore, it may be necessary to use matched samples or control groups to obtain valid and reliable follow-up data.

The methods used to evaluate a program should be especially selected or constructed in terms of the particular goals of that program and the situation in which the program effort is being made. Accordingly, evaluation plans should be developed along with program plans. This will help to assure that the goals are specific, that criteria of achievement adequately represent evidence of goal achievement, and that steps are taken to obtain an adequate baseline from which to measure change. Planning the evaluation in this way will also help to assure that the findings are tied closely to program needs, goals and methods. If so, they will be of maximum use in making future decisions.

4

Principles in the Evaluation of Community Mental Health Programs

**BRIAN MACMAHON, THOMAS F. PUGH, and
GEORGE B. HUTCHISON**

UNFORTUNATELY, there is no accumulated body of experience in the evaluation of community mental health programs from which governing or guiding principles can be drawn. Recently, there have appeared detailed accounts of two plans for the scientific evaluation of a community mental health program. However, one of these —the Milbank Memorial Fund's model for Syracuse[1]—was never intended to be put into effect, and although the other—the St. Louis School program[2]—has reached the operative stage, no results of the evaluation have yet been reported. Therefore, attempts at defining what constitute principles in the evaluation of community mental health programs must depend on knowledge gained from other areas, and discussion of the applicability of such principles in the evaluation of community mental health programs will perforce be theoretical.

Fortunately, we were asked to deal with principles, and not with practical problems. By comparison with the practical problems the principles involved are relatively simple, and briefly stated. They may be classed under one of three general headings.

1. The determination of what type of evaluation is required before designing the evaluatory plan.

2. The definition of the program, the population to be served, and the effects desired.

3. The choice of comparison groups which will permit the inferences required by the type of evaluation selected.

Types of Evaluatory Studies

According to the underlying purpose, evaluatory studies fall into one of two major categories. The first general category of evaluatory studies consists of those designed to test the hypothesis that a certain practice, if successfully carried out within specified limits, has a measurable beneficial outcome in the group on whom it is practiced; for example, to test the idea that surgical removal of the affected

breast leads to a lengthening of life among patients with breast cancer. This process we will refer to as evaluation of accomplishment.
Effective studies of this variety are by far the less common of the two
types of evaluation. In the field of community mental health they are
conspicuous by their absence. Meyer and Borgatta[3] have suggested
many reasons for this lack, but the most important appear to stem
from problems encountered in studying all cause-effect relationships,
exemplified in this instance by the desired cause-effect relationship
between the treatment and decreased disease prevalence. Unless the
beneficial effects of a therapy or preventive are startlingly obvious, a
situation which does not seem to be the case in most mental disorders, the evaluation of accomplishment requires formal experimental methods, including random or systematic allocation to treatment and comparison groups, objective assessment of results, and so
forth.

The second category comprises studies designed to find out whether
a supposedly therapeutic or preventive practice is in fact being carried out within specified limits—for example, are cancerous breasts
being removed in accordance with criteria established as "good surgical practice." This process we refer to as "evaluation of technic."
In evaluation of technic, cause and effect are not at issue—the procedure is concerned merely with the description of the quality of the
events of which the technic is comprised. Compared with evaluation
of accomplishment, evaluation of technic is relatively easy, and much
has been done in this area. In the field of surgery, for example, where
controlled evaluation of accomplishment is so rare, evaluation of
technic is highly developed. On the other hand there are still large
areas in which much remains to be done, as witness the singular
scarcity of studies such as that of Peterson[4] on the evaluation of the
technic of general medical practice.

Hutchison,[5] has previously drawn attention to the distinction
between these two types of evaluation, using a different terminology.
He distinguished "evaluation of intermediate objectives" (the
technic) from "evaluation of ultimate objectives" (the health benefits derived from the procedure). However, as he pointed out, while
physicians tend to regard health as an ultimate objective, not everybody shares this point of view; economists, for example, may regard health (including their own) as an objective intermediate to
the economic well-being of a country.

It is imperative to distinguish the purposes of these two types of
evaluatory study. Without any doubt, the first category—the con-

trolled evaluation of accomplishment—is the more vital. Unless it has been shown that the use of a certain technic is followed by beneficial results, what is the use of making sure that the technic is being followed? Once a technic has been shown to be of value, however, continuing studies designed to evaluate the application of the technic become crucial. The personnel and other facilities necessary to the controlled evaluation of accomplishment in a community program are so considerable that it is obviously impractical for them to be built into more than a few pioneering studies. Furthermore, once a technic has been clearly shown to be of value, further critical evaluations may be contra-indicated because of the undesirability of retaining untreated groups as controls. The importance of the initial controlled evaluations is evident since their results will be assumed to be applicable to much wider populations than those on which they were carried out. The subsequent evaluatory process is simply one to insure that in this wider application the technic as applied in a particular program is sufficiently similar to that applied in the original evaluations to justify the assumption that the same beneficial effects will occur as a result. Since the evaluation of technic does not require the identification of a cause-effect relationship, but merely the definition of the technic, and the observation, recording, and cataloguing of events of which it consists, it is a process that can be, and usually is, built into each individual program.

Before leaving the subject of categories of evaluation and their purposes, there is one concept that should be mentioned, if only to be dismissed. This is the idea that programs gaining "community acceptance" are, ipso facto, beneficial. That this reasoning is a non sequitur should be evident. It is demonstrated currently by the acceptance of well advertised nostrums, and historically by waves of enthusiasm that have been generated by a variety of medical cults.

Principle of Definition

Turning now to the second area of principle—definition—we have no intention of attempting to define community, mental, health or program. No such definition is needed here. What must be susceptible to definition, however, both as to what it is and as to what its intentions are, is the individual program that is to be evaluated. It is immaterial whether or not it falls into one's preconceptions of what the ingredients of a community mental health program ought to be.

A statement of the essence of a mental health demonstration used by Ernest Gruenberg, however, is particularly useful in identifying the type of program that seems capable of being evaluated.[6] From the context of the statement it does not appear that any distinction is intended between a demonstration and a program; indeed the statement might well be descriptive of a variety of service programs in the health field:

> "The essence of a mental health demonstration is that extra resources, extra interagency cooperation, extra consultative services from experts, etc., are made available to an entire population on a scale large enough that observable changes in the population's mental health can be anticipated."

We note from Gruenberg's statement that a community mental health program is made available to an entire population, and that changes are anticipated in the population's mental health. This population need not be defined as a whole population in the demographic sense, but may be restricted in terms of age, sex, occupation, club or school membership, or in some other way. Glidewell and his colleagues,[2] for example, are concerned with the evaluation of a program designed for school children in St. Louis. The Milbank Memorial Fund's model for Syracuse[1] was based on a program for recipients of Old Age Assistance. Depending on the nature of the program to be offered, there may be further specification of the group within the population that is expected to be the particular target of the preventive or therapeutic measures. This specification will usually be in terms of a particular illness or group of illnesses in the case of a treatment program, or of a particularly susceptible group of persons in the case of a preventive program.

Definition of the nature of the program is an area that may be more difficult in community mental health than in some other subject areas. This is unfortunate, because even if some intuitive procedure on the part of an individual or group is evaluated and found to be effective, there is little prospect for the more general application of the procedure until it can be defined in operational terms that are intelligible to a large body of professional workers. Also unfortunate is the fact that many community mental health programs employ a shot-gun approach in which a great number and variety of services are offered at the same time. If such a program is found effective, those who wish to emulate it are required to duplicate each of the component elements, unless they wish to undertake new evaluations involving particular components of the program. A procedure that seems more logical, although requiring greater patience on the part of the investigator, is the separate evaluation of the individual components of the larger program, if indeed these can be separated.

Next, in the context of definition, we come to definitions involved in the assessment of the effects of the program. To return, once again, to Gruenberg's statement, we note that observable changes can be anticipated. In order to evaluate a program it is necessary to state ahead of time the results which are anticipated, and to compare them with the results actually observed. Observation which makes note of all the observable changes which follow the introduction of a program, while useful as a method of formulating hypotheses, does not evaluate the program. Further studies will be required to test any hypotheses developed as a result of such a survey.

Measures of effectiveness may include such objective measures as mental hospital admission or discharge rates, length of stay, rates of truancy, delinquency, divorce, separation or suicide, and incidence of physical illnesses, such as cerebral syphilis and cerebral palsy. They may also include more complex, and at times subjective, psychologic and psychiatric assessments, provided that due precautions are taken to insure assessments that are replicable and are made independently of knowledge of the treatment group to which the patient belonged. Wherever opinion, whether of the patient or of a professional observer, forms part of the basis for evaluating the program, it is necessary for that opinion to be validated. It is not enough, for example, to take the patient's statement that he feels better at its face value. It is necessary to demonstrate that the holding of such an opinion is correlated with some change in the patient that can be objectively assessed as harmful or beneficial. The same is true of the feeling of a professional worker as to the benefit derived by the recipients of his service.

Gruenberg's concept that the results should be observable seems a very reasonable one, and yet one may wonder how far this principle has really been accepted in the community mental field. We cannot escape the impression that many of the practical problems in evaluating mental health activities, that one hears so much about, originate in the difficulty of identifying a characteristic (whether of people or of communities) that can be shown to change under the influence of a mental health program. From this difficulty it is inferred that our problem is one of identifying a "satisfactory" method of evaluation. We should not, however, overlook the alternative explanation—that the evaluation is in fact satisfactory but that there is no appreciable change to identify.

Certain concepts that are heard of with some frequency in the field of community mental health, although definable in the abstract, cannot be measured even in such simple terms as bigger or smaller, better or worse. Here also, difficulty in evaluation can be anticipated. Programs having as their objective a higher level of "positive mental health," for example, stand no more chance of being successfully evaluated than would a program of venereal disease control that was based on the objective of fostering positive genital health, however admirable such an objective may seem.

Principle of Comparison

An understanding of the principles underlying the selection of comparison groups is particularly important in studies that purport to evaluate accomplishment.

Ideally, we would like to know what would have happened to the population to whom a particular program was offered had there been some other program, or no program, during the same period. This is, of course, impossible to determine, and we must be satisfied with the assessment of the trend of events in some other population that has not been exposed to the program being evaluated but which is otherwise as similar as possible to the exposed group. This similarity, of the compared populations, the crux of the problem, can be assured only by random or systematic allocation of individuals or groups to treatment and comparison samples. Probably the most satisfactory procedure of all is the comparison of treatment and control groups randomly assigned from individuals offering themselves for the program. However, since the services in community mental health are frequently offered to groups rather than to individuals, this course may be impossible to put into practice. Where programs are restricted to small components of a population, such components may be randomized, as for example in the St. Louis study, where 15 schools have been assigned to various treatment and comparison groups in a systematic way. Another method, illustrated by the Milbank Memorial Fund's model for Syracuse, is that of comparing two or more large districts or cities, again selected randomly or systematically. This last method may be forced on us by the community-wide nature of many community mental health services, but it is less satisfactory that the others since there is the danger of changes occurring coincidentally with the program in one area but not in the other. However, as we have seen from the fluoridation experiments, the cumulative evidence from a number of such studies may be quite convincing.

In a large number of evaluatory studies use is made of data collected incidentally during, and without interference in, the course of a program. Comparison groups either are absent or consist of some readily available groups whose features of similarity to or difference from the experimental group are not precisely known. The attempt is to obtain some evaluatory information without the inconvenience of planning special evaluatory studies. To the extent that routine records are used for the purpose of evaluating technic or of describing prognosis for persons availing themselves of the service they may be perfectly satisfactory. In the minds of many investigators, however, it seems that estimates of prognosis among service participants are viewed as substitutes for the evaluation of accomplishment. While one would not discourage periodic analysis of individual program records at the present time, one should stress their limitations, and particularly discourage the idea that such analyses can be used to evaluate the accomplishment of a program.

Conclusion

Lemkau and Pasamanick,[7] preface their discussion of the problem of evaluation of mental health programs with the saying "Any fool can ask a question; the trick is to ask one that can be answered." We do not believe that we have been unrealistic in our statements as to what can and should be done. Rather, it seems to us that, despite the practical difficulties, community mental health programs are in many ways in unusually advantageous positions to be evaluated, particularly in terms of evaluation of accomplishment.

Of recent years serious doubts have been expressed by competent investigators as to the efficacy of surgical treatment of cancer in prolonging life. The accumulated cost of surgical therapy for cancer in money, personnel, and human misery (not to mention lives) over the past decades is astronomical. Regardless of whether such therapy is or is not effective, it is tragic that the evidence does not exist, and probably cannot now be obtained, to lay these doubts to rest. The organizers of mental health programs should not repeat the mistakes of our surgical predecessors. In the first place, they have before them the experience of the surgeons, and others, from which to learn. Second, mental health programs are being born into an era when critical evaluation is a recognized part of medical thought, and when the professional, technical, and financial help necessary to the operation of effective evaluatory studies is not difficult to obtain. Third, regardless of how firmly one is convinced of the effectiveness of a particular program, the ethics involved in leaving certain groups untreated do not arise, since there are not enough facilities to provide for everybody. Therefore, the major problem in evaluating the accomplishment of any health program—that of providing appropriate comparison groups—can readily be met, if an effort is made to select areas for application of such programs in a systematic and purposive way.

REFERENCES

1. Milbank Memorial Fund. "Model for a Project Which Would Demonstrate the Prevention of Mental Disorder in an Aged Population." In Planning Evaluations of Mental Health Programs. New York, N.Y.: Milbank Memorial Fund, 1958.
2. Glidewell, J. C., Mensh, I. N.; Domke, H. R., Gildea, M. C. L., and Buchmueller, A. D. Methods for Community Mental Health Research. Am. J. Orthopsychiat. 27: 38-54, 1957.
3. Meyer, H. J., and Borgatta, E. F. Paradoxes in Evaluating Mental Health Programs. Internat. J. Soc. Psychiat. 5: 136-141, 1959.
4. Peterson, O. L. An Analytical Study of North Carolina General Practice, 1953-1954. J. Med. Educ. 31: 1-165, 1956.
5. Hutchison, G. B. Evaluation of Preventive Services. J. Chronic Dis. 11: 497-508, 1960.
6. Gruenberg, E. M. "Progress Report to the Advisory Council on Mental Health Demonstrations; Development of the Concepts Underlying Mental Health Demonstrations." In Planning Evaluations of Mental Health Programs. New York, N. Y.: Milbank Memorial Fund. 1958.
7. Lemkau, P. V., and Pasamanick, B. Problems in Evaluation of Mental Health Programs. Am. J. Orthopsychiat. 27: 55-58, 1957.

This paper was presented before the Epidemiology and Mental Health Sections of the American Public Health Association at its annual meeting in San Francisco, Cal., November 1960.

5

Evaluation of Preventive Services

GEORGE B. HUTCHISON

DURING the past 50 years much of the world has experienced a dramatic change in its pattern of illness. By far the greatest part of this development has been the conquering of a wide spectrum of infectious diseases, and the key to this conquest has been increased understanding of the causative organisms. The earliest advances were dependent on attacking the organism outside the host, by general and specific sanitary measures. This was quickly followed by specific protection of the host by immunizations. Only relatively recently, highly effective methods of treating the established disease in the affected patient have been achieved.

With these developments firmly established as either past history or current practice, a new set of challenges predominates. The chief contenders are now the chronic degenerative diseases and malignancy. At present, control is far from satisfactory, whether related to treatment of established disease, protecting the individual, or attaching the etiological agent.

Although lack of basic knowledge of the processes involved in these diseases confounds the problem, it is widely felt that better application of presently available knowledge has great benefits to offer. In particular, it is felt that presently available therapy if applied at an earlier stage would greatly improve the picture. In line with this concept, preventive medicine has changed emphasis from activities with points of attack during prepathogenesis to early case-finding programs.

The prominent place of early case-finding in current thinking in preventive medicine is indicated by the following policy statement of the Health Insurance Plan of Greater New York: "The cornerstone of preventive medicine in group medical practice is the periodic health examination. The term 'periodic health examination' is used here to include all preventive health services to apparently well individuals ... at regularly stated intervals for the purpose of early detection of disease."[1]

Numerous reports have appeared urging increased early case-finding effort. These reports generally take the form of enumeration of conditions found or of review of follow-up. [2-4]

Other reports express some doubt as to the value of these findings in disease prevention. The editor of the *New England Journal of Medicine* writes, "The case for early detection ... is not completely open and shut.... The problem that confronts the physicians, patients and public alike is to decide how much value it has." [5] Crile [6] expresses a similar view: "I believe that the public and perhaps even the profession itself have been somewhat oversold on the importance of time in most diseases.... There are few diseases ... in which it makes any difference to the ultimate results whether the condition is recognized today or two weeks from today." A stronger comment is referred to in an editorial in the *Lancet*: "... several distinguished physicians declared that routine examinations of this kind are virtually useless for their intended purpose—namely, the detection and successful treatment of symptomless disease." [7] A somewhat more cautious statement suggests that the matter is not yet decided and that perhaps early case-finding is important in some but not all diseases. "We still do not know whether case finding and treatment in the presymptomatic stages of disease either diminish disability or postpone death for the majority of chronic diseases.... It may be that for some diseases, the diagnosis and treatment of early symptomatic disease will control such disease as effectively as its discovery and treatment in the presymptomatic stage." [8]

These conflicting views suggest the necessity of a careful evaluation of these programs. It is the purpose of this paper to describe the application of the principles of evaluation to preventive services. A generalized evaluation model applicable to all phases of preventive medicine will first be outlined. The specific application of the model in evaluating early case-finding programs will then be presented.

The Scope of Preventive Medicine

The term "preventive medicine" has been used in the previous section in connection with activities which prevent the initial occurrence of disease as well as with activities which prevent the progression of disease. If preventiveness is considered as a scalar quantity, it seems reasonable to speak of preventing the initial occurrence as being "more preventive" than preventing the progression of disease.

With this comparative concept in mind, all aspects of medical practice can be arranged in an ordered sequence, the position in the sequence representing the degree of preventiveness. This degree of preventiveness is defined by the extent to which the activity alters favorably the natural course of disease. The ultimate of this scale would be activities which completely eradicate the etiological agent of a disease, as, for example, malaria or yellow fever control programs. Specific vaccination would have only a slightly lower rating. Early treatment would in general rate higher on this scale than late treatment. As will be discussed later, however, this need not be so in every case, and both the natural course of a disease and the available therapy must be considered in determining the preventiveness of any program. Purely symptomatic or palliative therapy, although an important part of medical practice, has only minimal effect in changing the course of disease.

Following this line of thought, "preventive medicine" is understood to refer to a philosophy of medical practice which emphasizes methods which attack the natural course of a disease. This philosophy does not exclude any type of medical service but attempts to incorporate all appropriate services in coordinated programs which are effective in altering the course of diseases.

The term "preventive services" is generally used to refer to those services which are highest on this preventiveness scale, and these are the services of particular interest in this paper. However, the general outline for evaluation which follows is applicable to all medical services. The title of this paper, "Evaluation of Preventive Services," will then be understood to mean evaluation of the preventiveness of medical services.

Evaluation—General Model

A program evaluation, as the term will be used here, is a very special sort of research investigation and should be distinguished from demonstrations and program reviews. The latter two sorts of studies are similar in general purpose to the evaluation but less rigorous in design.

An evaluation answers one or more of the following questions with respect to an experiment:

(1) Does the program, as operating during the period of evaluation, accomplish the objectives set down prior to this period?

(2) To what degree does the program accomplish these objectives?

(3) What amount of effort is required by the program to achieve the objectives?

The steps basic to answering this set of questions are:

(1) Statement of objectives. Objectives are laid down before beginning the phase of the program to be evaluated. The statement of objectives includes a description of the measurements by which to gauge success.

(2) Program. The program is a procedure which is intended to alter existing behavior in such a way as to accomplish the stated objectives. The phase of the program being evaluated is designed specifically for the objectives and is hoped to be the best available method of accomplishing the objectives.

(3) Control. The control answers the associated implied question, "Would the objectives have been equally accomplished in the absence of the program?"

(4) Measurement of effect. The effect is measured with relation to the stated objectives and in terms of the initially prescribed gauge.

Application of the Model

The four steps of the model as applied to evaluating the preventiveness of medical services follow readily from the preceding discussion:

(1) The objective is to alter the natural course of disease in a favorable direction.

(2) The program is a medical service or coordinated group of services and is intended to be the best method, with current knowledge and available facilities, of accomplishing the objective. In the later sections the program discussed as illustrative of the method will be one of the early case-finding programs.

(3) The control is the natural course of disease as it exists with the normally available medical care of the community.

(4) The measure of effect is the extent to which the natural sequence of pathogenic events is favorably altered by the program.

Natural History of Disease

It will be apparent that an understanding of the natural history of disease is basic to the evaluation. The natural history of disease is used here to refer not only to the interrelation between the external etiological agents and the biologic response of the host but also to the effects of environmental factors, social and physical, to the community pattern of medical practice, and to the social and intellectual response of the host.[9] Thus the natural history of chronic pulmonary insufficiency may be quite different in certain urban areas with excessive industrial air pollution as compared with the course in relatively nonpolluted rural areas. Similarly, the natural history of disease in a highly literate and medically sophisticated area may be different from the sequence observed in a remote region with generally poor medical facilities and little education as to health principles.

These factors will be important in evaluations since the programs likely to be effective in altering the natural course will clearly be dependent on the characteristics of this course. In particular, some very simple programs may be highly profitable in the remote region mentioned above, but the same program might give no additional benefit to the natural course of events in the more advanced area.

In the following paragraphs a schematic representation of the natural course of disease is presented. This representation is adapted to the considerations of *early case-finding programs*. These programs are potentially useful only after the disease has begun and before it has been diagnosed in the natural course of events. An evaluation of other preventive activities, applicable in the prepathogenic period or in the period following diagnosis, would require a somewhat different scheme, emphasizing different portions of the disease course.

In Table I this natural sequence is indicated diagrammatically. A hypothetic disease as it affects an average individual in a specific environment is represented. Lengths of intervals along the sequence from A to D are proportional to the times between the indicated events. At the time of study, the most sensitive known detection device could detect this disease only after it had been present for a time AB. This average individual and his physician would not apply the detection test at B, so the diagnosis would not be known at this time. After an additional delay (BP), the disease would undergo some recognizable pathologic change. This might be the onset of symptoms, a change in some organ detectable on physical examination, or a change in some laboratory study. The event at point P

TABLE I. DIAGRAMMATIC REPRESENTATION OF
NATURAL HISTORY OF DISEASE

A	B	P	CRITICAL POINT	C	D
Biologic onset	Positive detection test possible	Pathologic change	X	Usual time of diagnosis	Final outcome

would also be overlooked or misunderstood, as a result of either patient or physician delay, and the diagnosis would be made only at point C.

Now let us suppose that at point X in this time sequence a critical event occurs in this disease. By a critical event it is meant that therapy instituted before this point is less difficult or more effective than therapy instituted after the point. More specifically, if the disease is curable, cure may be effected before the critical point but will be more difficult or impossible after the point. In the case of a self-limiting disease whose chief ill effect is a permanent deformity or other stigma, this permanent effect may be prevented by therapy before the critical point but is inevitable after this time. In the case of a chronic disease with no known cure, therapy before the critical point delays the progress of disease and postpones or lessens the severity of successive stages. Therapy begun after the critical point offers no advantage over the normal course, in which therapy is begun after point C, the time when the disease is diagnosed in its natural course.

The last example in the preceding paragraph indicates that the critical point is defined with relation to point C in the natural history of disease. It will be apparent that there may be an additional critical point (X') defined with relation to point X and falling to the left of point X (Table II). Therapy begun before X' would result in a more favorable sequence than therapy begun at point X, but therapy begun after X' and before X would offer no advantage over therapy begun at point X itself. Similarly there may be arbitrarily many critical points, each critical with respect to the next critical point to the right or to point C.

These points may correspond to recognizable pathologic changes as defined at point P (Table I), although this would not generally be the case.

The critical points together with point C divide the natural history of disease into a discrete set of segments. The concept of relative

TABLE II. MULTIPLE CRITICAL POINTS IN
NATURAL HISTORY OF DISEASE

B				C
Positive detection test possible	X''	X'	X	Usual time of diagnosis

potency of preventive activities discussed under the previous section, "The Scope of Preventive Medicine" may be defined in terms of these segments. Thus activities which cause therapy to be started during any time segment left of point X are effective preventive measures, and the farther the segment is to the left the more potent is the prevention. Within any segment, however, no point has any advantage over any other point.

A limiting case is that in which there are not discrete but continuous critical points. In such a disease, at every moment there is advantage to the future sequence of pathogenic events to begin therapy immediately.

Employing this schematic concept of natural history of disease we can state certain conditions which must be fulfilled if an early case-finding program is to be a successful preventive measure for a given disease.

(1) There must be a known effective therapy.

(2) There must be a diagnostic device capable of detecting the disease before its usual time of diagnosis in the community being studied.

(3) There must be one or more critical points, as defined above, in the natural history of the disease.

(4) Such a critical point must occur in the time sequence of the disease after the time when diagnosis first becomes possible and before the time when diagnosis is made under the usual disease pattern of the community.

In addition to these basic requirements some quantitative estimates can be made from the natural history diagram as to the probability of success of an early case-finding effort for a given disease.

(1) The longer the time between points B and C in Table I, the greater is the likelihood of diagnosing cases early by instituting a case-finding program. As an example, if some screening test is capable of detecting a disease more than a year before the time it is normally discovered, annual applications of the test will routinely discover disease earlier than usual. If, however, the test becomes positive only 3 months before symptoms would lead to its diagnosis, upon applying the test annually three-fourths of the cases will still be diagnosed as a result of symptoms which develop within a year following a negative test and only one-fourth will benefit by the screening. Here results could be improved by screening at more frequent intervals.

(2) The longer the time interval between points B and X'' in Table II, the greater likelihood there is of achieving the maximum

benefit possible from early case-finding approaches. The probability of achieving any prevention at all is proportional to the length of the interval BX. This probability is less than the probability of finding cases early, dependent on BC; that is, the number of cases found earlier than usual will in general be more than the number whose prognosis is benefited, since some may be found earlier than usual but still not early enough to be helped.

It should be noted again that the natural history events described are dependent on the environmental setting, including the generally available medical care, as well as on the biologic characteristics of the disease. In a specified community a new case-finding program may be unprofitable only because an equivalent procedure is already a generally accepted part of the community's natural disease course. The time of usual diagnosis, the sensitivity of screening tests, and the effectiveness of therapy will all vary with education of the population, alertness of physicians, and scientific developments in medicine.

The following conditions illustrate some of the patterns in which critical points may occur.

(1) Presbyopia is a disease in which there are no critical points, not because of lack of screening tests or lack of therapy, but because presently available therapy alleviates symptoms only and does not alter the course of the condition.[10]

(2) Carcinoma of the cervix is a disease in which there appears to be a single critical point occurring after the development of a positive screening test. The critical point occurs at the time when a distant metastasis becomes viable or when malignancy becomes inoperable as a result of local extension.[11]

(3) Carcinoma of the breast has proved particularly disappointing from the preventive medicine point of view. The mortality rate for carcinoma of this site in New York State remained virtually unchanged from 1931 to 1956 despite extensive efforts to educate the public as well as physicians to be alert to all suggestive lesions.[12] This and other similar observations have led some to the conclusion that certain malignant conditions are predetermined in their outcome and are not subject to any benefit from early case-finding efforts. In terms of the natural history diagram this would be described by considering that metastasis in breast cancer occurs either before point B or after point C. Early case-finding would be too late in the former type, since the disease is diffuse before any known test becomes positive. In the latter type, early case-finding would be unnecessary because diagnosis would be made soon enough without any

special effort. This result might hold true in areas with a good general level of health habits, while in a less alert area a preventive program might be indicated.

(4) Diabetes mellitus may be a disease in which progression of irreversible vascular change is continuous so that every improvement in time of starting therapy is beneficial in slowing this natural disease sequence. This would be represented by a continuous succession of critical points rather than a discrete set of such points.[13]

Analytic Study of Natural History

In order to make measurements of some of the intervals in the natural history of disease, it is first necessary to determine stages of disease which are identifiable in individual patients.

Identification of Stages of Disease. The interval from biologic onset to development of the first diagnostic indication (*AB* in Table I) is in most diseases a purely speculative time period. In some diseases its duration can be determined by identifying contact with an etiological agent. A known congenital disease, for example, Huntington's chorea, can be said to have had its biologic onset at time of conception.

Individuals with disease in the stage represented by the interval *BC* (from development of a positive test until time of usual diagnosis) can be identified by a screening survey of previously undiagnosed people. Similarly, individuals in the interval *CD* (from diagnosis to final outcome) can be identified from the medical history, and it is this interval that is most frequently discussed in disease descriptions.

The various critical points, *X*, *X'*, *X''*, etc., are in general not readily identified. Only when they coincide with some recognizable pathologic change is identification possible. Thus a critical point in most malignant conditions is identical with development of a metastasis. In the more common situation, when a critical point is not clearly related to an observable pathologic change, it is possible only to determine whether one or more critical points exist between two successive pathologic changes. As an example of this, it may be demonstrated in diabetes mellitus that treatment begun at the time of development of a positive glucose tolerance test is more effective in delaying late vascular change and death than treatment begun at the first appearance of a retinal vascular change. Therefore, there is at least one critical point between these two identifiable events in the disease course. We cannot say, however, whether a given patient has passed this point or not.

It will be apparent from the preceding paragraphs that it is of basic importance in describing natural history of diseases to have clearly defined stages of disease which can be identified by examination of individual patients. An example of such a staging is the now familiar use of retinal vessel changes for grading of hypertensive vascular disease. It is urged that similar stages be developed for all of the common chronic diseases as a first step in describing their natural histories. The more detailed a staging is developed, the more precisely can critical points be defined.

Determination of Duration of Stages of Disease. Two general methods for measuring the durations of identifiable stages of disease are commonly used. Either of the two methods may be used for any of these stages.

The one method follows a population longitudinally from the time one recognizable pathologic feature appears until a second feature appears. An example of this method is the recent study in Worcester, Massachusetts, of survival time following the first attack of cerebral thrombosis.[14] In this instance the second pathologic feature is death.

In the second method, the relationship: duration = prevalence/incidence is used. This approach generally involves a cross-sectional study to obtain prevalence and also reporting of new cases over some period of time to determine incidence. Dunn[11] has used this method for estimating the survival time of invasive uterine cancer.

The indications and contraindications for the two types of analysis will not be discussed here. Each involves certain assumptions which must be carefully considered when the findings of the study are to be generalized beyond the particular populations investigated. Either may be used when the natural history alone is to be investigated. In the type of problem of greatest concern in this paper, however, the chief interest is in a comparison of the natural history of disease with the course observed after introducing a new technique, namely, early case-finding efforts.

If the longitudinal study is used in connection with cases identified by a new technique, the results cannot strictly be considered to represent the natural history because of the effect of the study on the disease. However, with certain precautions the effect of detecting the cases early can be minimized by allowing all or a sample of cases to go untreated until the stage of disease at which diagnosis is normally established. This involves certain ethical problems but may be a feasible solution if there is no generally accepted opinion that early treatment of the disease in question is of known value. As an example, there is difference of opinion at the present time as to whether certain findings represent a precursor stage of classic diabetes. It may be acceptable to observe certain patients with these findings without recommending therapy until a diagnosis of classic diabetes can be made.

If the cross-sectional approach is applied to this same question, the average duration can be computed from prevalence and incidence data. The effect of the cross-sectional study itself on the course of the disease is relatively little as compared with the longitudinal approach.

Error of Interpretation. An error occasionally made in interpreting studies of the course of disease is to confuse the additional time of observation of the disease resulting from early case-finding with an added increment of life due to improved treatment. This fallacy is illustrated in Table III. In this table, two pathologic events are indicated—*P,* a recognizable clinical finding, and *D,* death. In the usual pattern of medical events diagnosis is made at *C* and death occurs at *D.* If an early case-finding program is applied, diagnosis is made at *C'.* Death is delayed to *D'* as a result of starting therapy early. The benefit due to early therapy is represented by the increment *DD',* and this can be measured by taking the difference between the two survival times *(PD* and *PD')* following clinical finding *P.* The common error is to compare the survival times *(CD* and *C'D')* from times of diagnosis *C* and *C',* respectively. This comparison clearly exaggerates the benefit of early case-finding, since the interval *CC'* is not an added length of life but simply an added time of recognized disease.

TABLE III. EFFECT OF EARLY CASE-FINDING ON SURVIVAL TIME

C	P	C	D	D'
Early diagnosis	Pathologic change	Usual diagnosis	Usual death	Delayed death

Level of Objectives

In the previous sections it has been stated that the common objective of preventive services is to interfere with the pathologic events in the natural history of disease. It is frequently useful to evaluate a program in terms of some more limited objective. As an example, it would seem reasonable to evaluate an early case-finding program by determining the frequency of finding cases early. Studies of intermediate objectives are, as a rule, far easier to carry out than studies of ultimate objectives. The information obtained is of correspondingly more limited value. The shortcut is justified only when the relationship between the intermediate and ultimate objectives has already been established or when it is anticipated that it will be established in a subsequent study. In an early case-finding effort it may have been clearly shown that finding cases of a specific disease in a given population leads to decreased mortality. It is then adequate to accept this information in evaluating various means of finding disease in the population and to confine these evaluations simply to determining appropriate case-finding rates.

It should be remembered that the original relationship between intermediate and ultimate objectives may change in time. Thus if the population and medical personnel become more alert to symptoms and signs over a period of time, they may improve the normal community level of early case-finding to such an extent that available diagnostic screening tests offer no additional value. Conversely, the development of a new case-finding test may make early detection efforts profitable in an area where they were previously unrewarding.

Levels of objectives form an extensive spectrum. The simplest level is the quantity of money spent. This may be the extent of evaluation required in certain administrative reports. More commonly it is required to show what services were performed, a second level of objective. Beyond this a third level would include some measure of the accomplishments of the service, such as numbers of patients contacted, numbers of positive cases discovered, or volume of treatment given.

All of the measures in the above paragraph may be considered intermediate in the sense that they do not measure the extent to which the natural history of disease is altered. This latter measure is the first level objective which is intrinsically valuable.

Higher and more complex levels exist in this spectrum. Thus, Baumgartner[15] has mentioned that in the Soviet Union health is considered a means rather than an end. A successful program would in that setting have to be measured in values to the state rather than the individual, as, for example, units of production output. Beyond this, theologians or philosophers could add more complex objectives of health services.

It is, then, to a certain extent arbitrary that improvement of health is accepted as an ultimate objective. It is felt that this is an objective that the medical profession generally accepts as intrinsically valuable, and lower level objectives are generally not acceptable, except insofar as they are felt to be indicators of health benefit.

Summary

A broad concept of preventive medicine has been described, embracing all phases of medical care. All medical services are preventive services to the extent that they are concerned with altering favorably the natural history of disease.

An evaluation model is described which is designed to answer the following questions with relation to health programs: (1) Does the program meet its objectives, or (2) to what degree does it meet the objectives, or (3) how efficiently are the objectives met?

A spectrum of intermediate and ultimate objectives is described. The ultimate objective of particular interest in preventive medicine is that objective which corresponds with the concept of prevention as an alteration of natural history of disease in a favorable direction. In order to measure this objective it is necessary to develop an analytic description of natural history of disease. A diagrammatic representation of such a description is presented.

It is urged that specific diseases be extensively studied to develop clearly definable phases of which reliable analytic description can be made.

The logical fallacy of confusing time of diagnosis with a pathologic change in disease history is discussed. It is pointed out that prolonged survival time following early diagnosis efforts may be due to two increments—one represents the additional portion of the early natural history brought under observation and the second represents the increased years of life attributable to beginning therapy at an advantageous time. It is necessary to distinguish these increments in evaluating preventive services.

It is urged that an evaluation not be accepted as complete until the correspondence of intermediate with ultimate objectives is established. In the case of early diagnosis programs, this requirement demands proof of the preventive medicine maxim, "The earlier the treatment the more effective the prevention." In order to predict benefit from early case-finding, a disease must have the following characteristics in the population in which it is being studied:

(1) There must be a known effective therapy.

(2) There must be a diagnostic device capable of detecting the disease prior to its usual time of diagnosis in the community being studied.

(3) There must be one or more critical points such that therapy instituted before the critical point is more effective in interfering with pathologic sequence than is therapy undertaken after the point.

(4) Such a critical point must occur in the time sequence of the disease after the time when diagnosis first becomes possible and before the time when diagnosis is made under the usual disease pattern of the community.

REFERENCES

1. Professional Standards for Medical Groups and Standards for Medical Centers. New York: Health Insurance Plan of Greater New York, 1959.
2. Tupper, C. J., and Beckett, M. D. Faculty Health Appraisal. Univ. of Michigan Med. Bull. 24: 35-43, 1958.
3. Prickman, L. E., Koelsche, G. A., Berkman, J. M., Carryer, H. M., Peters, G. A., and Henderson, L. L. Does the Executive Health Program Meet Its Objective? J.A.M.A. 167: 1451-1455, 1958.
4. Calabresi, P., Arvold, N. V., and Stovall, W. D. Cytological Screening for Uterine Cancer through Physicians' Offices. J.A.M.A. 168: 243-247, 1958.
5. Periodic Health Examination. New Eng. J. Med. 260: 559-560, 1959.
6. Massachusetts Memorial Hospitals Centennial Celebration: Health for the American People: A Symposium. Boston: Little, Brown & Co., 1956, pp. 5-6.
7. Routine Medical Examinations. Lancet, 1: 948-949, 1958.
8. Kruse, H. D., Baumgartner, L., Kolbe, H. W., and McCarthy, H. L. Public Health Aspects of Aging. Bull. N.Y. Acad. Med. 33: 493-518, 1957.
9. Leavell, H. R., and Clark, E. G. Textbook of Preventive Medicine. New York: McGraw-Hill, 1953, p. 9.
10. McLean, J. Eyeglasses as Therapeutic Agent. New York J. Med. 57: 3167-3173, 1957.
11. Dunn, J. E., Jr. Preliminary Findings of the Memphis-Shelby County Uterine Cancer Study and Their Interpretation. Am. J. Pub. Health. 48: 861-873, 1958.
12. Annual Report: Bureau of Cancer Control, New York State Department of Health, 1957.
13. Dolger, H. Vascular Complications of Diabetes Mellitus. Bull. N.Y. Acad. Med. 26: 779-785, 1950.
14. Robinson, R. W., Cohen, W. D., Higano, N., Meyer, R., Lukowsky, G. H., McLaughlin, R. B., and Mac Gilpin, H. H. Life—Table Analysis of Survival After Cerebral Thrombosis—Ten Year Experience. J.A.M.A. 169:1149-1152, 1959.
15. Minutes of Meeting: Committee on Preventive Medicine and Social Science Research of the Social Science Research Council, New York, Dec. 12, 1958. Unpublished.

6

Research in Large-Scale Intervention Programs

HOWARD E. FREEMAN and CLARENCE C. SHERWOOD

DISSATISFACTION with the social order and zealous efforts at community change have characterized the personal and academic lives of social scientists since their emergence as an identifiable group on the American scene.[1] In many ways, of course, the various disciplines and the persons that hold membership in them have changed markedly over the last several decades: the influence of visionary clergymen, guilt-ridden do-gooders, and political radicals —dedicated to projecting their own humanitarian views in the guise of scientific inquiry—has pretty well diminished.[2]

But the social scientist has expanded his role in the modification of community life and in the amelioration of social pathologies. He puts forth theories on which action programs may be based; he serves as expert and consultant to policy-makers; and he uses his research repertoire to guide program development. There are outstanding examples of such influence: the work of Stouffer and his associates on military problems, the studies of learning psychologists on educational practices, the manifesto of Clark and other social scientists in connection with the Supreme Court's integration decision, and most recently, the document of Ohlin and Cloward on delinquency programs.[3] Certainly much of social science activity is directed at understanding "basic" processes, but, whether by intent or not, social scientists serve as agents of social change; and, if one is willing to extrapolate from shifts in occupational settings, it appears that there is an increasing number of them who know full well the social-change potential of their work.[4]

Over the years social scientists, at least a small number of them, have been engaged in still another type of activity, the evaluation of health, education and welfare programs and interventions—in some instances by means of experimental designs that include control groups and pre-post-test measures. But up until recently the impact of their work and the findings of their studies on social policy and on community life has been minimal. This is so in spite of the fact that for 15 years or more there has been increased emphasis—particularly at the Federal level—on demonstration-research programs.

On paper, at least, there has been much concern with the assessment of therapeutic and rehabilitation efforts. Virtually all of the demonstration programs supported by public funds in the health and welfare field and many of the projects sponsored by philanthropic foundations include a requirement that the worth of the effort be assessed. For the most part, however, the evaluation requirement has remained a formality; granting agencies have tended to overlook it in their frenzy to implement programs intuitively believed worthwhile; statements and often elaborate designs for evaluation in demonstration-research programs have been included in proposals as a ritual with full knowledge that the commitment would not be met; and researchers have, on occasion, found it expeditious to accept evaluation assignments and then redirect the resources to another type of study.

Further, a significant proportion of studies that are actually initiated are not carried to completion. In part the failure to undertake and particularly to complete experimental investigations is related to the barriers put forth by practitioners. There is no need to underscore the difficulties of undertaking research when the cooperation of practitioners and flexibility on their part is necessary for the development and implementation of an adequate design; conflict between clinician and scientist pervades all fields and the difficulties that medical researchers have in undertaking experiments with human subjects are minimal in comparison with evaluation efforts in the community.[5] Also, of course, many social scientists engaged in evaluation studies regard them as a dilettante activity and their interest in such work continues only so long as they think they are testing a theory of concern to them or believe their work will provide scholarly publications or economic affluence.

As a consequence, adequately conceived efforts have in fact been undertaken only rarely and the sheer infrequency of completed investigations is a major reason for the minimal impact of evaluation research on social policy. Certainly it is difficult to point to many instances in which programs actually have been modified, expanded or terminated because of evaluation findings.

The multibillion dollar "War on Poverty" has intensified the demand for a concerted attempt to undertake broad-scale action-research demonstrations, and to engage in knowledge-seeking efforts evaluated in terms of effect—rather than merely in terms of whether or not the program proves workable administratively or whether or not so-called "experts" approve of it. Certainly, without efforts in this direction, literally billions of dollars may be spent without anyone knowing what works and, what is perhaps more frightening, without our being any better equipped to contribute to the next round of mass change efforts.

This situation would not be so serious if the social sciences had a significant reservoir of findings on which to base broad-scale intervention programs or had a wealth of experience in how to go about evaluating community-wide action programs in ways that provide "hard" findings on their worth. It also would not be so serious were there the opportunity to learn new methodological wrinkles or to develop a strategy for rendering the results of evaluation studies into a potent force in the determination of action programs and social policy. But we suddenly have a mandate to participate in massive social change, via community-wide efforts projected to restructure health and welfare activities and to reorient the efforts of practitioners. Despite the failure to work out methods and, most important, a strategy to influence policy on small-scale action programs, we now have been thrust into a prominent role in massive efforts designed to have an impact on virtually all community members and indeed on the very social order. It is simply not possible to retreat from this assignment, any more than it is for all physicists to avoid participation in the development and improvement of destructive devices.

The opportunity to participate carries with it great responsibility; our posture and pronouncements are likely to affect markedly the shape of future health and welfare programs and indeed of all community life. Although many individuals, for a variety of reasons, have decried so-called centralized programs of planned change and have expressed alarm over their control by public bodies and large foundations, there is little doubt that this is the direction that health and welfare activities are taking; and, the recent national election is clearly an overwhelming mandate for these efforts to continue.[6]

Perhaps those of us located in professional schools or employed directly by community-based programs are most sensitive to the stakes involved, but it is obvious that the comprehensive and massive character of projects sponsored by organizations such as the President's Committee on Juvenile Delinquency and Youth Crime, The Ford Foundation, and now the Office of Economic Opportunity are likely to rock the very foundations of our social system. If these observations are valid, we must rapidly accumulate an adequate technical repertoire for the task and explicate the conditions that must be met in order for our work to have social policy potential and to meet the demands of our times. It is essential that we understand better the environment in which we are being called upon to work; have a clearer understanding of the conceptual issues involved in measuring the impact of broad-scale programs; and recognize the knotty methodological problems that one encounters when participating in action-research demonstrations. In this paper we address ourselves to these issues and use portions of Action for Boston Community Development's (ABCD) delinquency action-research program to illustrate notions advanced in this paper.

The Research Environment

Since many social scientists have at one point or another been involved with large bureaucracies operating on a crash basis, certain rather obvious preliminary observations can be made most briefly. It is important to point out that dependence upon the legislative branch of our government or on whims of foundations for funds and the necessity to involve and obtain the cooperation of politically and ideologically antagonistic parties in local communities have and will continue to produce a considerable degree of disorder in most of the massive programs. The development of adequate staffs, personnel policies, and long range planning by community-based mass programs is difficult—some maintain almost impossible—given the condition of being affluent one minute and poverty-stricken the next and given the fleeting support of the various political forces involved. The shape, size, and goals of programs appear to change from day-to-day, and one of the difficulties of evaluation research in these settings stems from the high degree of organizational and interorganizational chaos.

Even in those efforts in which the over-all objectives remain relatively stable, the number of specific programs is large. Moreover most programs consist of a complex of multiple stimuli imposed over an extended period of time, and the goals of the individual programs are diverse. The situation is much too complex to fit the classical independent-dependent variable model. Therefore, action-research needs to be developed in terms of a series of staged inputs and outputs.

The juvenile delinquency action research demonstration project at ABCD which seeks to deal with this problem provides an illustration. It is based on three sets of variables: the dependent variable of the project is juvenile delinquency; more specifically defined as law-violating behavior of 12- through 16-year-old males residing in specific areas of Boston. The second set of variables are referred to as the intermediate variables; according to the three-step hypothesis, changes in the intermediate variables should produce desired change in the dependent variable. The third set are referred to as program variables: these are the specific interventions by which it is hoped to produce changes in one or more of the intermediate variables.

A brief description of one of the programs, the "Week-End Ranger Camp," may make the ABCD delinquency model clearer. At a regular summer-camp site, boys on probation participate each week-end in a series of activities such as discussion groups, council meetings, and work and recreational activities (the program variables). The model specifies that, as a result of these programs, shifts will occur in anomie, alienation and social values (the intermediate variables). The increased engagement of delinquent boys with the values and structural system of the society is held to lead to a reduction in delinquency (the dependent variable). In order to evaluate the program, the overall design specifies that local probation offices in parts of the city of Boston provide lists of names of boys eligible by reason of age, residence and other criteria for participation in the program. These boys were asked to come to the probation offices and participate in a study. At the office, the boys were pre-tested on several attitude measures—i.e., anomie, alienation and value scales. An attempt has been made to build procedures into the program which appear to have some hope of changing the attitudes of these youth and ultimately, according to the model, their on-the-street social behavior as well. After pretesting, the youth were randomly divided into two groups and the members of one group were invited to participate in the week-end program. The members of the other group were designated as ineligible for the program.

In order to undertake appropriately the evaluation of a mass program, it is necessary to develop an action-research design that includes a description of the interrelated elements: it must specify the ways the intermediate changes are expected to be produced, and provide hypotheses about the relationships between these changes and the dependent variable. Further, the design must outline the ways to determine, if such intermediate changes do occur, whether or not they are followed by the desired changes in the dependent variable.

A proper evaluation of the implementation of such a model requires not only knowing that certain effects were obtained but also

knowing with some degree of probability that the effects were sub-
stantively related to a particular set of stimuli. Consequently, one
major problem confronting efforts to evaluate programs of this type
is that of controlling the stimuli. Major strides toward the accumulation of definitive knowledge about the effects of programs will
not be made until we are able to think through and develop procedures for handling the problem of what constitutes the stimuli.
The basic question is what is it that should be repeated if the program appears to work?

There are two related but nevertheless operationally separate issues here. One is the design of the stimulus or intervention. The
other—and perhaps the more difficult one—is the problem of monitoring the intervention. Even if one begins with very definite and
clear cut intentions to conduct and evaluate "repeatable" programs,
it is possible to underestimate grossly the difficulties which are involved in both designing and monitoring programs with the goal
of repeatability in mind. It is clear that this problem cannot be
satisfactorily resolved simply by reducing it to a process of spelling
out procedures in great and specific detail, as difficult as even that
may be.

In an attempt to deal with this problem, the approach at ABCD
has been to move toward the development of principles rather than
procedures, toward a set of theoretical concepts or ideas which trace
the dynamics of how it is expected that the program will have the
desired effects, i.e., toward a theory which logically interrelates a set
of principles and procedures with desired outcomes. If such an impact model is sufficiently worked out, a set of working principles becomes available upon which practitioners can draw not only for the
design of programs but also to make practical decisions about day-
to-day program situations.

But unless the social science researcher participates, indeed leads
the dialogue and bargaining required for the development of an impact model—including the identification of goals, the description of
input-output variables, and the elaboration of a rationale that specifies the relationship between input variables and goals—these tasks
are likely to remain undone. Once the impact model is formulated,
the researcher must continue to remain within the environment,
like a snarling watchdog ready to oppose alterations in program and
procedures that could render his evaluation efforts useless.

It is only fair and from our view unfortunate to note that the researcher can expect little help or guidance from the funding groups

in these tasks. In part this is related to the lack of structured expectations of outcome on the part of these groups, but also because of an effort to maintain as non-directed a posture as possible in the light of accusations of authoritarian control over the programs, or the theories that underlie them, in individual cities. The various President's Committee on Delinquency projects illustrate this point well. From city to city, though the legislation directs attention to the reduction of youth crime and the amelioration of related problems, considerable latitude has been allowed individual cities not only in program development but in evaluation design. Thus, not only are there variations in whether one is concerned with area-crime rates, the police contacts of individual youths, or the reduction of deviant though not necessarily illegal behavior, but some cities apparently have not felt a need to be particularly concerned with any phenomenon of this sort. Unless the situation changes, the researcher is naive to expect that sanctions from above are going to provide him with much support in the specification of objectives, the identification of the intermediate variables (i.e., the goals of specific programs) or the outlining of the theoretical links between these intermediate variables and the over-all objectives.

The researcher has three choices: he can follow Hyman's recommendation and try to guess the intermediate and over-all goals, and later be told that the ones he selected were not relevant at all;[7] he can insist that program persons provide them in which case he should bring lots of novels to the office to read while he waits, or he can participate or even take a major responsibility for the development of the action framework. There is little likelihood of developing evaluation designs for these massive programs by either second-guessing the action people or by insisting upon their coming up with an appropriate and explicit flow-chart. Indeed, if the researcher is going to act responsibly as an agent of social change through his evaluation research, it probably is mandatory for him to engage himself in program development.[8] The task would be much easier if the sponsors of these massive programs would establish and enforce a requirement that the necessary specifications be part of any application and renewal of applications and that sanctions be exercised to prevent slippage.

Furthermore, the task would become more manageable if the sponsors provided a minimal set of outcome variables—uniform measurement would be most valuable for long-range program planning. It is most difficult, indeed probably impossible, to compare the

various delinquency prevention efforts of the last three years, the
various mental health reorganization attempts over the past ten
years and, unless there are marked changes in policy, only limited
likelihood of making city-to-city comparisons in the economic, educational, and occupational rehabilitation programs now underway as
part of the poverty package. Given the lack of structured directions
by the government and foundation granting programs, and the lack
of commitment to evaluation research on the part of many practitioners on the local level, it is not easy to manipulate the environment so the researcher can undertake his task.

Again, we must acknowledge that the researcher has not always
participated in these evaluation studies enthusiastically and with a
full sense of commitment; to argue that the problems of evaluation
research are solely due to the actions of others is as ludicrous as the
general who maintained that the high V.D. rate among his troops
was due to the promiscuity of the civilian population. Participation
within the action environment obligates the researcher to bring to
bear his substantive knowledge in the design of programs; to be a
positive influence in their development and to recommend or con-
demn program plans or at least forcefully report and interpret findings from other research that have a bearing on program development. This we often fail to do. If we did exercise our responsibility,
we probably would have built into these massive efforts more attempts
to use physical means such as brighter street lights to prevent delinquency and have exerted more pressure for coercive programs
such as forced literacy training as a condition of probation and
parole in contrast with increased numbers of therapeutic communities and the burgeoning of street-worker projects.[9]

Conceptions of Evaluations

In order to influence social policy, findings from social-action experiments must provide a basis for the efficient allocation of financial
and human resources in the solution of social problems. It is this
notion of the efficient allocation of resources that is the key to the
whole problem of planning and choosing among social-action
programs.

Traditionally service has been viewed—and in a vague way measured—in terms of that which is offered such as counseling, guidance,
therapy, advice and the like. Good service is therefore that which
is offered in a professional manner by a qualified person who in
turn is supervised by a qualified supervisor. But service needs to be

viewed not only in terms of process but of impact as well. In the final analysis, success must be viewed in terms of outcome rather than in terms of the supposed quality of the procedures used. The implications of this shift in view are considerable:

1. It forces those responsible for program design to clearly specify their objectives, to define what it is they are trying to achieve, what specific changes they are trying to effect. At the very least, it requires them to cooperate in efforts to operationalize what they have in mind.

2. It shifts the emphasis from "procedure as an end" to "procedure as a means." Program personnel must then consider the relationship between the procedures it recommends and the defined outcomes that have been chosen.

3. It leads to a reconsideration of the whole notion of cost of service. Currently, we are in the grip of the proponents of the "per capita cost of service" point of view. If programs were to compete on the basis of how much it costs to achieve one unit (however that may be defined) of desired outcome, the ultimate selection of programs would be very different.

4. And, finally, this view forces the inclusion of solid, empirical research into the over-all planning and program operation, because the decisions as to the optimum allocation of the resources available can, within this view, only be made on the basis of empirical evidence.

The first requirement of evaluation research is the determination of efficacy. Evaluation research efforts must, therefore, seek to approximate the experimental model as much as possible—we do not do so often enough and some of the so-called evaluation designs of the current mass programs have completely forgone an experimental or quasi-experimental approach. Admittedly, there is a limit to the extent controlled experiments can be conducted within these programs. Nevertheless it is possible in most instances to make use of at least rudimentary or quasi-designs to approximate the conditions of the before-after and/or pre-post test designs, be it through randomization or statistical procedures.

The situation is exceedingly complex because of the previously discussed need to evaluate a series of input-outputs rather than just examining specific independent-dependent variable relationships. The kinds of massive efforts going on are of a linked input-output type and it is necessary to assess the efficacy of each of the specific programs, to measure the interactions among programs, and to tie together by means of relational analysis the impact that changes due to sub-programs have on the over-all program objectives. For example, an educational program may be designed to improve reading and this must be assessed, but if the over-all objective of the community project is to reduce school drop-outs, the relationship between reading improvement and drop-outs must also be demonstrated.

Of the many problems confronting the utilization of experimental models, the linking issue seems to be the most difficult. There is too great a tendency to use assumed reflectors of change rather than direct measures of desired change, such as shifts in attitudes toward Negroes when the program is concerned with reducing discrimination. The problem is most serious when attitude scales are used as substitutes for measures of overt behavior. Most of us are aware of the limited correlations often found between attitudes and behavior, but as a recent paper points out, the situation may be worse than that: re-analysis of several studies suggest that changes in attitudes may be *inversely* correlated with changes in behavior. Thus, if one may extrapolate, reducing prejudice may indeed lead to increasing discrimination.[10] Use of attitudinal reflectors instead of the direct behavioral measures specified in an impact model may therefore render impossible the linking process.

Given the size of community efforts under the poverty program, assessing the efficacy of each sub-program in every city is pretty well impossible. Even assuming the availability of research funds, the problem of obtaining necessary professional manpower renders this unworkable. Consequently, a more practical approach would be to sample programs in various cities and this raises knotty problems because of the already-made observations of the linked input-output character of these programs. Sampling must be attempted in terms of the selection of linked programs and the sampling unit needs to be a sub-system of linked programs, analytically if not actually distinct. For example, if one of the goals of a day-care program is to free unmarried mothers so they may receive literacy training to be eligible for employment counseling and training, this "sub-system" of programs must constitute the sampling unit. It is worth emphasizing again that in order to sample such linked programs, it is necessary to have explicit statements of the goals and linkages of the various parts of the community-wide efforts and emphasizes the need for well formulated conceptual frameworks (impact models) for current efforts.

But, we have no alternative to experimental evaluation. Should we demand less in terms of the treatment of community problems than we call for in the provision of medical care for ourselves or our pets? Despite the problems of limited sampling and of validity and reliability in assessing consumer goods, many of us read *Consumer Reports* before making major purchases and a few of us even query our physicians about the efficacy of his intended therapies. We reject notions of "intuitive reasonableness" and "impressionistic worth" and seek out comparative assessments in making many personal decisions and we have the responsibility to insist on such evaluation in these mass programs as well.

At the present time even the most basic aspects of these community-wide programs are open to question. Many of the mass efforts, for example, are heavily committed to community organization programs and to the stimulation of expressive actions on the part of the so-called deprived populations. These programs have, as in the case of New York City's Mobilization for Youth, been a major source of controversy and yet, despite the resources expended and the conflict occasioned by them, at present they cannot be condemned or condoned in terms of objective evidence.[11] It is possible to mass opinions pro and con but such major issues cannot be settled on the basis of evidence though it is thirty years ago that community experiments were attempted by a social scientist in Syria.[12]

It is possible, despite the difficulties, to conduct reasonably well-controlled experiments in the community, even ones which require the cooperation of a number of individuals and agencies. At ABCD it has been found possible to institute studies with the random allocation of subjects to treatment and non-treatment groups. These designs usually must be modified because not all of those randomly selected for the experimental groups agree to participate in the programs and therefore the exposed and the unexposed populations do not constitute truly random samples from the same population. In addition, it is possible to obtain the necessary cooperation for rather extensive pre-testing of both experimental and control youth. It is likely that some version of a pre- post-test design is going to be necessary in such experiments because of this element of voluntary self-selection to participate on the part of the experimental group. Thus we are eventually going to have to (and because of this cooperation we will be able to) rely on covariance adjustments to bring the experimental and control groups back into line.

It is worth noting, however, that a main reason we were able to get support for the randomization procedures was because of the limited number of openings in the programs. But there is still great public resistance to and a considerable lack of understanding about randomization. This problem is likely to be even more serious in the case of really massive programs in which there appears to be room for everybody. This is likely to be particularly true where randomization to non-treatment groups is involved.

Furthermore, in addition to the ever present abhorrence of "denial of service" there is a very strong proclivity on the part of practitioners to believe that they know which type of person will benefit most from a particular program. Therefore, co-operating practitioners designate more people for a program than there are openings only with great reluctance. There is a related tendency for practitioners to want the most deserving youth to receive the opportunity to participate in special programs. Unfortunately, in many programs, it is impossible to determine the extent to which these two tendencies are operating in the selection of candidates for the program. But if only the most deserving are selected—even from among say probationers—the possibility of program impact may be lessened because both the experimental and the control subjects may fare very well according to the outcome criterion. Another problem is that when the selection is left to the personal preference of the practitioners the representativeness of the demonstration population relative to some larger population will be unknown.

There are two lessons here of relevance to the evaluation of antipoverty programs. One is that random allocation to treatment and *non-*treatment groups is not likely to be possible frequently. But, random allocation to alternative treatments is feasible more of the time. This means, however, if such an approach is to be carried out well, the alternative treatments should be thought through very carefully so that at a minimum they are different and not camouflaged versions of the same basic idea. The impact model—the set of theoretical concepts or ideas which trace the dynamics of how it is expected that the program will have its desired effects—again rears its annoying head, and in turn a hard look at what the goals, the outcome variables, of such programs are and how to measure them will be required.

The second is that these broad scale anti-poverty programs are not likely to be well-off with regard to knowledge of the representativeness of population treated; it is necessary to face the problem of self-selection for participation and thus extensive pre-testing with sound instruments is going to be essential if anything resembling definitive findings is to emerge. Not only should there be common use of some of the same instruments across similar programs within communities but also across similar programs between communities. For the first time we might have some cross-country comparative material concerning the populations being reached and the changes being observed.

Accountability is the second requirement of evaluation research. By accountability we refer to evidence that there is indeed a target population that can be dealt with by means of a program; that this population is important either because of its size or the intensity of pathology; and that the project program for the target population actually is undertaken with *them*.

It is not enough to evaluate efficacy—the outcomes of programs. The massive efforts now underway need to be evaluated in terms of accountability as well. While one might be accused of being inhuman for saying it, given the needs, there is little excuse for sanctioning action programs that affect insignificant portions of the population. One of the aspects of accountability is the estimation of the incidence and prevalence of problems. Oftentimes programs are developed to deal with problems that exist in the minds of practitioners or because of stereotypes held by the public. To cite one illustration, consider drug-addiction; despite newspaper and public alarm, the incidence in many urban centers is so low that on accountability grounds these efforts hardly merit the attention of so many or the utilization of extensive research resources to evaluate them. If small-size programs use up all the potential clients and thus there are no cases left for assignment to control groups, then only under very unusual circumstances may the researcher be justified in collaborating in their evaluation or even attempting to do so. If the programs are of a large-scale type, then the denial of services or at least the provision of "ordinary" treatment to a few for control purposes and subsequent estimation of worth is entirely necessary.

Accountability, however, has to do with more than the number of clients served and the size of the potential aggregate of them. Evaluation researchers, in addition to a responsibility for determining efficacy, must deal with the implementation of the prescribed process. In many instances we have engaged in outcome studies without having any knowledge of whether or not what program people maintain is going on actually takes place. It is clear that in many of the sub-programs being implemented as part of these massive efforts—even when evaluation studies of the finest design are accompanying them—we are estimating the utility of programs that never get off the ground, evaluating programs in which volunteers do no more than sign up or week-end educational camping programs in which kids have a good time and do nothing more than play ball or eat marshmallows around the fireside. To say a program fails when it is not truly implemented is indeed misguided, and the evaluation researcher's responsibility here is one of providing evidence and information that permits an accounting of what took place as well as what was the result.

Finally, what we hardly ever worry about, to our knowledge, is efficiency.[13] The various specific programs that are linked together on these massive packages differ extensively in target groups, use of scarce resources and duration. At the risk of being ludicrous, suppose *neither* individual psychotherapy *nor* group psychotherapy has any impact on the lives of persons but the former costs ten times that of the latter, given such a situation there is little doubt where one should put his money. In certain fields of medicine and in certain areas of welfare there is literally no way, given the community's ideological outlook, to cease all treatment even if no efforts are efficacious. But without being too cynical, even when we know this is the case, we refuse to employ a concept of efficiency. Suppose short-term treatment institutions for de- linquent offenders do no better than long-term ones, if they are more economical is this not something that the evaluation researcher has a responsibility to take into account?[14]

In terms of all programs, the efficient one is that which yields the greatest per unit change not the one that can be run at the least cost per recipient. What costs the most, takes the longest, and involves the greatest amount of manpower in gross terms may have the greatest net efficiency.[15] Decisions on the continuance of various programs beyond trial-demonstration periods require that we think in these terms. In most evaluation efforts we fail to relate units of change to economic, or manpower or time expenditures.

We contend that concepts of *accountability* and *efficiency* as well as *efficacy* need to be implemented in order for evaluation research to be undertaken properly. Admittedly, we ought to seek out efficacious programs. But these programs are or at least should be accountable in order for policy and program persons to make rational decisions, and we must also concern ourselves with efficiency of operations.

Problems of Measurement

In previously discussing the impact model notion, we have suggested that in the design of these community programs the premise is that certain changes will be followed by other changes. Programs are designed to expose members of a target population to procedures that hopefully will produce changes in the individual or his environment.

These individual or environmental changes are expected to produce improved behavior, for example less law violation on the part of the individual in the ABCD delinquency project. It is hoped that a significantly greater proportion of the experimentals in each program than their controls will experience the desired change and those experiencing such change, whether they are experimentals or controls, will manifest a reduction in law-violating behavior. It should be re-emphasized that the hypothesis asserts a relationship between two sets of changes, not between two static conditions.

The problem of obtaining reasonably reliable change measures precedes the problem of relating change measures, since attempting to relate sets of unreliable change scores does not appear to be too promising a game to play. There has been, of course, a long-standing concern for the problem of the reliability of scores. Interest in the reliability of *change* scores is somewhat more recent and is only now receiving attention among statisticians and psychometricians.[16] Problems arising out of the mathematically demonstrated greater unreliability of change scores relative to the reliability of the scores from which they were derived and problems arising out of demonstrated regression to the mean tendencies in test-re-test situations are likely to remain central as well as difficult issues for those who are brave or foolish enough to pursue this change problem.

The problem of the measurement of the relationship between sets of change scores involves serious statistical and mathematical difficulties. Measurements of each variable at a minimum of three points in time are required to provide some estimate of the shape of the curves involved. Two of the problems involved are: (1) the relationship between the shapes of the curves—the change curve for the intermediate variable and the change curve for the dependent variable—and (2) the question of the time lag throughout the series and between the two sets of changes. When are the presumed effects of the program on the intermediate variable expected to take place: while the program is going on or after participation in the program has terminated? And for how long are the effects supposed to last? How long a time is expected to lapse between the changes in the intermediate variable and their presumed effects on the dependent variable? What are their relative rates of change? These and similar questions are directly related to some very practical issues such as the amount of success a project can possibly have during some specified demonstration period. If there is considerable lag or the rate of change in the dependent variable is relatively low, much of the effects of the demonstration may take place after the cut-off point for the evaluation of the project. Again the need for a theoretically-based impact model is, it seems to us, underscored.

Of the many other problems which beset efforts to conduct and evaluate large-scale action programs, there are two more that should be noted. One is the problem of the meaning of change in the dependent variable—in our case, a reduction in law-violating behavior—and the other is the problem which arises from the fact that members of the target population may, in fact undoubtedly will, be involved with more than one of the programs and such multiple involvement is nonrandom.

The first decision made at ABCD concerning the definition of change in the dependent variable was that we could not use comparisons over time of area rates of delinquency as a basis. ABCD's aims were to change behavior, not to move law-violating people out of an area and non-violating people into it. Therefore an area delinquency-rate comparison over time was rejected as a basis for measuring change since wide variations in delinquency rates may occur over time simply because of changes in the constituency of the population. It was decided that a reduction in law-violating behavior would have to be measured in terms of the behavior of a specified population—that is, a cohort of individuals. The same issue confronts the Office of Economic Opportunity's community-action programs and the decision on evaluations must be the same.

Another major problem in defining how change in the dependent variable is to be measured is that of shifts in the character of the target population such as the known relationship between age and delinquency. Beginning around 10 or 11, age-specific delinquency rates increase rather sharply up into and through the late teens. Therefore to simply compare a given individual's behavior at age 15 with his behavior at age 14, 13, 12 and so on would lose sight of the fact that the probability of a delinquent act increases as he gets older. If a cohort of 15-year-olds committed the same number of delinquent acts at age 15 as they did at age 13, for example, this might not look like a reduction —and in terms of absolute numbers it is not—but in terms of what might have been expected of them it is. Therefore, within the framework of ABCD's approach, a reduction of law-violating behavior must be defined in terms of a comparison of an observed measure with an expected measure. That is, a prediction instrument is required to provide an estimate of the law-violating behavior which would have occurred had there been no intervention.

A very similar problem will arise if efforts are made to take a hard look at the possible effects of various components of large-scale community efforts to deal with poverty. For example, employability—which is central to most of the poverty proposals—is also a function of age. It is quite well known that the great bulk of the very difficult to employ 16- to 21-year-olds begins to disappear into the job market and from the unemployment rolls as they approach their middle twenties. Therefore, if evaluations of community programs dealing with this particular segment of the population are based upon observations of their employment history subsequent to exposure to one or more anti-poverty programs, the success observed may be much more apparent than real. What is needed is a measure of their employment status and prospects at some point in time as compared with estimates of what would have been the case at that same point in time had there been no intervention.

A second issue that requires comment is that of multiple-exposure to programs. This has presented the ABCD project with distinct methodological difficulties. It is likely to be an even greater problem for any effort to evaluate the effects of anti-poverty programs. Two tendencies combine here, we believe, to aggravate the problem. One is the inclination on the part of practitioners to want to shower programs on the members of the target population. The other is the sheer amount of money that is involved and the resulting large number of programs that are likely to be conducted. This is an extremely important issue if we are serious in our desire to ultimately acquire knowledge concerning the most efficient allocation of human and financial resources. For if the members of the target population participate in a number of different programs and even if desired change occurs and is measured, a way must be devised to sort out the relative contributions of the different programs to the outcome. Otherwise, in order to produce the same results again the whole menagerie of programs would have to be repeated even though only a relatively few of the programs may have actually contributed to the desired outcome. Again, a prediction instrument appears to be indispensable to the solution of this problem. Individuals must be grouped according to the programs they have participated in—in our approach, according to the intermediate variable changes they have experienced—and then the groups compared on the differences between observed dependent variable and expected dependent variable behavior.

Concluding Comments

These remarks, though not entirely original, of course, may prove relevant for researchers who have occasion to participate in the evaluation of community-wide programs. The need to become engaged in the action environment, to look at a linked input-output system, to develop impact models, and to insist on experimental designs, and the necessity to assess efficiency and to recognize the accountability function in evaluation are, to our minds, key points and ones not well-documented in our methods books and not always held to by persons participating in the evaluation of these massive efforts.

But we would like to feel that we have communicated more than some specific observations—that we have conveyed the potential and importance of the evaluation researcher's role and the sense of conviction, commitment, and responsibility required. At no other point in time have we had so great an opportunity to have an impact on the social order; if we are to realize our potential within our current stance as social scientists, however, we need more than additional technical innovations. An outlook, an ideology almost a morality if you will, must be developed in order to function appropriately as agents of social change.

NOTES AND REFERENCES

1. Odum, H. American Sociology. New York: Longmans Green, 1951.
2. Stein, M. Sociology on Trial. New York: Prentice-Hall, Inc., 1963.
3. Cloward, R. A., and Ohlin, L. E. Delinquency and Opportunity. Glencoe, Ill.: The Free Press, 1960 and Clark, K. B. (Ed.) Desegregation in the Public Schools. Soc. Probl. 2, 1955.
4. Sibley, E. Education of Sociologists in the United States. New York: Russell Sage Foundation, 1963.
5. Fox, R. C. Experiment Perilous: Physicians and Patients Facing the Unknown. New York: The Free Press, 1959.
6. Seeley, J. R. Central Planning: Prologue to a Critique. In Morris, R. (Ed.) Centrally Planned Change: Prospects and Concepts. New York: National Association of Social Workers, 1964, pp. 41-68.
7. Hyman, H. Applications of Methods of Evaluation for Studies of Encampment for Citizenship. California: University of California Press, 1962.
8. Freeman, H. E. The Strategy of Social Policy Research. In the Social Welfare Forum 1963. New York: Columbia University Press, 1963, pp. 143-156.
9. Admittedly, the evidence about the latter two approaches is fragmentary but nevertheless hardly in the direction to encourage the current expansion efforts. See Perrow, C. Hospitals: Goals, Structure and Technology. In March, J. (Ed.) Handbook of Organizations. Chicago: Rand McNally, 1964; Miller, W. B. The Impact of a Total-Community Delinquency Control Project. Soc. Problems, 10: 168-191, 1962.
10. Festinger, L. Behavioral Support for Opinion Change. Publ. Opin. Quart. 28: 404-417, 1964.
11. Warren, R. L. The Impact of New Designs of Community Organizations. Paper presented at the annual meetings of the National Social Welfare Assembly, November 30, 1964, New York City.

12. Dodd, S. C. A Controlled Experiment on Rural Hygiene in Syria. Beirut, Lebanon: American Press, 1934.
13. An illustration of a study that does consider this problem is Jahn, J., and Bleckner, M. Serving the Aged. (Methodological Supplement—Part I). New York: Community Service Society of New York, 1964.
14. Freeman, H. E., and Weeks, H. A. Analysis of a Program of Treatment of Delinquent Boys. Amer. J. Sociol. 62: 56-61, 1956.
15. Sherwood, C. C. Social Research in New Community Planning Organizations. Paper read at National Conference of Social Welfare, Cleveland, 1963.
16. Harris, C. W. Problems in Measuring Change. Madison: University of Wisconsin Press, 1963.

This paper draws heavily on material presented by the authors in separate papers at the 1964 meetings of the American Statistical Association, Chicago, Ill.

7

Evaluation Research Programs in Public Health Practice

ANDREW C. FLECK

EVALUATION is a verbal symbol much in vogue in public health administration circles. Its popularity is a result of its ambiguity. Like most ambiguous sacred symbols, the term can be widely shared. Trouble starts only when believers in ambiguous symbols try to impose their definitions on others. Hence, my usage of the term is not being presented as the only one which is proper. Variation in viewpoints and methods should be expected.

Lack of agreement as to the content of evaluation should not prevent us from understanding how evaluation relates to other equally ambiguous word symbols. Appreciation of a logical form should not require common understanding of its parts. For example, the proposition that "*A*" is bigger than "*B*" conveys meaning, yet the symbols "*A*" and "*B*" mean nothing that we can agree on at present.

Let us start by accepting the terms evaluation, knowledge and action as "givens." We can then examine the implications of Clarence Lewis's proposition about the relationship between evaluation, knowledge, and action, since it serves as the basis for our methodology. He said:

> Knowledge, action and evaluation are essentially connected. The primary and pervasive significance of knowledge lies in its guidance of action: knowing is for the sake of doing. And action, obviously, is rooted in evaluation. For a being which did not assign comparative values, deliberate action would be pointless; and for one which did not know, it would be impossible.[1]

The sequence of knowledge, assignment of comparative values, and deliberate action tells us that we are not interested in knowledge for its own sake, no matter how highly society may value this type of pursuit. The value is placed on the deliberate action. The distinguishing feature converting a search for knowledge into an evaluation project is the presence of a purpose that the knowledge sought is to be used as a guide for practical action.

The knowledge needed for the evaluation process depends upon the level of the evaluation project. James has proposed that "in order to evaluate a program completely, evaluation should begin at the lowest level objective."[2] Perhaps dissection of the whole into manageable parts facilitates precision, but the knowledge obtained may not be applicable as a guide for action if it ignores as irrelevant the factors which are most important in bringing about action in a formal organization. A priori dissection of the whole into manageable parts assumes coincidence of stated and actual objectives.

James' "efficiency" approach works well if the alternative courses of action are at a technical level, such as the choice of an immunizing agent to be used in a clinic—although not always here either. The rub comes in if the alternatives considered require alteration in the organizational structure through which the action must be implemented. If the evaluator is to function in a proper staff role to management, he should consider at the outset more than technical efficiency.

"It is difficult to criticize on logical grounds the concept of increased productivity—getting all you can for your money. However, ... the word efficiency has acquired a stigma ... in many circles [management theorists], principally because of its association with the single value system ... which viewed labor as a commodity.... Under this single system of values, ... managers ... regarded themselves and their enterprises as insulated from the broad problems of human welfare."[3]

The kind of knowledge needed to evaluate public health practice must go beyond the confines of scientism and become truly scientific, embracing all values relevant to formal organizations. The overwhelming fact of life today is the growing dominance of large formal organizations as a means for action. Disregard of this fact tends to lead to an evaluation which is precise, applauded, but filed and forgotten by the organization.

Evaluation staff work must not be based on the assumption that change will occur through peremptory decisions. Folsom has remarked that in his experience, staff work influencing future action of organizations is based upon an ability to persuade,[4] and a sympathetic understanding of the conditions which evoke loyalty and employee participation. This is a good guide for the staff evaluator. Folsom's full description of the qualities of the chief executive could serve as a job description for a staff evaluator.

Experiences such as those advanced by Folsom should receive serious consideration by all public health administrators. Our descriptive knowledge of organizations has been provided by the historical and biographical records of these successful business administrators and executives. Social psychologists, sociologists, economists, political scientists, and so-called scientific managers have attempted to systematize this information, or supplement it, by case studies. But variation in the background of the systematizers has produced conflict of theoretical opinion. However, the *ad hoc* evaluator can select from among two "classical" theories and one newer "behavioral model" to guide his approach to the study of his organization.

The two classical theories are the "physiological organization theory" which follows engineering principles, viewing the participant as an extension of his physical task or machine, and the "departmental division theory" which tends toward the search for optimal task assignment, with the total set of tasks given in advance.[5,6] The theory which we have found most useful is the behavioral model which encompasses some features of the classical theories plus study of the motivational base of the participants who are performing tasks within an organization.[6]

Formal Organizations

One of the business managers who contributed to the development of organization theory was Chester Barnard. His definition of a formal organization which incorporates the behavioral features stated that:

> An organization comes into being when (1) there are persons able to communicate with each other (2) who are willing to contribute to action (3) to accomplish a common purpose.[7]

Since there can be no organization without persons, the evaluator who fulfills his staff role must select his method to accommodate the study of the factors which bear on the willingness of the participants to act.

Description of the patterns of interaction, individual motives, and collective purpose of the organization is the methodological step of first importance if not in sequence. Avoid over-simplification of this task. Produce more than a chart of the organization which can be published. Most of the facts you will need can be published only after you or the organization has ceased to exist. The common tendency to dispose of an organization with an organization chart perhaps results from the fact that a good chart always lends an air of authority. Indication of staff and line relationships, compounded by three-dimensional overlays and charting of the informal communication "short-circuits" that occur in an organization always conveys the impression that the problem, if not actually solved, is at least clearly understood.

It has been my observation that public health administrators like to draw these organization charts but never follow them, preferring to operate on an intuitive or informal basis. The evaluator's methods should improve on the usual intuitive method of understanding the organization he seeks to guide.

"Selznick has suggested that organizations should be regarded as 'natural communities.' As such, they are subject to the same kinds of influences, pressures, prejudices, and biases as any of the social organisms. A structuring of legitimate authority relationships is not enough."[8]

Provision of a method for identification of an organization and definition of all the factors operative within it, is an uncomfortable problem. March and Simon sidestepped this issue. I quote: "For present purposes we need not trouble ourselves about the precise boundaries to be drawn around an organization or the exact distinction between an 'organization' and a 'non-organization.' We are dealing with empirical phenomena, and the world has an uncomfortable way of not permitting itself to be fitted into clean classifications."[9]

Describing the Organization

Nevertheless, guidelines for description of the living organization can be offered. Identification of the individuals interacting to produce the organization's action is your first step. This is not a simple task. Success depends upon your having a right of access to all information without providing a justification. Source material which serves as the means to identify the participants and provides you with clues about behavior, comes from examination of correspondence, expense account claims, and the historical record of the previous incumbents' behavior and statements. Your review is supplemented by subsequent personal interviews. Frank discussion should be encouraged by developing the art of listening. From this data it is sometimes immediately possible to draw an inference as to the purpose toward which the collective effort is directed. This may not be the same as the purpose established by management or the legislature.

The method resembles the technique for program auditing described by Flook and Mountin.[10] Our modification is the reversal of the order. We audit history and activity first, form inferences as to purpose and roles, and then review the plan of allocation of tasks among the organization's members. The variances between the paper plan and the inferences derived from observation are very instructive.

The final set of interviews is reserved for those individuals who appear on the paper plan as participants, but not in the observable action. Mark these individuals off for special examination since their failure to appear on the record of interaction may indicate that they are not a part of the organization even though they appear on the formal structure. Their special status deserves considerable study since a group of persons carrying out an organization's purpose are interdependent. Their collective actions are independent of external contingencies except for interactions involving service to their clientele. Relatively high degrees of self-containment are both a distinguishing mark and a variable characteristic of formal organizations.

Carry-over of interdependency into the participants' social life should not be overlooked. The development of social self-containment as a feature of organizational life can lead to institutional forms which are analagous to the immunological mechanisms characteristic of biological organisms. Extreme rigidity can be expected if social interdependency is present.

At this point you are ready to draw a publishable organization chart and describe the plan for allocation of tasks, channels of communication, and the mechanisms for coordination. If your study of the organization is complete, you will complete this step with "tongue in cheek."

Selection of a Method for Intra-organization Evaluation

Selection of a method to measure input and output is your next step. Completion of a series of evaluation studies has convinced me that any formal organization or suborganization is influenced by two antithetical needs—stability and survival. The need for short-term stability requires routine, and the need for long-range survival requires change. The selection of an intra-organizational evaluation method depends on whether short-term stability or long-term survival is more highly valued. If you have studied your organization you can answer this question.

An organization or suborganization which values short-term stability will tolerate only two of the methods, the ritualistic and the operational, but will act only on recommendations which do not disturb the organization. Conversely, an organization or suborganization which places a high value on change for the sake of survival, will require a behavioral method to insure that changes in routine will take place at all levels in the organization.

A good evaluator should give management what it needs. Extra-organizational evaluators need not consider this rule. They need not consider organizational stability and short-run values. However, outsiders never really understand the organization as well as a generalist insider. The insider is in a better position to help with the difficulties encountered by policy-makers in influencing bureaucratic action. Selznick has described this frustration of policy by a suborganization which continues existing routines serving anachronistic goals. However, anachronistic administrations die out if they do not adapt to great changes of political climate and public needs. This process is the ultimate evaluation.

Ritualistic Evaluation Methods

If your organization values short-run stability, use the ritualistic method. The basis for the method is the development of "health practice indices." The American Public Health Association indices, not yet published (1963), are derived from so-called "evaluation schedules." A range of normative standards are expressed as numerical units. The units measure things which should be influenced by public health organizations. The things measured may or may not be relevant to the self-contained interaction of an organization aimed at serving a clientele.

To illustrate, in the American Public Health Association's 1961 Guide to Community Health Study, one inquiry is directed at the percentage of known cases of tuberculosis under medical supervision. This is a useful index; however, if an organization has a bad score, it can be explained away by showing that the score is the resultant of many contingencies external to the organization.

Organizational changes need not take place if the factors that produce the index are to a large extent irrelevant to the organization. This is what makes the ritualistic method popular if one wishes to continue existing routines. A bad score still leaves the option of increasing the intensity at which the same routines are carried out. A bad score can be used to justify adding more staff and spending more dollars. Organizations are seldom disturbed by this prospect of more money and more staff.

Ritualistic evaluations are useful if properly used; their principal deficiency lies in their failure to *force* critical examination of organization.

Operational Methodology

Operational methodology has been used in upstate New York to evaluate the mass radiographic survey tuberculosis case-finding program. Organizational needs for stability are ignored and only a few of the factors involved in organizational survival are considered. Alternative combinations of manpower, technology, materials, place and time were examined to identify what were maximum yields per unit of cost. Efficiency was the only value considered.

The mass radiographic survey objective was viewed as the discovery of unknown potentially communicable cases of tuberculosis. And it was against this standard that efficiency was measured—cost factors were balanced against numbers of cases found. Methodological problems were encountered, the most important of which was the need for a precise definition of what constituted a case. The practice of reporting results on the basis of provisional findings, requiring retroactive review of records, was the second important problem. Completion of these steps and analysis of the data resulted in the issuance of interdicts against continuation of surveys in selected types of areas. However, we failed to consider all the organizational values creating the need for continuation of present routines, particularly in terms of interdepartmental relationships. As a result, the organization refused to carry out all of the recommendations.[11] Proper attention to the description of the organization, guided by organizational theory, could have forecast this failure to follow through on the recommendations.

The examination of results against a preconceived scheme of technical values is not without its hazards. The unequivocal precision obtainable by the operational method is more than offset by its failure to describe accurately the conditions under which an organization will act. Consideration of technical efficiency as the only value can lead to seriously defective evaluation studies.

A recently published history of the Atlantic slave trade underscores the true nature of the operational type of evaluation.[12] The objective of the Atlantic slave trade was to transport marketable flesh to Atlantic seaports. The objective could be measured in terms of hundredweight delivered per dollar expended. The principal cost, transportation, was fixed. The variable under control was the number of individuals transported per square foot of ship space. Constraints were the mortality rates among the cargo from communicable and other disease, the speed at which the vessel could move in order to be free from apprehension by coastal patrols and other factors, all functions of load. The managerial staff debated whether it was better to ship the cargo with standing room only or with reclining space. Modern operational evaluation techniques could have resolved this problem with a great deal of precision by the construction of a mathematical model accommodating the more significant variables. However, presence of the cargo's un-questioning obedience to orders is the assumption underlying the operational method. In public administration, the participants are not cargo, and the assumption of obedience to peremptory orders is not valid.

Behavioral Model

The behavioral model was used in the evaluation of the New York State program for rehabilitation of crippled children. By this time our evaluation group had acquired enough experience to realize that more variables than just those which measure efficiency toward the stated purpose had to be taken into account. Legislative and programmatic statements of purpose were not accepted at face value. The field survey identified all significant participants. A tentative statement of program purpose was reached inferentially from the facts gained by observing the behavior of the participants.

The next step was an historical review of all documents describing the relationship of the state to the physically handicapped covering the 19th and 20th centuries. The last step was the analysis of the case load, the costs, and the revenue sources. The entire study took 18 months.

The basic discovery was that collective behavior was directed toward the goal of a system of social insurance to supplement private resources for the purchase of medical care for children. This comprehensive medical care purpose contrasted with the stated purpose of rehabilitation of selected cases, with adult economic and social self-sufficiency as the goal for these children.

Within four months of circulation of a first draft of the study, top management recommended that the Governor's Office take steps to implement the report recommendations.

Concomitantly, twelve meetings were held with the program operators to reach agreement on the final report's content and format. The final report was issued ten months after the first draft was released. At this time the Governor announced the master plan looking toward a broad program of medical aid for the children of the state. The evaluation study revealed a great trend and provided guidelines for deliberate action which are now being used.

Summary

Research in the evaluation of public health practice involves the study of formal organizations. Evaluation studies are successful if they produce deliberate action. The methodology and acceptability of results of intra-organizational evaluation depend primarily on the presence or creation of acceptance at all organizational levels that change in routines is necessary for organizational survival.

REFERENCES

1. Lewis, C. I. An Analysis of Knowledge and Valuation. The Paul Carus Foundation Lectures VII. LaSalle, Ill.: Open Court Publishing, 1946, p. 3.
2. Confrey, E. A. (Ed.) Administration of Community Health Services. Chicago: International City Managers Assn., 1961, p. 125.
3. Pfiffner, J. M., and Sherwood, F. P. Administrative Organization. Englewood Cliffs, N.J.: Prentice-Hall, Inc., 1960, pp. 98-99.
4. Folsom, M. B. Executive Decision Making: Observations and Experience in Business and Government. McKinsey Foundation Lecture Series, New York: McGraw-Hill, 1962, p. 22.
5. March, J. G., and Simon, H. A. Organizations. New York: John Wiley. 1958, pp. 12-33.
6. Koontz, H. Making Sense of Management Theory. Harvard Bus. Rev. 40: 24-46, 1962.
7. Barnard, C. I. The Functions of the Executive. Cambridge, Mass.: Harvard University Press, 1938, p. 82.
8. Pfiffner and Sherwood, op. cit., p. 13.
9. March and Simon, op. cit., p. 1.
10. Flook, E. and Mountin, J. W. Program Audit—a Device for Reflecting Public Health Performance. Amer. J. Publ. Hlth. 37: 1137-1142, 1947.
11. Fleck, A. C., Hilleboe, H. E., and Smith, G. E. Evaluation of Tuberculosis Case-finding by Mass Small Film Radiography. Publ. Hlth. Rep. 75: 805-813, 1960.
12. Mannix, D. P., and Cowley, M. Black Cargoes: A History of the Atlantic Slave Trade 1518 to 1865. New York: Viking Press, 1962.

8

Two Approaches to
Organizational Analysis:
A Critique and a Suggestion

AMITAI ETZIONI

ORGANIZATIONAL goals serve many functions. They give organizational activity its orientation by depicting the state of affairs which
the organization attempts to realize. They serve as sources of legitima-
tion which justify the organization's activities and its very existence, at
least in the eyes of some participants and in those of the general public
or subpublics. They serve as a source for standards by which actors
assess the success of their organization. Finally, they serve as an important starting point for students of organizations who, like some of the
actors they observe, use the organizational goals as a yardstick with
which to measure the organization's performance. This paper is devoted to a critique of this widespread practice and to a suggestion
of an alternative approach.

Goal Model

The literature on organizations is rich in studies in which the criterion for the assessment of effectiveness is derived from organizational
goals. We shall refer to this approach as the goal model. The model
is considered an objective and reliable analytical tool because it omits
the values of the explorer and applies the values of the subject under
study as the criteria of judgment. We suggest, however, that this model
has some methodological shortcomings and is not as objective as it
seems to be.

One of the major shortcomings of the goal model is that it frequently makes the studies' findings stereotyped as well as dependent
on the model's assumptions. Many of these studies show (a) that the
organization does not realize its goals effectively, and/or (b) that the
organization has different goals from those it claims to have. Both
points have been made for political parties,[1] trade unions,[2] voluntary associations,[3] schools[4] mental hospitals,[5] and other organizations. It is not suggested that these statements are not valid, but it

101

seems they have little empirical value if they can be deduced from the way the study is approached. [6]

Goals, as norms, as sets of meanings depicting target states, are cultural entities. Organizations, as systems of co-ordinated activities of more than one actor, are social systems.

There is a general tendency for cultural systems to be more consistent than social systems. [7] There are mainly two reasons for this. First of all, cultural images, to be realized, require investment of means. Since the means needed are always larger than the means available, social units are always less perfect than their cultural anticipations. A comparison of actual Utopian settlements with descriptions of such settlements in the books by the leaders of Utopian movements is a clear, although a somewhat disheartening, illustration of this point. [8]

The second reason for the invariant discrepancy between goals and social units, which is of special relevance to our discussion, is that all social units, including organizations, are multifunctional units. Therefore, while devoting part of their means directly to goal activities, social units have to devote another part to other functions, such as the creation or recruitment of further means to the goal and the maintenance of units performing goal activities and service activities.

Looking at the same problem from a somewhat different viewpoint, one sees that the mistake committed is comparing objects that are not on the same level of analysis as, for example, when the present state of an organization (a real state) is compared with a goal (an ideal state) as if the goal were also a real state. Some studies of informal organizations commit a similar mistake when they compare the blueprint of an organization with actual organizational practice and suggest that an organizational *change* has taken place. The organization has "developed" an informal structure. Actually, the blueprint organization never existed as a social fact. What is actually compared is a set of symbols on paper with a functioning social unit. [9]

Measured against the Olympic heights of the goal, most organizations score the same—very low effectiveness. The differences in effectiveness among organizations are of little significance. One who expects a light bulb to turn most of its electrical power into light would not be very interested in the differences between a bulb that utilizes 4.5 per cent of the power as compared with one that utilizes 5.5 per cent. Both are extremely ineffective. A more realistic observer would compare the two bulbs with each other and find one of them relatively good. The same holds for organizational studies that compare actual states of organization to each other, as when the organizational output is measured at different points in time. Some organizations are found gradually to increase their effectiveness by improving their structure and their relations with the environment. In other organizations effectiveness is slowly or rapidly declining. Still others are highly effective at the initial period, when commitments to goals are strong, and less effective when the commitment level declines to what is "normal" for this organization. These few examples suffice to show that the goal model may not supply the best possible frame of reference for effectiveness. It compares the ideal with the real, as a result of which most levels of performance look alike—quite low.[10] Michels, for example, who applied a goal model, did not see any significant differences among the trade unions and parties he examined. All were falling considerably short of their goals.

When a goal model is applied, the same basic mistake is committed, whether the goals an organization claims to pursue (public goals) or the goals it actually follows (private goals) are chosen as a yardstick for evaluation of performance. In both cases cultural entities are compared with social systems as if they were two social systems. Thus the basic methodological error is the same. Still, when the public goals are chosen, as is often done, the bias introduced into the study is even greater.[11] Public goals fail to be realized not because of poor planning, unanticipated consequences, or hostile environment. *They are not meant to be realized.* If an organization were to invest means in public goals to such an extent that it served them effectively, their function, that is, improving the input-output balance, would be greatly diminished, and the organization would discard them.[12] In short, public goals, as criteria, are even more misleading than private ones.

System Model

An alternative model that can be employed for organizational analysis is the system model.[13] The starting point for this approach is not the goal itself but a *working model of a social unit which is capable of achieving a goal.* Unlike a goal, or a set of goal activities, it is a model of a multifunctional unit.[14] It is assumed a priori that some means have to be devoted to such nongoal functions as service and custodial activities, including means employed for the maintenance of the unit itself. From the viewpoint of the system model, such activities are functional and increase the organizational effectiveness. It follows that a social unit that devotes all its efforts to fulfilling one functional requirement, even if it is that of performing goal activities, will undermine the fulfillment of this very functional requirement, because recruitment of means,[15] maintenance of tools, and the social integration of the unit will be neglected.[16]

A measure of effectiveness establishes the degree to which an organization realizes its goals under a given set of conditions. But the central question in the study of effectiveness is not, "How devoted is the organization to its goal?" but rather, "Under the given conditions, *how close does the organizational allocation of resources*[17] *approach an optimum distribution?*" "Optimum" is the key word: what counts is a balanced distribution of resources among the various organizational needs, not maximal satisfaction of any one activity, even of goal activities. We shall illustrate this point by examining two cases; each is rather typical for a group of organizational studies.

Case 1: Function of Custodial Activities

One function each social unit must fulfill is adjusting to its environment. Parsons refers to this as the "adaptive phase" and Homans calls the activities oriented to the fulfillment of this function "the external system." This should not be confused with the environment itself. An organization often attempts to change some limited parts of its environment, but this does not mean that adjustment to the environment in general becomes unnecessary. The changes an organization attempts to introduce are usually specific and limited.[18] This means that, with the exception of the elements to be changed, the organization accepts the environment as it is and orients its activities accordingly. Moreover, the organization's orientation to the elements it tries to change is also highly influenced by their existing nature. In short, a study of effectiveness has to include an analysis of the environmental conditions and of the organization's orientation to them.

With this point in mind let us examine the basic assumptions of a large number of studies of mental hospitals and prisons conducted in recent years on the subject "from custodial to therapeutic care" (or, from coercion to rehabilitation). Two points are repeated in many of these studies: (1) The *goals* of mental hospitals, correctional institutions, and prisons are therapeutic. "The basic function of the hospital for the mentally ill is the same as the basic function of general hospitals . . . that function is the utilization of every form of treatment available for restoring the patients to health."[19] (2) Despite large efforts to transform these organizations from custodial to therapeutic institutions, little change has taken place. Custodial patterns of behavior still dominate policy decisions and actions in most of these organizations. "In the very act of trying to operate these institutions their *raison d'être* has often been neglected or forgotten."[20] Robert Vinter and Morris Janowitz stated explicitly:

> Custody and care of delinquent youth continue to be the goals of correctional agencies, but there are growing aspirations for remedial treatment. The public expects juvenile correctional institutions to serve a strategic role in changing the behavior of delinquents. Contrary to expectations, persistent problems have been encountered in attempting to move correctional institutions beyond mere custodialism. . . . Despite strenuous efforts and real innovations, significant advances beyond custody have not been achieved.[21]

The first question the studies raise is: What are the actual organizational goals? The public may change its expectations without necessarily imposing a change on the organization's goals, or it may affect only the public goals. As Vinter and Janowitz suggest, much of the analysis of these organizations actually shows that they are oriented mainly to custodial goals, and with respect to these goals they are effective.[22]

But let us assume that through the introduction of mental health perspectives and personnel—psychiatrists, psychologists, social workers—the organization's goal, as an ideal self-image, changed and became oriented to therapy. We still would expect Vinter's and Janowitz's observation to be valid. Most prisons, correctional institutions, and mental hospitals would not be very effective in serving therapy goals. Two sets of reasons support this statement. The first set consists of internal factors, such as the small number of professionals available as compared to the large number of inmates, the low effectiveness of the present techniques of therapy, the limitations of knowledge, and so on. These internal factors will not be discussed here, since the purpose of this section is to focus on the second set, that of external factors, which also hinder if not block organizational change.

Organizations have to adapt to the environment in which they function. When the relative power of the various elements in the environment are carefully examined, it becomes clear that, in general, the subpublics (e.g., professionals, universities, well-educated people, some health authorities) which support therapeutic goals are less powerful than those which support the custodial or segregating activities of these organizations. Under such conditions, most mental hospitals and prisons must be more or less custodial. There is evidence to show, for example, that a local community, which is both an important segment of the organizational environment and which in most cases is custodial-minded, can make an organization maintain its bars, fences, and guards or be closed.

> The [prison] camp has overlooked relations with the community. For the sake of the whole program you've got to be custodially minded.... The community feeling is a problem. There's been a lot of antagonism.... Newspapers will come out and advocate that we close the camp and put a fence around it.[23]

An attempt to change the attitudes of a community to mental illness is reported by Elaine and John Cumming. The degree to which it succeeded is discussed by J. A. Clausen in his foreword to the study. "The Cummings chose a relatively proximate goal: to ascertain whether the community educational program would diminish people's feelings of distance and estrangement from former mental patients and would increase their feelings of social responsibility for problems of mental illness." They found that their program did not achieve these goals.[24] It should be noted that the program attempted by education to change relatively abstract attitudes toward *former* mental patients and to mental illness in general. When the rumor spread that the study was an attempt to prepare the grounds for the opening of a mental hospital in the town, hostility increased sharply. In short, it is quite difficult to change the environment even when the change sought is relatively small and there are special activities oriented toward achieving it.[25] D. R. Cressey, addressing himself to the same problems, states: "In spite of the many ingenious programs to bring about modification of attitudes or reform, the unseen environment in the prisoner's world, with few exceptions, continues to be charged with ideational content inimical to reform."[26]

This is not to suggest that community orientation cannot be changed. But when the effectiveness of an organization is assessed at a certain point in time, and the organization studied is not one whose goal is to change the environment, the environment has to be treated as given. In contemporary society, this often means that the organization must allocate considerable resources to custodial activities in order to be able to operate at all.[27] Such activities at least limit the means available for therapy. In addition they tend to undermine the therapeutic process, since therapy (or rehabilitation) and security are often at least partially incompatible goals.[28] Under such circumstances low effectiveness in the service of therapeutic goals is to be expected.

This means that, to begin with, one may expect a highly developed custodial subsystem. Hence it seems justifiable to suggest that the focus of research should shift from the problem that, despite some public expectations, institutions fail to become primarily therapeutic to the following problems: To what degree are external and internal[29] organizational conditions responsible for the emphasis on security? Or are these conditions used by those in power largely to justify the elaboration of security measures, while the real cause for that elaboration is to be found in the personal needs or interests (which can be relatively more easily changed and for which the organization is responsible) of part of the personnel, such as guards and administrators? To what degree and in what ways can therapy be developed under the conditions given? Do external conditions allow, and internal conditions encourage, a goal cleavage, i.e., making security the public goal and therapy the private goal of the organization or the other way around?

We have discussed the effect of the two models the researcher uses to study the interaction between the organization and its environment. We shall turn now to examine the impact each model has on the approach to the study of internal structure of the organization.

Case 2: Functions of Oligarchy

The study of authority structure in voluntary associations and political organizations is gradually shifting from a goal model to a system model. Michels' well-known study of socialist parties and trade unions in Europe before World War I was conducted according to a goal model.[30] These parties and unions were found to have two sets of goals: socialism and democracy. Both tended to be undermined: socialism by the weakening of commitments to revolutionary objectives and overdevotion to means activities (developing the organization) and maintenance activities (preserving the organization and its assets); democracy by the development of an oligarchic structure. A number of studies have followed Michels' line and supplied evidence that supports his generalizations.[31]

With regard to socialism, Michels claims that a goal displacement took place in the organizations he studied. This point has been extensively analyzed and need not be discussed here.[32] Of more interest to the present discussion is his argument on democracy. Michels holds that an organization that has *external* democracy as its goal should have an *internal* democratic structure; otherwise, it is not only diverting some of the means from goal to nongoal activities, but is also introducing a state of affairs which is directly opposed to the goal state of the organization. In other words, an internal oligarchy is seen as a dysfunction from the viewpoint of the organizational goals. "Now it is manifest that the concept *dictatorship* is the direct antithesis of the concept *democracy*. The attempt to make dictatorship serve the ends of democracy is tantamount to the endeavour to utilize war as the most efficient means for the defense of peace, or to employ alcohol in the struggle against alcoholism."[33] Michels goes on to spell out the conditions which make for this phenomenon. Some are regarded as unavoidable, some as optional, but all are depicted as distortions undermining the effectiveness of the organization.[34]

Since then it has been suggested that internal oligarchy might be a *functional* requirement for the effective operation of these organizations.[35] It has been suggested both with regard to trade unions and political parties that conflict organizations cannot tolerate internal conflicts. If they do, they become less effective.[36] Political parties that allow internal factions to become organized are setting the scene for splits which often turn powerful political units into weak splinter parties. This may be dysfunctional not only for the political organization but also for the political system. It has also been pointed out that organizations, unlike communities and societies, are segmental associations, which require and recruit only limited commitments of actors and in which, therefore, internal democracy is neither possible nor called for. Developing an internal political structure of democratic nature would necessitate spending more means on recruitment of members' interests than segmental associations can afford. Moreover, a higher involvement on the part of members may well be dysfunctional to the achievement of the organization's goals. It would make compromises with other political parties or of labor unions with management rather difficult. This means that some of the factors Michels saw as dysfunctional are actually functional; some of the factors he regarded as distorting the organizational goals were actually the mechanisms through which the functions were fulfilled, or the conditions which enabled these mechanisms to develop and to operate.

S. M. Lipset, M. A. Trow, and J. S. Coleman's study of democracy in a trade union reflects the change in approach since Michels' day.[37] This study is clearly structured according to the patterns of a system model. It does not confront a social unit with an ideal and then grade it according to its degree of conformity to the ideal. The study sees democracy as a process (mainly as an institutionalized change of the parties in office) and proceeds to determine the external and internal conditions that enable it to function. It views democracy as a characteristic of a given system, sustained by the interrelations among the system's parts. From this, a multifunctional theory of democracy in voluntary organizations emerges. The study describes the various functional requirements necessary for democracy to exist in an organization devoted to economic and social improvement of its members and specifies the conditions that have allowed these requirements to be met in this particular case.[38]

Paradox of ineffectiveness. An advantage of the system model is that it enables us to conceive of a basic form of ineffectiveness which is hard to imagine and impossible to explain from the viewpoint of the goal model. The goal approach sees assignment of means to goal activities as functional. The more means assigned to the goal activities, the more effective the organization is expected to be. In terms of the goal model, the fact that an organization can become more effective by allocating less means to goal activities is a paradox. The system model, on the other hand, leads one to conclude that, just as there may be a dysfunction of underrecruitment, so there may be a dysfunction of overrecruitment to goal activities, which is bound to lead to underrecruitment to other activities and to lack of co-ordination between the inflated goal activities and the depressed means activities or other nongoal activities.

Cost of system models. Up to this point we have tried to point out some of the advantages of the system model. We would now like to point out one drawback of this model. It is more demanding and expensive for the researcher. The goal model requires that the researcher determine the goals the organization is pursuing and no more. If public goals are chosen, they are usually readily available. Private goals are more difficult to establish. In order to find out how the organization is really oriented, it is sometimes necessary not only to gain the confidence of its elite but also to analyze much of the actual organizational structure and processes.

Research conducted on the basis of the system model requires more effort than a study following the goal model, even when private goals are chosen. The system model requires that the analyst determine what he considers a highly effective allocation of means. This often requires considerable knowledge of the way in which an organization of the type studied functions. Acquiring such knowledge is often very demanding, but it should be pointed out that (*a*) the efforts invested in obtaining the information required for the system model are not wasted since the information collected in the process of developing the system model will be of much value for the study of most organizational problems; and that (b) theoretical considerations may often serve as the bases for constructing a system model. This point requires some elaboration.

A well-developed organizational theory will include statements on the functional requirements various organizational types have to meet. These will guide the researcher who is constructing a system model for the study of a specific organization. In cases where the pressure to economize is great, the theoretical system model of the particular organizational type may be used directly as a standard and a guide for the analysis of a specific organization. But it should be pointed out that in the present state of organizational theory, such a model is often not available. At present, organizational theory is dealing mainly with general propositions which apply equally well but also equally badly to all organizations.[39] The differences among various organizational types are great; therefore any theory of organizations in general must be highly abstract. It can serve as an important frame for specification, that is, for the development of special theories for the various organizational types, but it cannot substitute for such theories by serving in itself as a system model, to be applied directly to the analysis of concrete organizations.

Maybe the best support for the thesis that a system model can be formulated and fruitfully applied is found in a study of organizational effectiveness by B. S. Georgopoulos and A. S. Tannenbaum, one of the few studies that distinguishes explicitly between the goal and system approaches to the study of effectiveness.[40] Instead of using the goals of the delivery service organization, they constructed three indexes, each measuring one basic element of the system. These were: (a) station productivity, (b) intraorganizational strain as indicated by the incidence of tension and conflict among organizational subgroups, and (c) organizational flexibility, defined as the ability to adjust to external or internal change. The total score of effectiveness thus produced was significantly correlated to the ratings on "effectiveness" which various experts and "insiders" gave the thirty-two delivery stations.[41]

Further development of such system-effectiveness indexes will require elaboration of organizational theory along the lines discussed above, because it will be necessary to supply a rationale for measuring certain aspects of the system and not others.[42]

Survival and effectiveness models. A system model constitutes a statement about relationships which, if actually existing, would allow a given unit to maintain itself and to operate. There are two major subtypes of system models. One depicts a *survival model,* i.e., a set of requirements which, if fulfilled, allows the system to exist. In such a model each relationship specified is a prerequisite for the functioning of the system, i.e., a necessary condition; remove any one of them and the system ceases to operate. The second is an *effectiveness model.* It defines a pattern of interrelations among the elements of the system which would make it most effective in the service of a given goal.[43]

The difference between the two submodels is considerable. Sets of functional alternatives which are equally satisfactory from the viewpoint of the survival model have a different value from the viewpoint of the effectiveness model. The survival model gives a "yes" or "no" score when answering the question: Is a specific relationship functional? The effectiveness model tells us that, of several functional alternatives, some are more functional than others in terms of effectiveness. There are first, second, third, and *n* choices. Only rarely are two patterns full-fledged alternatives in this sense, i.e., only rarely do they have the same effectiveness value. Merton discussed this point briefly, using the concepts functional alternatives and functional equivalents.[44]

The majority of the functionalists have worked with survival models.[45] This has left them open to the criticism that although society or a social unit might change considerably, they would still see it as the same system. Only very rarely, for instance, does a society lose its ability to fulfill the basic functional requirements. This is one of the reasons why it has been claimed that the functional model does not sensitize the researcher to the dynamics of social units.[46]

James G. March and Herbert A. Simon pointed out explicitly in their outstanding analysis of organizational theories that the Barnard-Simon analysis of organization was based on a survival model:

> The Barnard-Simon theory of organizational equilibrium is essentially a theory of motivation—a statement of the conditions under which an organization can induce its members to continue participation, and hence assure organizational *survival*. ... Hence, an organization is "solvent"—and will continue in *existence*—only so long as the contributions are sufficient to provide inducements in large enough measure to draw forth these conditions.[47] [All italics supplied.]

If, on the other hand, one accepts the definition that organizations are social units oriented toward the realization of specific goals, the application of the effectiveness model is especially warranted for this type of study.

Models and Normative Biases

The goal model is often considered as an objective way to deal with normative problems. The observer controls his normative preferences by using the normative commitments of the actors to construct a standard for the assessment of effectiveness. We would like to suggest that the goal model is less objective than it appears to be. The system model not only seems to be a better model but also seems to supply a safety measure against a common bias, the Utopian approach to social change.

Value Projection

In some cases the transfer from the values of the observer to those of the observed is performed by a simple projection. The observer decides a priori that the organization, group, or public under study is striving to achieve goals and to realize values he favors. These values are then referred to as the "organizational goals," "public expectations," or "society's values." Actually they are the observer's values projected onto the unit studied. Often no evidence is supplied that would demonstrate that the goals are really those of the organization. C. S. Hyneman pointed to the same problem in political science:

A like concern about means and ends is apparent in much of the literature that subordinates description of what occurs to a development of the author's ideas and beliefs; the author's ideas and beliefs come out in statements that contemporary institutions and ways of doing things do not yield the results that society of a particular public anticipated.[48]

Renate Mayntz makes this point in her discussion of a study of political parties in Berlin. She points out that the functional requirements which she uses to measure the effectiveness of the party organization are derived from *her* commitments to democratic values. She adds: "It is an empirical question how far a specific political party accepts the functions attributed to it by the committed observer as its proper and maybe noblest goals. From the point of view of the party, the primary organizational goal is to achieve power."[49]

There are two situations where this projection is likely to take place: one, when the organization is publicly, but not otherwise, committed to the same goals to which the observer is committed; the other, when a functional statement is turned from a hypothesis into a postulate.[50] When a functionalist states that mental hospitals have been established in order to cure the mentally ill, he often does not mean this as a statement either about the history of mental hospitals or about the real, observable, organizational goals. He is just suggesting that *if* the mental hospitals pursued the above goal, this *would be* functional for society. The researcher who converts from this "if-then" statement to a factual assertion, "the goal is . . ." commits a major methodological error.

But let us now assume that the observer has determined, with the ordinary techniques of research, that the organization he is observing is indeed committed to the goals which he too supports, for instance, culture, health, or democracy. Still, the fact that the observer enters the study of the organization through its goals makes it likely that he will assume the position of a critic or a social reformer, rather than that of a social observer and detached analyst. Thus those who use the goal model often combine "understanding" with "criticizing," an approach which was recommended and used by Marx but strongly criticized and rejected by Weber. The critique is built into the study by the fact that the goal is used as the yardstick, a technique which, as was pointed out above, makes organizations in general score low on effectiveness scales.[51]

Effects of Liberalism

The reasons why the goal model is often used and often is accompanied by a critical perspective can be explained partially by the positions of those who apply it. Like many social scientists, students of organizations are often committed to ideas of progress, social reform, humanism, and liberalism.[52] This normative perspective can express itself more readily when a goal model is applied than when a system model is used. In some cases the goal model gives the researcher an opportunity to assume even the indignant style of a social reformer.

Some writers suggested that those who use the system models are conservative by nature. This is not the place to demonstrate that this contention is not true. It suffices to state here that the system model is a prerequisite for understanding and bringing about social change. The goal model leads to unrealistic, Utopian expectations, and hence to disappointments, which are well reflected in the literature of this type. The system model, on the other hand, depicts more realistically the difficulties encountered in introducing change into established systems, which function in a given environment. It leaves less room for the frustrations which must follow Utopian hopes. It is hard to improve on the sharp concluding remark of Gresham M. Sykes on this subject:

> Plans to increase the therapeutic effectiveness of the custodial institution must be evaluated in terms of the difference between what is done and what might be done—and the difference may be dishearteningly small.... But expecting less and demanding less may achieve more, for a chronically disillusioned public is apt to drift into indifference.[53]

Intellectual Pitfall

Weber pointed out in his discussion of responsibility that actors, especially those responsible for a system, such as politicians and managers, have to compromise. They cannot follow a goal or a value consistently, because the various subsystems, which they have to keep functioning as well as integrated, have different and partially incompatible requirements. The unit's activity can be assured only by concessions, including such concessions as might reduce the effectiveness and scope of goal activities (but not necessarily the effectiveness of the whole unit). Barnard made basically the same point in his theory of opportunism.

Although the structural position of politicians and managers leads them to realize the need to compromise, the holders of other positions are less likely to do so. On the contrary, since these others are often responsible for one subsystem in the organization, they tend to identify with the interests and values of their subsystem. From the viewpoint of the system, those constitute merely segmental perspectives. This phenomenon, which is sometimes referred to as the development of departmental loyalties, is especially widespread among those who represent goal activities. Since their interests and subsystem values come closest to those of the organization as a whole, they find it easiest to justify their bias.

In systems in which the managers are the group most committed to goal activities (e.g., in profit-making organizations), this tendency is at least partially balanced by the managers' other commitments (e.g., to system integration). But in organizations in which another personnel group is the major carrier of goal activities, the ordinary intergroup difference of interests and structural perspectives becomes intensified. In some cases it develops into a conflict between the idealists and the compromisers (if not traitors). In professional organizations such as mental hospitals and universities, the major carriers of goal activities are professionals rather than administrators. The conflict between the supporters of therapeutic values and those of custodial values is one case of this general phenomenon.[54]

So far the effect of various structural positions on the actors' organizational perspectives has been discussed. What view is the observer likely to take? One factor which might affect his perspective is *his* structural position. Frequently, this resembles closely that of the professional in professional organizations. The researcher's background is similar to that of the professionals he studies in terms of education, income, social prestige, age, language, manners, and other characteristics. With regard to these factors he tends to differ from managers and administrators. Often the researcher who studies an organization and the professionals studied have shared years of training at the same or at a similar university and have or had friends in common. Moreover, his position in his organization, whether it is a university or a research organization, is similar to the position of the physician or psychologist in the hospital or prison under study.[55] Like other professionals, the researcher is primarily devoted to the goal activities of his organization and has little experience with, understanding of, or commitment to, nongoal functions. The usual consequence of all this is that the researcher has a natural sympathy for the professional orientation in professional organizations.[56] This holds also, although to a lesser degree, for professionals in other organizations, such as business corporations and governmental agencies.

Since the professional orientation in these organizations is identical with the goal orientation, the goal model not only fails to help in checking the bias introduced by these factors but tends to enhance it. The system model, on the other hand, serves to remind one (*a*) that social units cannot be as consistent as cultural systems, (*b*) that goals are serviced by multifunctional units, and hence intersubsystem concessions are a necessary prerequisite for action, (*c*) that such concessions include concessions to the adaptive subsystem which in particular represents environmental pressures and constraints, and (*d*) that each group has its structural perspectives, which means that the observer must be constantly aware of the danger of taking over the viewpoint of any single personnel group, including that of a group which carries the bulk of the goal activities. He cannot consider the perspective of any group or elite as a satisfactory view of the organization as a whole, of its effectiveness, needs, and potentialities. In short, it is suggested that the system model supplies not only a more adequate model but also a less biased point of view.

NOTES AND REFERENCES

1. Michels, R. Political Parties. Glencoe: Free Press, 1949. Ostrogorski, M. Democracy and the Organization of Political Parties. New York: Macmillan, 1902.
2. Michels, op. cit. Foster, W. Z. Misleaders of Labor. Chicago: Trade Union Educational League, 1927. Kopald, S. Rebellion in Labor Unions, New York: Boni & Liveright, 1924.
3. Seeley, J. R., Junker, B. H., Jones, R., Jenkins, N., Haugh, M., and Miller, I. Community Chest. Toronto: Toronto University Press, 1957.
4. A nonscientific discussion of this issue in a vocational school is included in Evan Hunter's novel, *The Blackboard Jungle*. New York: Simon and Schuster, 1956.
5. Belknap, I. Human Problems of a State Mental Hospital. New York: McGraw-Hill, 1956, esp. p. 67.
6. While such studies have little empirical value, they may have some practical value. Many of the evaluation studies have such a focus.
7. Parsons, T. The Social System. Glencoe: Free Press, 1951.
8. Buber, M. Paths in Utopia. Boston: Beacon Hill, 1958.
9. Actually, of course, in order for a blueprint to exist, a group of actors—often a future élite of the organization—had to draw up the blueprint. This future élite presumably itself had "informal relations," and the nature of these relations undoubtedly affected the content of the blueprint as well as the way the organization was staffed and so forth.
10. Harrison, P. M. Authority and Power in the Free Church Tradition. Princeton: Princeton Univ. Press, 1959, p. 6. Harrison avoids this pitfall by comparing the policy of the church he studied (The American Baptist Convention) at different periods, taking into account, but not using as a measuring rod, its belief system and goals.
11. Some researchers take the public goals to be the real goals of the organization. Others choose them because they are easier to determine.
12. Public goals improve the input-output balance by recruiting support (inputs) to the organization from groups which would not support the private goals. This improves the balance as long as this increase in input does not require more than limited changes in output (some front activities). An extreme but revealing example is supplied in Philip Selznick's analysis of the goals of the Communist Party. He shows that while the private goal is to gain power and control, there are various layers of public goals presented to the rank and file, sympathizers, and the "masses." Selznick, P. The Organizational Weapon. New York: Free Press, 1952, pp. 83-84.
13. Compare with a discussion of the relations between a model approach and a system approach in Meadows, P. Models, Systems and Science. Amer. Sociol. R. 22: 3-9, 1957.
14. For an outline of a systems model for the analysis of organizations, see Parsons, T. A Sociological Approach to the Theory of Organizations. Admin. Sci. Quart. 1: 63-85, 225-239, 1956.
15. The use of concepts such as goals, means, and conditions does not imply the use

of a goal model as defined in the text. These concepts are used as defined on the more abstract level of the action scheme. On this scheme see Parsons, T. The Structure of Social Action. Glencoe: Free Press, 1937.

16. Gouldner distinguished between a rational model and a natural-system model of organizational analysis. The rational model (Weber's bureaucracy) is a partial model since it does not cover all the basic functional requirements of the organization as a social system—a major shortcoming, which was pointed out by Robert K. Merton in his "Bureaucratic Structure and Personality," Social Theory and Social Structure, rev. ed. Glencoe: Free Press, 1957, pp. 195-206. It differs from the goal model by the type of functions that are included as against those that are neglected. The rational model is concerned almost solely with means activities, while the goal model focuses attention on goal activities. The natural system model has some similarities to our system model, since it studies the organization as a whole and sees in goal realization just one organizational function. It differs from ours in two ways. First, the natural system is an observable, hence a "natural" entity, while ours is a functional model, hence a construct. Second, the natural system model makes several assumptions that ours avoids, as, for example, viewing organizational structure as "spontaneously and homeostatically maintained," etc. See Alvin W. Gouldner, "Organizational Analysis," in Merton, R. K., Broom, L., and Cottrell, L. S.., Jr. (Eds.). Sociology Today. New York: Basic Books, 1959, pp. 404 ff.

17. "Resources" is used here in the widest sense of the term including, for example, time and administration as well as the more ordinary resources.

18. One way in which organizations can change their environment, which is often overlooked, is by ecological mobility, e.g., the textile industry moving to the less unionized South. But this avenue is open to relatively few organizations.

19. Quoted from Greenblatt, M., York, R. H., and Brown, E. L. From Custodial to Therapeutic Patient Care in Mental Hospitals. New York: Russell Sage Foundation, 1955, p. 3. See also Smith, H. L. and Levinson, D. J. The Major Aims and Organizational Characteristics of Mental Hospitals, in Greenblatt, M., Levinson, D. J., and Williams, R. H. (Eds.). The Patient and the Mental Hospital. Glencoe: Free Press, 1957, pp. 3-8.

20. Greenblatt, York, and Brown, op. cit., p. 3.

21. Effective Institutions for Juvenile Delinquents: A Research Statement. Social Service Rev. 33: 118, 1959.

22. R. H. McCleery, who studied a prison's change from a custodial to a partially "therapeutic" institution, pointed to the high degree of order and the low rate of escapes and riots in the custodial stage. See his Policy Change in Prison Management. East Lansing: Governmental Research Bureau, 1957. See also Cressey, D. R. Contradictory Directives in Complex Organizations: The Case of the Prison. Admin. Sci. Quart. 4: 1-19, 1959; and Achievements of an Unstated Organizational Goal: An Observation on Prisons. Pacific Sociol. Rev. 1: 43-49, 1958.

23. Grusky, O. Role Conflict in Organization: A Study of Prison Camp Officials. Admin. Sci. Quart. 3: 452-472, 1959, quoted from p. 457. McCleery shows that changes in a prison he analyzed were possible since the community, through its representatives, was willing to support them, op. cit., pp. 30-31.

24. See Cumming, Elaine, and Cumming, J. Closed Ranks. Cambridge: Harvard University Press, 1957, p. xiv.

25. Ibid. It is of interest to note that the Cummings started their study with a goal model (how effective is the educational program?). In their analysis they shifted to a system model (p. 8). They asked what functions, manifest and latent, did the traditional attitudes toward mental health play for the community as a social system (ch. vii). This explained both the lack of change and suggested possible avenues to future change (p. 152-158).

26. Preface to the 1958 Reissue, in Clemmer, D. The Prison Community. New York: Rinehart, 1958, p. xiii.

27. Grusky, op. cit.; see also Cressey, "Foreword," to D. Clemmer, op. cit.

28. See Cressey, Contradictory Directives.

29. It seems that some security measures fulfill internal functions as well. They include control of inmates till the staff has a chance to build up voluntary compliance and safety of other inmates, of the staff itself, of the inmate in treatment, of the institutional property, as well as others. These internal functions are another illustration of the nongoal activities that a goal approach tends to overlook and that a system approach would call attention to.

30. Michels, op. cit.

31. See Garceau, O. The Political Life of the American Medical Association. Cambridge: Harvard University Press, 1941; McKenzie, R. T. British Political Parties. London: Heinemann, 1955. See also note 2.

32. Merton, R. K. Social Theory and Social Structure, rev. ed. Glencoe: Free Press, 1957, pp. 199-201. Blau, P. M. The Dynamics of Bureaucracy. Chicago: University of Chicago Press, 1955, see index; Sills, D. L. The Volunteers. Glencoe: Free Press, 1957, pp. 62-69.

33. Michels, op. cit., p. 401.

34. The argument over the compatibility of democracy and effectiveness in "private government" is far from settled. The argument draws from value commitments but is also reinforced by the lack of evidence. The dearth of evidence can be explained in part by the fact that almost all voluntary organizations, effective and ineffective ones, are oligarchic. For the most recent and penetrating discussion of the various factors involved, see Lipset, S. M. "The Politics of Private Government," in his The Political Man. Garden City: Doubleday, 1960, esp. pp. 360 ff. See also Fisher, L. H. and McConnell, G. Internal Conflict and Labor Union Solidarity, in Kornhauser, A., Dublin, R., and Ross, A. M. (Eds.) Industrial Conflict. New York: McGraw-Hill. 1954, pp. 132-143.

35. For a summary statement of the various viewpoints on the effect of democratic procedures on trade unions, see Kerr, C. Unions and Union Leaders of Their Own Choosing. New York: Fund for the Republic, 1957.

36. Ibid.

37. Union Democracy. Glencoe: Free Press, 1956. See also Lipset, S. M. Democracy in Private Government. Brit. J. Sociol. 3: 47-63, 1952; The Political Process in Trade Unions: A Theoretical Statement, in Berger, M. et al. Freedom and Social Control in Modern Society. New York: Van Nostrand, 1954, pp. 82-124.

38. Limitations of space do not allow us to discuss a third case of improved understanding with the shift from one model to another. Although apathy among members of voluntary associations as reflecting members' betrayal of their organizational goals and as undermining the functioning of the organization has long been deplored, it is now being realized that partial apathy is a functional requirement for the effective operation of many voluntary associations in the

service of their goals as well as a condition of democratic government. See Jones, W. H. M. In Defense of Apathy. Political Studies. 2: 25-37, 1954.

39. The point has been elaborated and illustrated in Etzioni, A. Authority Structure and Organizational Effectiveness. Admin. Sci. Quart. 4: 43-67, 1959.

40. Georgopoulos, B. S., and Tannenbaum, A. S. A Study of Organizational Effectiveness. Am. Sociol. Rev. 22: 534-540, 1957.

41. For a brief report of another effort to "dimensionalize" organizational effectiveness, see Kahn, R. L., Mann, F. C., and Seashore, S. Introduction to a special issue on Human Relations Research in Large Organizations: II. J. Soc. Issues. 12: 2, 1956.

42. What is needed from a methodological viewpoint is an accounting scheme for social systems like the one Lazarsfeld and Rosenberg outlined for the study of action. See Lazarsfeld, P. F. and Rosenberg, M. (Eds.). The Language of Social Research. Glencoe: Free Press, 1955, pp. 387-491. For an outstanding sample of a formal model for the study of organizations as social systems, see Barton, A. H. and Anderson, B. "Change in an Organizational System: Formalization of a Qualitative Study," in Etzioni, A. Complex Organizations: A Sociological Reader. New York: Holt, Rinehart & Winston, 1961.

43. For many purposes, in particular for the study of ascriptive social units, two submodels are required: one that specifies the conditions under which a certain *structure* (pattern or form of a system) is maintained, another which specifies the conditions under which a certain level of activities or *processes* is maintained. A model of effectiveness of organizations has to specify both.

44. Merton, R. K. Social Theory and Social Structure, rev. ed. Glencoe: Free Press, 1957, p. 52. See last part of E. Nagel's essay, A Formalization of Functionalism, in Logic without Metaphysics. Glencoe: Free Press, 1957.

45. One of the few areas in which sociologists have worked with both models is the study of stratification. Some are concerned with the question: is stratification a necessary condition for the existence of society? This is obviously a question of the survival model of societies. Others have asked: which form of stratification will make for the best allocation of talents among the various social positions, will maximize training, and minimize social strains? Those are typical questions of the effectiveness model. Both models have been applied in enlightening debate over the function of stratification; see Davis, K. A. Conceptual Analysis of Stratification. Am. Sociol. Rev. 7: 309-321, 1952; Davis, K., and Moore, W. E. Some Principles of Stratification. Ibid. 10: 242-249, 1954; Tumin, M. W. Some Principles of Stratification: A Critical Analysis. Ibid. 18: 387-394, 1953; Davis, K. Reply. Ibid. 394-397; Moore, W. E. Comment. Ibid. 397. See also Schwartz, R. D. Functional Alternatives to Inequality. Ibid. 20: 424-430, 1955.

46. For a theorem of dynamic functional analysis see Etzioni, A. and Lazarsfeld, P. F. The Tendency toward Functional Generalization, in Historical Materials on Innovations in Higher Education. Collected and interpreted by Stern, B. J.

47. Organizations. New York: Wiley, 1958, p. 84. See also Gouldner, op. cit., p. 405, for a discussion of "organization strain toward survival." Theodore Caplow developed an objective model to determine the survival potential of a social unit. He states: "Whatever may be said of the logical origins of these criteria, it is a reasonable assertion that no organization can continue to exist unless it reaches a minimal level in the performance of its objective functions, reduces spontaneous conflict below the level which is distributive, and provides sufficient

satisfaction to individual members so that membership will be continued."
The Criteria of Organizational Success. Soc. Forces. 32: 4, 1953.

48. Hyneman, C. S. Means/Ends Analysis in Policy Science. PROD. 2: 19-22, 1959.

49. Party Activity in Postwar Berlin, in Marvick, D. (Ed.) Political Decision
    Makers. New York: Free Press, 1961.

50. On this fallacy, see Zetterberg, H. L. On Theory and Verification in Sociology.
    New York: Tressler Press, 1954, esp. pp. 26 ff.

51. One of the reasons that this fallacy does not stand out in organizational
    studies is that many are case studies. Thus each researcher discovers that his
    organization is ineffective. This is not a finding which leads one to doubt the
    assumptions one made when initiating the study. Only when a large number of
    goal model studies are examined does the repeated finding of low effectiveness,
    goal dilution, and so on lead one to the kind of examination which has been
    attempted here.

52. A recent study of social scientists by Lazarsfeld, P. F. and Thielens, W., Jr.
    demonstrates this point. The Academic Mind. Glencoe: Free Press, 1958. Some
    additional evidence in support of this point is presented in Lipset, S. M., and
    Linz, J. The Social Bases of Political Diversity in Western Democracies. (In
    preparation.) Ch. xi, pp. 70-72.

53. Sykes, G. M. "A Postcript for Reformers," in The Society of Captives. Princeton:
    Princeton University Press, 1958, pp. 133-134.

54. Another important case is the conflict between intellectuals and politicians in
    many Western societies. For a bibliography and a recent study, see Wilensky, H.
    L. Intellectuals in Labor Unions. Glencoe: Free Press, 1956.

55. These similarities in background make communication and contact of the re-
    searcher with the professionals studied easier than with other organizational
    personnel. This is one of the reasons why the middle level of organizations is
    often much more vividly described than lower ranking personnel or top man-
    agement.

56. Arthur L. Stinchcomb pointed out to the author that organizations whose
    personnel includes a high ratio of professionals are more frequently studied
    than those organizations which do not.

9

Professional Communities and the Evaluation of Demonstration Projects in Community Mental Health

BERNARD J. BERGEN

IT is still undoubtedly true, as Kotinsky and Witmer had occasion to remark in 1955,[1] that the field of community mental health lacks a high degree of "coherence" and organization. There is a notable lack of clarity, and often sharply conflicting views about such fundamental matters as the meaning of "preventing" mental illness; the appropriate conditions for practicing different methods of treatment and care of patients; and not least of all, what the community itself can offer and how it can be successfully used in programs directed toward these ends. It may be naive to expect a unified viewpoint at this time when the field is being pushed forward with an intense sense of urgency that involves reshaping much of the traditional ideas about preventing and caring for emotional disorders. Nevertheless, there has hardly even begun to emerge the clear guidelines that are essential if we are to sort out and pick our way through the heterogeneous perspectives that exist on these and similar matters.

While it is neither a particularly fresh nor enlightening notion, it seems nonetheless true that this lack of coherence is the result of difficulties experienced in mounting and implementing a vigorous research program. Although the problems requiring solution in the community mental health field place the burden of research on "demonstration projects," efforts to evaluate the accomplishments of these are, as MacMahon, Pugh and Hutchison have recently pointed out, "conspicuous by their absence."[2]

A demonstration project, defined in "ideal" terms by Elizabeth Herzog, is one which "... tests out a hunch or conviction based on experience or practice and systematically builds up evidence designed to show whether the hunch or conviction stands up to the test. The demonstration project combines the world of research and the world of practice."[3] The question we ask, as the basis for this paper, is why the diverse "hunches and convictions" that have been and are currently being carried into practice in the field of community mental health, whether bearing the arbitrary label of "demonstration" or not, are rarely designed as empirical "tests?"[4]

While the observation that more systematic evaluations of demonstrations are badly needed is fairly commonplace and frequently reiterated, less frequent are attempts to identify the factors that make this a problem. What is needed is a way of looking at Herzog's "ideal" definition of demonstration projects not only in terms of the methodological issues implied by this definition, but also in terms of the social-psychological issues that are present. The evaluation of demonstrations should be seen as a *social* process, the organization and implementation of which simply cannot be taken for granted. Few more pressing needs exist at this time, than to analyze and understand our own activities from this viewpoint.

The present paper proposes to take some steps in this direction. The purpose is to formulate the problem in social-psychological terms, and identify some of the stresses which may be associated with the requirement that demonstrations evaluate themselves. In the absence of systematic empirical data, this analysis must be regarded as suggestive. It is our primary hope, however, that pulling together even limited and consequently selective experiences into a general frame of reference, will serve to open fruitful lines of approach that will stimulate broader and systematic research efforts.[5]

Formulating the Problem

The last part of Herzog's definition, "The demonstration project combines the world of research and the world of practice" is particularly crucial, since not every project constructed to test a hunch or a conviction must necessarily be concerned with practice as part of the test. Demonstration projects, however, provide innovating services which are felt to be necessary for meeting otherwise neglected mental health needs. Innovation always implies an element of uncertainty and the concomitant requirement for evaluating the usefulness of the service provided. It is for this reason that demonstration projects have been described as "field experiments."[6]

Although a fairly extensive literature exists describing the formal logical requirements for evaluative research,[7, 8, 9-12] rarely is systematic evidence presented about the failure or success of the demonstration itself. This literature, often directed toward practitioners rather than researchers, conveys the impression that it is the former's combined lack of knowledge about and sympathy for research that is the primary cause of the problem. These factors unquestionably operate, but it is difficult to believe that they are pervasive as is sometimes implied. The problem rather seems to be that the requisites for systematic research, which are often obvious enough, meet inordinate difficulties being accepted and carried out. There often seems to be, for lack of a better term, a "defensiveness" associated with carrying them through. In a sense, demonstration projects do not often seem to "jell" in a way that supports systematic self-evaluation. This, we suggest, is rooted in the one feature which sets demonstration projects off from other types of projects: the attempt to organize both practice and research to achieve a single common goal.[13] Our understanding of what is entailed by this collaboration is, to date, very limited. Much has been written, on the other hand, about the problems of collaboration between professional disciplines on exclusively research projects.[15] On these projects, however, disciplines that are traditionally associated with service, such as psychiatry and social work, do not participate in a research capacity. Demonstrations present, therefore, as Luszki has noted,[16] qualitatively different kinds of problems and represent a special type of social climate for pursuing research.

From both personal experience and the few who have touched on the matter in print, it is difficult to avoid the impression that this climate often produces or exacerbates conflicts and tensions between the major disciplines involved. Practitioners see researchers having different "long term" goals while they themselves are interested in the immediate patient and his situation. The researcher is accused of "callously" subjecting people to experimental manipulation which, as one practitioner, quoted by Luszki, eloquently put it, "produces the kind of humanitarianism which has been characteristic of the most idealistic totalitarian experiments to which individual lives have been ruthlessly sacrificed."[17] The researcher accuses the practitioner of being unable and unwilling to admit failure while the practitioner accuses the researcher of being extremely rigid and unwilling to bend his research design. Both practitioners and researchers deplore in the other a perceived lack of respect for other points of view.[18]

Beneath their ad hominem coloration, these themes reflect real issues. They underscore as well, however, a peculiar paradox. As vigorously and as often as the conflicts betweeen research and practice are stressed, their necessary inter-relatedness is equally stressed. Practice depends upon research, and research has no meaning unless it can be converted into actual practice. In the field of mental health, a pervasive theme is the broad communality of interests, goals and sentiments shared by research and practice. It is, perhaps, precisely the obviousness of this which has led to emphasizing, as the source of the conflicts between researchers and practitioners, individual personality and temperament. Luszki has summarized this point of view: "No clear-cut statement can be made of the extent to which the differences and resulting conflicts are disciplinary. Undoubtedly, many are a consequence of individual personality and temperament rather than a direct result of disciplinary differences."[19]

Factors of idiosyncratic personality and temperament, though undoubtedly present, are, at best, only a partial explanation and should not divert us from investigating the role that the demonstration project, as an organization, may play in the problem. From a social-psychological point of view, demonstration projects are organized attempts to order the social relations of its participants for purposes of achieving specified goals. In this sense, they are more than simply collections of individuals who happen to be engaged in roughly similar pursuits because they have roughly similar interests. Implementing the goal which MacMahon, Pugh and Hutchison have called the "evaluation of accomplishment"—i.e., testing ". . . the hypothesis that a certain practice . . . has a measurable beneficial outcome in the group on whom it is practiced," [20] depends upon fulfilling certain logical requirements. These are so familiar by now that they require only brief mention:

A control group is necessary in order to compare experimental effects with those that occur without experimental intervention. Comparison populations ". . . can be assured only by random or systematic allocation of individuals or groups to treatment and comparison samples." The goals of the demonstration and its procedures must be capable of being objectively assessed and measured. The services provided must be defined operationally so that they can be clearly identified and communicated to others. Experimental procedures must be standardized over time, so as to constitute a "series of trials" from which evidence about their effects can be accumulated and analyzed. These constitute the fundamental considerations that enter into formulating a "research design," without which objective evaluation is impossible.

Granting their logical importance, research designs also have social-psychological significance. When translated from the abstract language in which they are often couched into actual interpersonal operations, research designs can be seen to be no less than normative proscriptions that define for each practitioner his role on the project. A design constitutes a set of demands as to how he should relate to which clients or patients; to his fellow staff members, and most importantly, to himself. Demands of this scope, despite their logical necessity, must invariably be accompanied by strains and conflicts which, as Luszki[21] and more recently, Meyer and Borgatta have noted[22] can impede the movement of the demonstration project toward a goal of self-evaluation. They are particularly problematic because of a characteristic which demonstration projects share with all service organizations: being staffed by persons who bring with them and maintain an important identification with a specific professional community. In this sense, demonstration projects can be thought of as communities within a community. Before analyzing some of the concrete ways in which the elements of a research design come into conflict with this, it proves necessary to define in more detail what is meant by a "professional community."

The Concept of "Professional Community"

To talk about "professional communities" is possible, as Goode has pointed out,[23] primarily because members of a profession are bound together by a common identity, values and language. The "distinctive focus" of these is the "possession of some specific skill or cluster of skills."[24] In other words, a professional is one who possesses competence in some area shared only by the other members of his own profession. It is this unique competence which determines the relations of professional communities to the larger society. While the professional community cannot exist unless the larger society recognizes it as legitimate, the professional community controls its own standards of recruitment and evaluation.

It is of vital importance, in this respect, that the process of training a professional entails more than transmitting technical skills. It is, in the strictest sense, a process of adult socialization where the values of the professional community are made a part of the person. Professionalization, for the individual recruit, means involvement with a community way of life that ". . . provides life goals, determines behavior and shapes personality."[25] To put it more succinctly, becoming a professional implies incorporating important features into one's personal identity. As such, the professional, as in the case of anyone else, can be expected to seek experiences that will be compatible with his sense of identity and which will reinforce and confirm it.

The larger society depends upon this in the face of its inability to judge or evaluate the competence and reliability of what "it is buying."[26] In addition to whatever formal mechanisms a professional community may set up to maintain professional standards, the most important mechanism is the professional's own inner controls through his sense of personal identity. In the face of this intimate connection between one's profession and one's self, we could expect that any conditions that make demands incidental to or in conflict with a professional's sense of what is important to his identity would fail to gain his full commitment and possibly lead him to actively oppose them.

This may seem like an obvious point, but it is easy to overlook when dealing with professional practice in the field of mental health. The significance that research designs can have as constituting precisely such conditions is not often explicit discussed. One reason may be that providing service to persons in need is based on rational procedures—i.e., it involves a commitment to knowledge discovered and supported by rational or scientific procedures as distinct, let us say, from pure tradition or mysticism. The "natural" connection between this and the rational utility of research designs may easily obscure looking for a conflict between a person's commitment to rationality as a value, and his ability to conform behaviorally to some kinds of demands that may reflect these values. For persons to adequately play roles proscribed by norms based on rational, or for that matter, any other kind of values, requires being able to formulate and sustain perceptions of themselves and their relations to others that do not arouse immobilizing conflicts and anxieties. We suggest that the basic elements of a research design do constitute a set of conditions which easily provoke such conflict and anxieties among professional mental health practitioners, and as such, contribute to making effective evaluative research problematic. These rational "elements" tend to make the practitioner's role on the project marginal, in the sense of reducing opportunities for professional, hence personal rewards, while at the same time conforming to these demands would not be identical with attaining a new identity as a professional researcher.

The remainder of the paper will be concerned with suggesting some of the concrete ways this operates and in showing how the demands implicit in a research design have a different and often opposite meaning for professional researchers.

Sources of Conflict and Strain

Perhaps the most fundamental demand made by a research design is that the practitioner subject his activities to public scrutiny. At first glance, this does not seem to be a unique state of affairs. Undue secrecy is rarely part of the values of any professional community, and most professionals, during the course of their careers are exposed to one or another form of evaluation and criticism. The prototype of this occurs, of course, during their training period when it is particularly intense. But the demands of a research design go beyond this kind of "professional" evaluation. The practitioner is expected to conceive of his activities as data—i.e., as an object of research. The sense in which accepting such a role imposes special strains and anxieties is best appreciated by reviewing certain aspects of his professional activity.

Providing help to persons in psychological need is recognized as more than a matter of simply applying general rules to a specific situation. The idea of "clinical service" implies an intimate bond between the practitioner as a person and his client. Particularly in the area of mental health, the role which knowledge as such is acknowledged to play in the helping process is less than that of the way the practitioner uses it and himself in an ongoing relationship. Few professions of any sort emphasize, as do those in the area of mental health services, the importance to the practitioner of having an understanding of himself and his feelings as they bear on the "treatment" situation. Although the very nature of his clinical activity and his own professional values make it virtually impossible to separate the practitioner as a person from his activities, he is expected by the research design to expose himself to the kinds of objective judgments generally reserved for impersonal "data"—judgments of failure and success. It is not unreasonable, given this, to suggest that he is likely to view these expectations as an open challenge to his sense of worth and self-esteem. This kind of challenge is not easily or lightly taken up.

However, one may argue, the professional researcher is also subject to the objective verdicts of failure or success to be yielded by his own design. Indeed, the researcher, as part of his professional career, seems to be required to consistently expose himself to this kind of challenge. One might ask why he seems to accept it as a necessary concomitant of the vital business of gaining knowledge, while the professional practitioner seeks to obstruct this business by keeping his "risks" low?

The question, reasonable on the surface, is based, however, on a false premise. The terms "failure and success" have a different significance for the professional identity of the researcher who is bound to his research operations in a totally different way than the practitioner to his professional activities. This is best understood by seeing science as a system of advocacy with the researcher playing an advocate's role. Ernest Nagel has phrased this neatly:[27] "The practice of scientific method is the persistent critiques of arguments, in the light of tried canons for judging the reliability of the procedures by which evidential data are obtained, and for assessing the probative force of the evidence on which conclusions are based."

The professional identity of the researcher is, in effect, linked more to the structure of his arguments than to the substance of what he argues about. By definition, the results of an experiment—i.e., its success or failure, are not predictable at the outset. The fact that data may fail to support a particular hypothesis is not a reflection on the personal and professional competence of the researcher. It is simply "a fact of nature," and clearly out of his control. Indeed, in a very real sense, it is not a failure at all but a special, albeit limited kind of "success." What would threaten his professional identity is to advocate something that is false. This depends, to a large extent, upon matters that are his professional duty to control—the method of the experiment itself. It is for this reason that the researcher places such a great emphasis on a "tight" research design often, as practitioners are quick to point out, to the extent where the total effort seems out of proportion to the results that would be yielded.

Practitioners, however, are not advocates, and their personal identities are not bound to the advocate's problems. More to the point, their different professional "needs" are likely to be in opposition. The more rigorous the design, the sharper the demands on the practitioner to conform to and sustain a perception of himself as a datum. The more he rejects this impersonal image, the less able is the researcher to implement a stringent design. It would be hard to find conditions less suitable for working out a reasonable *modus vivendi*.

This, however, is not the only way in which the research design and the needs of the professional practitioner may find themselves in active opposition. The practitioner is expected to organize his relations to patients or clients in highly specific ways as reflected in such requirements as the random assignment of service to experimental and control populations and providing services to all comers in a predefined way over a specified series of trials. The strains of complying with these demands seem to derive less from questions of their ethicality than from the practitioner's having to abandon important ways of obtaining psychological gratification and support for his professional identity. The fact that these "artificial" procedures will ultimately benefit patients, even these self-same patients, is not a difficult point to grasp intellectually. However, it is much more difficult for the practitioner to commit himself in a total way to this abstract conception when the rewards that nourish his professional identity accrue from highly individualized experiences with patients.

The particular patient in his particular situation is the focus for the major values of practitioners' professional communities, regardless of how sympathetic they may otherwise be to research. This is well illustrated by the fact that the professional image of the psychiatric community is not severely undermined by its well known difficulties in agreeing on general criteria for defining a psychiatric case. As long as psychiatric illness in an individual can be identified in a clinical setting (and simply presenting oneself as having psychological problems makes one a suitable candidate for psychiatric care), then the ambiguities presented by attempting to generally classify psychiatric illness are difficulties that can be lived with, albeit not always comfortably. In this sense, the term "clinical judgment" for the practitioner is a highly valued notion that advertises his competence and it is not merely fortuitous that "interesting" cases, defined as those which present idiosyncratic features that do not fit general principles, are also highly valued. Nor is it fortuitous that the care and treatment of patients is often regarded, with pride, as an art as much as a science.

The personal meaning which individual patients have for practitioners has no counterpart for professional researchers. The researcher, trained to the task of seeking general order from the confusion and complexity presented by the particular, is concerned with abstracting from a particular situation those features it has in common with other situations. His purpose is to generalize about the conditions under which these features will vary. The complex imponderables in the clinical situation that present stimulating challenges to the ingenuity of the individual practitioner are harrowing problems in reduction and conceptual organization to the professional researcher. The idea both of control groups and of thinking of clinical situations as a series of trials to be "run out" afford him the possibility of making generalizations but require control, as far as possible, over the practitioner's individuated response to each specific case as it presents itself. The researcher is thus prone to divide analytically the practitioner into one or more separate sets of "operations," defined in a way that would allow them to be duplicated by others in different contexts. This may be conceptually possible to accomplish, but it is another matter for the practitioner to be able to accept the routinized and impersonal image of himself and his relationship to his clients that is demanded.

It is important to stress that the issue in conflict is not whether generalizations should or should not be established about experience. The logical necessity of generalizing is inescapable as long as one's professional activities are committed to a rational frame of reference. Practitioners are generally well aware of this. The problem concerns the tensions associated with their being expected to mobilize motivational resources to support a role that is at odds with what is central to their own professional self-image.

There is, in addition to these demands made by a research design, another aspect to demonstration projects that may produce the kinds of strains that impede evaluative research. These projects which often, although not always, involve the collaboration of several different professional communities require, in the very least, some formal way of allocating and coordinating functions and duties. They require, in effect, some minimum authority structure in order to function as an ongoing concern. The most prominent feature of this has already been implied by all of our previous discussion—namely, the subordination of the practitioner to the researcher through conforming to the research design. It is easy to see from this point of view how the practitioner would be prone to feel that this is a situation where the standards for his own professional functions have been made contingent on the sanctions and mandates of a related but different profession. Smith has noted that in the relations between professional communities, this is not a particularly infrequent state of affairs; but he has also noted that where it does occur, it is accompanied by uncomfortable tensions, anxieties and conflicts.[28]

The problems of organizing inter-profession relations, along these and other lines have been commented on and studied in a variety of contexts.[29-31] If there is one thing that stands out, it is that relations are not openly fluid, but are rather carefully structured. Greenwood has pointed out that, for the most part, professional collaboration is carried on through the mechanisms of consultation and referral.[32]

Both of these mechanisms function to guard the autonomy of the professions by protecting their option to refuse to become involved or by giving them leeway to negotiate the ground rules for collaboration. They are protected, as well, from having to become involved in situations which might compromise their image of unique competence through exposure to situations where the risk of failure is high and the possibility of rewards low.

The coordination of professional relations on an organizational basis must always entail, on the other hand, some degree of loss of freedom or autonomy. It is not unreasonable to expect that this loss would be particularly difficult to tolerate where the professions in question, such as those in the field of mental health and the social sciences have only recently gained or are still struggling to attain a secure professional status in their own eyes and in the eyes of the public. We must not forget that such matters as the prevention and care of psychiatric disorders, the limits of therapy, and even the nature of mental illness, all constitute to one degree or another, open subjects for research and demonstration that may well reveal the limitations of both professional competence and the unique worth assigned to some professional functions. Every profession rests to some extent on a set of fictions,[33] and demonstration projects may well exacerbate the role these fictions play in barring effective coordination.

The research professional, who often shows too little sympathy for these problems, is not immune from them. He is generally careful to guard his own sense of unique competence by rarely seeing research, unlike, for instance, practice, as a subject suitable for interprofessional collaboration. His defensiveness is often manifested through confusing a technical knowledge of statistics with the definition of research itself.

These problems, centering on the collaboration of research and practice, are undoubtedly not exhaustive of all those that can be cited. They do serve to indicate, however, that the demonstration project, which might appear on the surface to be easily integrated around procedures that are hardly disputable in the light of rational values, can be in reality a complex social organization whose integration is not simply to be taken for granted.

Summary and Discussion

We have indicated that the importance of demonstration projects is derived in part from the commitment of the practicing professions to a rational frame of reference—i.e., to basing their practices upon knowledge accumulated through research activity. We have suggested, however, that even as rational systems for acquiring such knowledge, these projects, through their research designs, are capable of making demands that are not entirely congruent with the values of the professional community of practitioners. A commitment to rationality does not describe the nature of the practicing professions in the same sense in which it describes the nature of the research professions. These differences in values reflect themselves in a differential ability between researchers and practitioners to make commitments to the roles and self-perceptions necessary to the organized pursuit of such knowledge.

It has been our major contention, tentatively presented and which must itself be subjected to systematic investigation, that this produces strains and conflicts that serve as major hindrances to implementing evaluative research. It is difficult not to infer that some of the arguments often directed against evaluative research, such as the "impossibility" of measuring patient improvement or the "self-evident" nature of the demonstration in question, which often fly in the face of logic and reason, are defensive measures against the conflicts and tensions imposed by research demands on professional practice. Indeed, Mitchell and Mudd have gone so far as to call the anxiety observed in practitioners who were asked to adopt certain research techniques, "neurotic anxiety" because of its inordinate persistence in the face of rational arguments.[34] We have suggested that this kind of "explanation" is too simplistic and does not take into account important factors in the social organization of research and the nature of professional identity. Nevertheless, it is of vital importance to study further reactions of this sort, which we hypothesize is the reason that demonstration projects do not function effectively as the major research instrument in community mental health.

The study of professionalization and the problems involved in professional collaboration is, unfortunately, in its infancy, although its importance for understanding organizational behavior has already been shown, especially in the area of the treatment and care of mental disorders.[35, 36] We cannot, however, say to what extent the kinds of problems suggested as important in this paper are indigenous to all situations of collaboration, or specify the conditions under which they can be expected to be minimal or disappear. We must keep in mind that research and practice have not been historically prepared for the kind of organized collaboration represented by demonstration projects and time may be an important element in solving the problem. Researchers, trained to the values of a system of advocacy, are not usually prone to sympathize with the practitioner's values that the care and treatment of persons in distress is itself *sui generis*—i.e., needs no justification in terms of some larger, more general issue, or for that matter, needs no justification in terms of the eventual outcome for the patient himself. The professional practitioner is prone to overlook what seems, on the face of it, to be an academic point but which is rather absolutely basic—the goal of demonstration projects is not to provide service at all, but to produce propositions about service. These are two different matters involving different kinds of organized efforts.

On the other hand, because the problem of evaluating demonstration projects may be rooted in some of the processes of human functioning that are difficult to reach, then possibly neither the passage of time nor simply understanding the problem, by itself, will result in a solution. The solution may well lie in the process of professional training itself. Perhaps, this must be altered so that individuals can be trained to identify their professional image with both service and research in a new and admittedly, as yet undefined way. This does not seem to be outside the realm of possibility.

In any event, the demonstration project undeniably remains one of the sharpest and most difficult challenges faced by professional researchers and practitioners. The dilemmas it faces in the course of evaluating itself must be more fully explored before they can be fully solved.

NOTES AND REFERENCES

1. Kotinsky, R., and Witmer, H. L. Introduction in Kotinsky, R., and Witmer, H. L. (Eds.) Community Programs for Mental Health. Cambridge: Harvard University Press, 1955, p. xv.
2. MacMahon, B., Pugh, T. F., and Hutchison, G. B. Principles in the Evaluation of Community Mental Health Programs. Am. J. Publ. Hlth. 51: 963-968, 1961.
3. Herzog, E. Research, Demonstrations and Common Sense. Child Welfare, 61: 243-247, 279, 1962.
4. For purposes of this paper, it is largely irrelevant whether projects are specially funded by foundations, government or otherwise, for specific periods of time or whether they are simply part of the activities of an existent agency undertaken because of a perceived need for changing or adding to its procedures. In this sense, we are using the term "demonstration" in a less restricted way than it is sometimes used.
5. This analysis draws upon the relevant literature, the author's observations and experiences while research director of a demonstration project and subsequently consultant to another, and interviews with both researchers and practitioners with demonstration project experience.

6. Proceedings of the Thirty-Fourth Annual Conference of the Milbank Memorial Fund, Part II. Planning Evaluation of Mental Health Programs. New York: Milbank Memorial Fund, 1958.

7. MacMahon, Pugh, Hutchison, op. cit.

8. Herzog, op. cit.

9. Howe, L. P. Problems in the Evaluation of Mental Health Programs, in Kotinsky, R. and Witmer, H. L. (Eds.), op. cit.

10. Herzog, E. Some Guide Lines for Evaluative Research. U.S. Department of Health, Education and Welfare, 1959.

11. Group for the Advancement of Psychiatry. Some Observations on Controls in Psychiatric Research, Report No. 42, 1959.

12. Glidewell, J. C. Methods for Community Mental Health Research. Am. J. Orthopsychiat. 27: 38-54, 1957.

13. This collaboration can take a number of forms—e.g. the functions of research and practice can be combined in the same individuals, or may be distributed among separate individuals in a division of labor. The former introduces complications not found in the latter. Some of these have been discussed by Perry and Wynne.[14] The discussion following in this paper is applicable to the general problem of research-practice collaboration regardless of the particular form it may take. For the sake of avoiding undue complications, however, I have had in mind throughout, a model of a demonstration project consisting of separate "staffs" of researchers and practitioners with mutually exclusive functions.

14. Perry, S. E., and Wynne, L. C. Role Conflict, Role Redefinition and Social Change in A Clinical Research Organization. Soc. Forces. 38: 62-65, 1959.

15. Clausen, J. A. Selected Bibliography—Discussions of Interdisciplinary Collaboration in Sociology and the Field of Mental Health. New York: Russell Sage Foundation, 1956, p. 61.

16. Luszki, M. B. Team Research in a Social Science: Major Consequences of a Growing Trend. Hum. Org. 16: 21-24, 1957.

17. Luszki, M. B. Interdisciplinary Team Research: Methods and Problems. New York: New York University Press, 1958.

18. Fringe, J. Research and the Service Agency. Soc. Casewk. 33: 343-348, 1952.

19. Luszki, 1958, op. cit.

20. MacMahon, Pugh, Hutchison, op. cit. These authors also define a type of evaluative study they call "evaluation of technic." This is ". . . designed to find out whether a supposedly therapeutic or preventive practice is in fact being carried out within specified limits. . . ." Both this and the evaluation of accomplishment have important contributions to make to the field of community mental health. While they must stand in a logical relationship to each other, since demonstrating what is known requires, first, knowing something, they can conceivably require different kinds of organization. This paper is concerned only with the "evaluation of accomplishment."

21. Luszki, 1958, op. cit.

22. Meyer, H. J. and Borgatta, E. F. Paradoxes in Evaluating Mental Health Programs. Int. J. Soc. Psychiat. 5: 136-141, 1959.

23. Goode, N. J. Community Within A Community: The Professions. Am. Soc. Rev. 22: 194-200, 1957.

24. Smith, H. L. Contingencies of Professional Differentiation, in Nosow, S. and Form, W. H. (Eds.) Man, Work, and Society. New York: Basic Books, 1962.

25. Greenwood, E. Attributes of a Profession. Ibid., p. 206.

26. Goode, op. cit.

27. Nagel, E. The Structure of Science. New York: Harcourt, Brace & World, 1961, p. 13.

28. Smith, op. cit.

29. Vinter, R. D. The Analysis of Treatment Organizations. Paper presented at the 57th annual meeting of the American Sociological Association, 1962. (mimeo.)

30. Levine, S., and White, P. E. Exchange as a Conceptual Framework for the Study of Interorganizational Relationships. Admin. Sci. Quart. 5: 583-601, 1961.

31. Weiner, L., and Bergen, B. J. Psychiatric Home Treatment: Problems of Innovation in Community Psychiatry. Inter. J. Soc. Psychiat. 9: 200-207, 1963.

32. Greenwood, op cit.

33. Smith, op. cit.

34. Mitchell, H. E., and Mudd, E. E. Anxieties Associated with the Conduct of Research in a Clinical Setting. Am. J. Orthopsychiat. 27: 310-330, 1957.

35. Vinter, op. cit.

36. Weiner, op. cit.

Section II

Research Designs

10

Toward a "Theory of Method" for Research on Organizations

JOSEPH E. MCGRATH

Introduction

Organization research is a meeting ground (and, hopefully, a melting pot) for the sociologist, the economist, the political scientist, the operations researcher, the mathematician, the social psychologist, and the engineer. Men from each of these fields, and others, have contributed much to our current state of knowledge about the nature and dynamics of organizations.

But because the field of organization research is inherently as well as historically an interdisciplinary field, it is marked by great diversity in concepts, terms, and methods of study. Since the men who do organization research come from a variety of backgrounds, they tend to bring with them different tools, different concepts, and different methodological approaches. Consider, for example, the extreme differences in methodology between Mesarović, Sanders, and Sprague,[1] and Bass[2] and contrast them further with Seashore and Bowers[3] in their studies of organizational effectiveness; or consider the differences between Guetzkow, et al.'s[4] and Jenson's[5] approaches to the study of internation tensions; similarly, notice the differences between Cyert and March's,[6] and Likert's[7] and Homan's[8] empirically derived organization theories. Even when these sets of studies deal with the "same" problem in the field of organization research, the methodological differences among them seem about as great as the differences between the methodologies of totally separate scientific disciplines.

Such diversity has both positive and negative effects on the field. On the plus side, diversity of concepts and methods insures a dynamic, searching, pluralistic growth for the field, which probably offers a substantial safeguard against conceptual stagnation. On the other hand, diversity of theoretical concepts—and above all, diversity in the use of methods—leads to considerable malcommunication within the field, which doubtless decreases the efficiency with which we can advance our knowledge.

Furthermore, it is apparent that every methodology has some limitations in terms of what it *cannot* do (or cannot do efficiently), as well as some advantages in terms of what it *can* do. Hence, methods are not totally interchangeable, and the choice of methodology in any given case should be made on the basis of the possibilities and limitations of that methodology *vis à vis* the research problem to which it is to be applied.

This chapter is written on the assumption that differences in research methodology *do* make a difference in the yield of research. In other words, when we choose one methodology over others in a study of organization, we are thereby affecting the kinds and amount of information which we can obtain from results of that study. If this assumption is true, it follows that we should choose the methodology that we will use in a given case on the basis of the kinds of information we are seeking (i.e., the nature of the problem we are studying), and we should choose so as to maximize the amount of information which we will gain about that problem. It also follows that when we choose our methodology for reasons of personal preference, familiarity, or operational expediency, we are changing the nature of the problem about which we will be gaining information, as well as altering the amount of information which we can gain from our study.

If we are to make "rational" choices of methodology, so as to maximize the amount of information relevant to our purposes, we must be able to do at least two things. First, we must be able to compare alternative approaches in terms of their relative effectiveness in providing the desired information. This, in turn, requires ability to specify what we mean by "research information," and how we will assess the efficiency of a research approach for generating such information. In short, if we are to make rational choices of method, we need a "theory of method" to guide us in those choices.

This chapter is an attempt to take some first steps toward the development of such a "theory of method" for the study of organizations. Our presentation falls naturally into three stages which constitute the three sections of the chapter. First, we will consider methodologies that have and/or can be applied to the study of organizations, and attempt to place them in a framework within which they can be related to one another. Secondly, we will attempt to define certain key concepts—"research information," "information potential" and "information yield"—and from them formulate what we mean by "comprehensiveness," "efficiency," and "effectiveness" of a study. Then, in the final section, we will try to apply these concepts to compare and contrast different methodologies, and will consider some of the implications of these comparisons for programmatic planning of organization research.

It should be pointed out here that we doubt if any of the concepts presented in this chapter will in themselves be new or startling to the reader. Nor will our conclusions likely offer the reader profound new insights. The contribution which this chapter makes, if any, lies in its attempt to formulate some well-recognized concepts and distinctions in a fairly systematic and rigorous way. Hence, this chapter will not particularly add to "what we know," but, hopefully, it will add to our appreciation of the import of "what we know" for "what we do," when we set out to do research on organizations.

A Classification of Data-Collection Methods Used in Organization Research

Many streams of endeavor contribute to the current field of organization research, and studies based on many different methodological approaches form part of the body of knowledge of that field. The methodology used in studies of organizations range from carefully delimited, laboratory-controlled studies, such as those on communication networks by Bavelas,[9] Leavitt,[10] Guetzkow and Simon[11] and others, to broad and sweeping conceptual analyses of large organizations, and even total societies (e.g., Homans,[8] Merton,[12] Parsons[13]). Organization research includes intensive case studies of single organizations (e.g., W. F. Whyte,[14] Selznick[15]) broad surveys of many organizations of a single type, journalistic analyses based on anecdotal evidence (e.g., W. H. Whyte,[19] Riesman[20]) true "field experiments" which involve experimental manipulations of an entire large-scale organization (e.g., Morse and Reimer,[21] Seashore and Bowers [3]) man-computer simulation studies (e.g., Guetzkow,[4] Bass,[2] Rome and Rome, [22]) all-computer simulations and use of formal mathematical models.[23] At a superficial glance, it would appear that the only common feature of all these approaches is that they are—or are intended to be—applicable to the study of some aspect of organizations.

We can begin to see some common elements among these methodologies, however, when we consider each of them in terms of the nature of the setting within which data-collection takes place and in terms of the extent to which activities of the investigator intrude upon, or are responsible for, the nature of that setting. Viewed in

these terms, in fact, most of the types of methodology used in organization research seem to fit within one of four major classes. We will
label these four classes of research settings as field studies; experimental simulations; laboratory experiments; and computer simulations.

Field Studies

Field studies are those research investigations which take place
within "natural" or "real-life" social situations. This category includes all types of empirical investigations which use data from real,
existing organizations. Within this category we include a number of
types of research which are heterogeneous in many respects. For example, one kind of "field study," as the term is used here, are those
"studies" which consist only of casual or anecdotal observations.
Another kind of field study would be the systematic and intensive
case study of existing or past organizations, including those done
primarily through analysis of records and documents (e.g., Selznick,[15] Alger[26]). Broad surveys are also included,[27] as are both
the so-called natural experiments and the carefully planned, delib-
erately-executed field experiments (e.g., Seashore and Bowers,[3]
Morse and Reimer,[21] Coch and French[29]).

The kinds of research here included within the over-all category
of field studies show marked variations in method. They are listed
here in a generally increasing order of rigor of procedure. At the
same time, they are here classed together on the basis of one crucial
common feature. All of these types of field studies are investigations
which obtain their data directly from real, existing organizations of
the kind to which results are intended to apply. That is, all field
studies are direct studies of (members of) the class of phenomena
with which the investigation is concerned, namely, real "flesh-and-
blood" organizations. One important feature of data obtained from
a "real-life" situation is that the humans in that situation are operating under natural (not necessarily stronger) motivational forces,
since the phenomena being studied are a part of their actual lives.

Experimental Simulations

The term "experimental simulations" is used here to refer to empirical investigations which attempt to create a relatively faithful
representation of "an organization" under quasi-laboratory conditions, set that simulated organization "in motion," and study the
operation of that organization as it is expressed in the behavior of
humans who are assigned roles within it (e.g., Bass,[2] Guetzkow, et al.,[4]

Rome and Rome[22]). This category is roughly equivalent to Guetz-kow's category of "man-computer simulations" (Guetzkow[30]).

In such studies, many features of the structure and process of the organization are simulated, often by the use of computers, to study the process and consequences of behavior of human subjects who operate the simulated system. These studies are distinguished from laboratory experiments (Class 3 in our present classification) in several respects. First, the stimulus situation within which the individual is operating is more or less continuous in an experimental simulation, in contrast to the laboratory experiment which usually consists of a series of discrete trials. Secondly, as a part of the continuous nature of experimental simulations, participants' responses at any particular point in time partly determine (along with the "rules of the game") the stimulus situation in which they will be operating at subsequent points in time. Finally, experimental simulations differ from laboratory studies in that they attempt to simulate or model properties of "real-life" organizations, which is the key defining property of this class of methods in the present schema.

However, experimental simulations vary considerably in terms of the degree of fidelity of the simulation involved. They also vary in terms of the complexity of the simulation, and in terms of whether the particular simulation is intended to represent a generic type of organization or some particular type of organization. All three of these distinctions go together to determine whether the simulation presents the participants with a "bare-bones," fairly abstract representation of only the key processes felt to be important (e.g., Guetz-kow et al.'s internation simulation[4]) or whether it attempts to provide them with a content-enriched stimulus situation which "seems" very similar to the "real" situation (e.g., see discussion on realism in Bass[2]). Experimental simulations also vary in terms of how "open" or "closed" they are; that is, in terms of how much of the total operation of the organization is simulated and how much is left to determination by the performance of the human participants.

Laboratory Experiments

Laboratory experiments are those studies in which the investigator does not attempt to recreate "reality" in his laboratory, but rather tries to abstract variables from real life situations and represent them in a more fundamental form. His purpose is to study the operation of these more fundamental processes under highly controlled conditions. He is not so much interested in making his laboratory situation a "greenhouse" for the study of some particular class of organizations. Rather, he is interested in studying fundamental processes which presumably underlie the behavior of humans in a broad range of organizational (and other) settings.[31]

Perhaps the essential features of laboratory experiments as they relate to the field of organization research can best be presented by using the studies of communication networks (Bavelas,[9] Christie, et al.,[39] Guetzkow and Simon,[11] Leavitt,[10] Shaw,[40] and others) as illustrations of this class of method. The communication net studies isolate one fundamental feature common to *all* organizations, namely, the pattern of communication linkages between organizational components and study the effects of variations in this pattern under laboratory conditions. Neither the specific nets studied (four and five node nets, of various patterns ranging from highly centralized to highly decentralized) nor the tasks being performed (symbol-identification problems, simple arithmetic problems, etc.) were meant to "simulate" real organizational structures or real organizational tasks. Rather, the purpose of the communication net studies was to determine how variations in highly abstract and basic patterns of communication influenced certain basic kinds of human activities (e.g., transmission and reception of messages, deductive problem-solving, organizational planning) and certain classes of human reactions (felt satisfaction, attraction to the group, job satisfaction), which presumably operate in *all* human organizations.

This attempt to create and study generic structures or processes is one of several features which distinguish laboratory experiments from experimental simulations as discussed previously. Other distinguishing features are the frequent use of a series of discrete, independent "trials," for which the stimulus conditions are entirely preprogrammed by the investigator, rather than using a continuous stimulus situation which is partly determined by prior responses of participants. This pattern of procedure gives the laboratory experimenter greater control over the stimulus situation and reduces confounding between different stages of performance, although it also reduces the continuity and the "felt realness" of the situation for the participant.

Computer Simulations

This class of methods should more properly be called "mathematical models." It is here referred to as computer simulations, both in order to contrast it with experimental simulations (Class 2 in the present schema) and because the special kind of logical or mathematical model which we call computer simulations is frequently used in the study of organizations. Guetzkow[30] designates this class of studies as "all-computer" studies. Computer simulations are also sometimes referred to as "Monte Carlo" studies, because they generally utilize the procedure of random selection from predetermined probability distributions as a means of "simulating" specific behaviors of parts of the system on specific occasions.

Computer simulations are distinguished from experimental simulations because they are closed or logically complete models of the class of phenomenon being simulated. *All* variables, including the "dependent variables" or "output variables" which result from operation of the system, are built into the formulation of the simulation model itself. Thus, the model does not involve or require performance by human participants. Performance or output variables are "contained" within the model, most often as stochastically determined consequences of the computerized "operation" of the simulated organization.[41]

Computer simulations can represent either a generic class or a particular class of organizations. Computer simulations vary considerably in the "richness" and complexity with which they simulate the (class of) organizations being studied. They vary, in particular, in the extent to which the simulation tries to represent "depth" characteristics of the human components of the organization (e.g., values, attitudes, norms, conformity pressures) as well as their superficial "output" characteristics. They also vary, of course, in the "validity" or "reasonableness" of the assumptions by means of which such representations of human behavior are inserted into the model.

Models do not necessarily have to make use of computers to belong in the computer simulation class as here defined. In fact, an interesting example of a simple and low-cost model, which "runs" without the use of any major computational aids but which nevertheless has all of the essential characteristics of this class of research methods, is presented in Guetzkow.[30] The essential feature of this class of research is that *all* structures and processes which are to be dealt with in the investigation are represented in the simulation model itself either as parameters, as operating rules, or as stochastic processes.

Relations Between the Four Classes of Methods

These four classes of methods appear to be more or less ordered along a continuum which has several facets. The ordering continuum can be thought of as proceeding from concrete (at the field study end) to abstract (at the computer simulation end). Alternatively, we can label the ends of the continuum as realism versus artificiality, or we can label them as going from "open" to "closed" settings, or from "loose" to "controlled" conditions.[42]

Regardless of how we designated the underlying continuum, the four different classes of methods which we have identified along that continuum differ markedly from one another in terms of the advantages which they offer the researcher and in terms of the limitations which they impose upon him. At the field study end of the continuum, for example, the investigator has the substantial advantages of "felt realism" and of the operation of inherent motivational forces. As pointed out previously, this does not necessarily mean that human participants are operating at higher levels of motivation. Rather, it means that they are operating under more "natural" kinds of motivations, since the study itself is an integral part of their lives. These advantages of the field study are gained at the cost of less precision, less control, and less freedom to manipulate variables whose effects may be of central concern. Research methods at the other end of the continuum—laboratory experiments and computer simulations—have as their major advantages precisely those characteristics which are the major disadvantages of the field study: precision, control of variables, and considerable freedom to manipulate variables of central concern. However, they also have the complementing disadvantage of lack of realism.

These and many other advantages and disadvantages of various research settings make it very clear that the four classes of methods are not at all interchangeable. Rather, they seem to offer complementary approaches, and the choice of the best approach in a given case must reckon with the *relative* importance of realism, precision of measurement, opportunities to manipulate variables, and many other features of the research situation. Our purpose here is to work toward development of some guide rules for making these comparisons, hence for making our choices of method more nearly "rational."

Development of such guide rules requires that we establish a network of basic methodological concepts—a theory of method—in terms of which we will "calculate" the relative efficiency, comprehensiveness, and effectiveness of various research approaches, so that their relative usefulness to us in a given case can be determined with some rigor. Accordingly, we will interrupt our consideration of different classes of research methods temporarily to establish some basic tools for methodological comparisons in the next section of this presentation. Then, in the final section of the chapter, we will return to a comparison of advantages and disadvantages of different research settings armed with more adequate tools for making such comparisons.

Some Concepts for Assessing the Adequacy of Research Methods

The Nature of a Research Problem

Research has to do with identification and measurement of variables thought to be relevant to a certain problem or phenomenon and determination of the interrelationships among those variables. When we do research, we ask three basic questions: (a) What are the important or relevant variables (conditions, parameters, properties, etc.) of the phenomenon I wish to study? (b) How does each of them vary (in nature); what range of values can each of them assume? (c) How do they co-vary; is the value of one variable predictable from (or predictive of) the value of one or more other variables?

Let us consider a "research problem" as a set of variables, descriptive of some phenomenon which is of interest to us, whose covariations we are going to attempt to describe. The variables in such a set include: (a) properties of the class of object or entity being studied (e.g., individuals, organizations, etc.), including properties that have to do with relations between parts; (b) properties of the environment, situation, or setting within which that class of objects exists (including suprasystems to which the objects are organic, their physical environments, their tasks); and (c) properties of the action or behavior of the objects in relation to the environment.

A variable of any of the above types is *relevant* to the research problem if its variation has an (appreciable) effect on, or is (detectably) affected by, variations in one or more of the other variables of the set.

We will assume that, in any given case, there are a *finite* number of relevant variables in the set to be studied. (Variables which are determinable mathematical functions of one another—such as the radii and diameters of a given set of circles—are considered collectively as a unitary variable.) *All* of the relevant variables are always present at *some* value (including "zero" or "absent") in a research situation, whether their presence is recognized by the researcher or not. Hence, the research problem always concerns the total set of variables V. We cannot reduce the number of relevant variables in the situation; we can only limit the scope of our study by restricting variation of

some of them, or reduce the precision of our study by ignoring variation of some of them.

Alternative Treatments of Variables

We must do something about each of the relevant variables in a
research problem. Basically, any one variable can be treated in one
of four mutually exclusive ways:

Treatment W. We can *control* a certain variable V_j so that all of
its values except one, k_i, are *prevented* from occurring. We can do
this in several ways: by selective sampling of cases, by arrangement
of conditions, etc.

Treatment X. We can *manipulate* a certain variable V_j so that a
certain value k_i is *required* to occur. This operation can also be performed by a number of techniques, including design or assembly of
parts, induction of conditions, and so forth.[43]

Treatment Y. We can deal with a given variable V_j by *permitting it
to vary freely and measuring* the values of it which do occur. Such
measurement can take various forms, including the use of physical
instruments, the use of human observers, the use of self-reports by
the objects of study.

Treatment Z. We can *ignore* a variable V_j by permitting it to vary
freely, but failing to determine what values *do* occur. This treatment
is applied to all variables which are *in* the relevant set V, but which
are not dealt with by Treatments $X, Y,$ or Z.

In any given research situation, *every* relevant variable is handled
by one and only one of these four treatments. These four ways of
treating variables are used with differential frequency in studies
conducted in different types of research settings. For example, Treatments W and X are the hallmarks of laboratory studies and are used
seldom or not at all in field studies. The use of Treatment Z is more
or less inevitable in field studies, but its use can be minimized in
the laboratory.

These four ways of treating variables have different implications
for the scope, precision, and effectiveness of study design, because
they have different effects on the amount of research information
which inheres in a study design and the amount of information which
can be extracted from that study. So, before returning to a discussion
of research settings and their uses, let us consider the concepts of
research information, information potential and information yield
within a research design.

Research Information, Information Potential, and Information Yield

Research information has to do with the specification of relationships between variables. We have gained research information when we ascertain *whether or not* the occurrence of a particular value of a variable V_1 is predictive of (or predictable from) the value(s) which obtain for variable V_2 (V_3, . . ., V_N). As a convention, we will say that we gain research information from determination of *whether or not* two (or more) variables vary together, while we will say that we gain *positive research information* when we discover that two such variables *do,* in fact, vary together predictably.

The amount of information which *can* be gained about any given situation is a function of the amount of "uncertainty," or *potential information,* which is inherent in that situation. The *potential information* contained in a situation depends on the number of (relevant) variables and the number of values which each variable can assume. If there are V variables relevant to a situation, and each has k values, then for *any given instance* (trial, event, etc.) of that situation there are k^v possible combinations of values of the variables involved. That term k^v represents the *total information potential* of a situation.[44]

We gain *positive research information* to the extent that we reduce the number of possible combinations of values of variables k^v by ascertaining that two or more variables vary concomitantly. That is, we gain *positive research information* when we can predict that the occurrence of a certain value k_1 of variable V_1 will be accompanied by the occurrence of a certain value k_i (or a *restricted* range of values, less than the total range) of another variable V_2, *under conditions where values of V_2 other than the predicted value(s) are free to occur* (insofar as the study operations are concerned). Hence, we gain positive research information *when and only when* something that is *free to happen* predictably *does not.*

On the other hand, when we *reduce the potential information* of a situation by deliberately precluding the occurrence of certain values of a variable (as we do when we "experimentally control" a variable, as in Treatment W), we have not gained any research information by so doing. Rather, when we *alter* what values of a variable can occur—either by preventing some values from occurring (as in experimental control of a variable, Treatment W), or by insuring that a certain value of the variable does occur (as in experimental manipulation, Treatment X)—we *reduce* the potential information which our study situation contains below that which is contained in the "real-world" situation. For example, if one variable is controlled at a single value, its range of occurrence is reduced from k to 1 value, and the total information potential is reduced from k^v to k^{v-1}. If there are five variables, each with ten possible values, $k^v = 100,000$, $k^{v-1} = 10,000$, a reduction by $9/10$ in this particular case.

This reduction of potential information represents a restriction of the scope of our study and a limitation on the generality of our findings. We can represent the scope or generality of a given study in terms of the ratio of the information potential of the study to the information potential of the "real-world" situation to which it refers (and to which its results are intended to apply) k^{v-w}/k^v, where w refers to the number of variables which were *made to occur* at one particular value.

The total potential information in a study situation sets the upper limit for the total research information which that study *can* yield, just as the amount of uncertainty associated with a message limits the amount of information which the message can convey. Within this limit, study procedures affect the extent to which that potential information is realized as research information. By definition, research information involves statements about the covariation (or lack of it) between two or more variables, at least one of which is free to vary "at will." Determination of such covariation, or its absence, requires: (*a*) that at least one of the variables being related be free (insofar as our study procedures are concerned) to take on any of a range of values, *and* (*b*) that we identify (measure) what value of all of the variables being related *actually obtained* in each of a given set of instances. When we permit a variable V_j to vary freely, but do not determine what values it assumes (Treatment Z), we do *not* reduce the information potential inherent in the situation (i.e., the number of alternative combinations of values of variables which can occur), but we greatly reduce the information which we can *extract* from the situation (i.e., the *information yield* of our study). Variables which are uncontrolled but unmeasured (Treatment Z) generate *noise* in our data. Extending the previous illustration: If we have five variables, each with ten values, $k^v = 100,000$. If one of the five variables is controlled at a single value, but a second variable is ignored, the total information potential of the *study* remains $k^{v-1} = 10,000$; but the accountable or specifiable information is reduced to k^{v-2}, which equals 1,000. If *accountable* information is considered *information yield,* and effects of variables which are uncontrolled but ignored are considered *noise,* the ratio $k^{v-(w+z)}/k^{v-w}$ expresses the *precision* of a study in terms of the ratio of *accountable information* (*information yield*) to *potential information*.[45]

Efficiency, Comprehensiveness, and Effectiveness

One might consider that the *efficiency* of a study is reflected in its precision as defined above; that is, the ratio of accountable information to potential information, $k^{v-(w+z)}/k^{v-w}$. One might further view the *comprehensiveness* of a study in terms of its scope or generality, expressed as the relation between information potential of the study and information potential of the referent situation, k^{v-w}/k^{v}, as previously discussed. However, we should probably view the *over-all effectiveness* of a study by comparing its *information yield* to the *total potential information of the referent situation*. Hence, effectiveness of a study can be expressed as $k^{v-(w+z)}/k^{v}$. In this view, we lose "comprehensiveness" when we control variables (i.e., restrict their range of values, by Treatments W or X); we lose "efficiency" when we ignore variables (i.e., let them vary but fail to measure them, Treatment Z); and we lose "effectiveness" when we do *either* of these.

Since different types of research settings vary in their relative uses of Treatments W, X, Y, and Z, as previously noted, these settings also differ, in an orderly way, in the extent to which they are limited in comprehensiveness, efficiency, and effectiveness. We shall examine these differences in the next section.

Comparison of Research Methods

Let us return now to consideration of the four classes of research settings previously described. As already noted, these four classes of research settings differ in the extent to which they utilize the four treatments of variables (see Table 1). Hence, they differ in their potential information and their information yield. Let us consider the four classes of methods comparatively, in terms of the way they use the four different treatments of variables, and the consequences of that use.

Treatment W: Experimental Control

The use of Treatment W, control of a variable by experimental means, tends to increase as we move along the continuum of methods from field studies to computer simulations. This occurs in two ways. First, the laboratory or computer investigator uses Treatment W deliberately to hold certain of the relevant variables in the problem at a

TABLE 1. RELATIVE FREQUENCY OF USE OF DIFFERENT TREATMENTS OF VARIABLES IN THE FOUR CLASSES OF RESEARCH SETTINGS

Classes of Research Settings	Alternative Treatments of Variables			
	Treatment W Excluded by Control	Treatment X Made to Occur by Experimental Manipulation	Treatment Y Varying Freely and Measured	Treatment Z Varying Freely but Ignored
Field studies	Low or no use	Low or no use	High or low use, gross measurement	Very high use
Experimental simulations	Medium to high use	Moderate use	High or low use, moderately precise measurement	High use
Laboratory experiments	High use	High use	High or low use, precise measurement	Low use
Computer simulations	Very high use	Very high use	Not possible	Not possible

single, constant value so that they will not confound effects of other variables which are of more central concern to him. In doing so, he deliberately reduces the scope or comprehensiveness of his study—he cuts down the potential information in it—as a price for excluding "noise" from it. However, the laboratory or simulation investigator also often uses Treatment W *unwittingly.* That is, in the process of simulating or recreating the class of phenomena being studied, he is likely to overlook important features of the real life situation which he is modeling. Hence, he applies Treatment W to these variables by holding them at a single constant value ("zero" or "excluded"). These exclusions also reduce the information potential of the study, even though they are not done on the basis of deliberate choice by the investigator. In the field study, the investigator usually does not have an opportunity to control variables, either deliberately or unwittingly. Hence he avoids both the problems and the advantages involved in use of Treatment W.

The use of Treatment W has positive and negative effects on a study design. On the positive side, to control a variable (Treatment W), rather than permitting it to vary freely without measuring it (Treatment Z), prevents a loss of efficiency in the study by reducing the "noise." On the other hand, to control a variable at a single value (Treatment W), rather than making it occur at each of a series of specific values (Treatment X) or letting it vary but measuring its variation (Treatment Y), reduces the information potential of the study below the information potential of the referent situation and thus reduces the scope or comprehensiveness of the study.

Results of a study only refer to the specific combinations of conditions used. They might or might not hold if one or more of those variables to which Treatment W has been applied had been held at some *different* value. Such a situation would occur in all cases where a variable that is held constant has *interactive* effects with other variables in the problem. It is often said that systems in general, and organizations in particular, are complexes of *interactive* variables. If so, then we need to be very careful not to violate that concept of organizations by choosing to control key *interactive* variables at a single value in order to make our study design more feasible.

We should also be concerned, it would seem, about selection of the *particular value* at which we will control a variable to which we have decided to apply Treatment W. If we *must* limit a relevant variable to a single value, hence limit the applicability of our results to combinations of conditions which include that value, we probably ought to choose the natural modal value of that variable as it occurs in the referent situation rather than some value which gives us "baseline" information, or a "cleaner" (looking) design, or a study plan that is easy to implement.

As a rather simple illustration, suppose we wish to simulate or do experiments pertaining to an organization whose subsystems have a mixture of male and female members. We might want to do a laboratory study of the effects of group communication processes on the performance effectiveness of such groups. A study using uniformly male groups (or uniformly female groups), or using a constant ratio of males and females in each group, would seem on the surface to offer a "cleaner" design (and perhaps a design that is easier to implement). However, such designs may very well not be as useful as a design which determines male-female composition of groups on a random basis. Sex differences (and especially *sex composition* differences) may very well *interact with* communication patterns in affecting task performance.

That is, the "best" communication pattern for task effectiveness may be quite different in all-male, all-female, and mixed-sex groups. If this were true, results obtained from study of all-male groups just simply would not apply to mixed-sex groups even if all other features of the study were well executed. In fact, trying to apply results of such a study to real life organizations which have mixed-sex work groups would *systematically* lead us to the *wrong* answer (i.e., we would be led to select as optimal a communication pattern which was definitely *not* optimal for task effectiveness).

If we found it necessary to do our experiment with groups of only one sex composition, we would be better off using the composition pattern that is modal for those groups (or organizations) to which we want to apply our findings. If we used randomly composed groups, or groups with the male-female proportion which was most predominant in the referent organizations, we still would not gain information about other sex composition patterns, of course. Nor would we avoid the problems posed by the interaction effects of the variable we chose to control. But at least we would obtain results which, when applied, would lead us to be *systematically right* in our choice of optimal communication patterns.

Treatment X: Experimental Manipulation

In Treatment X, we use experimental manipulation to insure that a certain value k_i of variable V_j will occur on a certain occasion (or trial). Most often, we are manipulating circumstances so that different values of V_j occur on different trials according to a predetermined schedule. If only one value of a variable is used for *all* trials, treatment X becomes identical with Treatment W, and has the same restrictive effects on the study design. If the variable is manipulated so that every one of its possible values occur on some trials, then Treatment X does not place any limitation on the information potential of the study. In most cases, however, experimental manipulations use more than one, but less than all values of the variable; hence they lead to some restriction in scope.

The use of Treatment X tends to increase as we go from field studies to computer simulations. Furthermore, there tends to be an increase in the number of values of a variable which are utilized when a variable is manipulated. For example, when a field study does manage to include an experimentally manipulated variable it is almost always necessary to limit the manipulation to two, or at the most, three, levels of the variable (including control groups, e.g., Seashore and Bowers,[3]

Morse and Reimer[21]). In laboratory experiments, on the other hand, it is often possible to vary systematically one or more variables at each of a series of values. To the extent that this can be done, we can then determine the functional relationships between the manipulated variables and other "free-but-measured" variables (Treatment Y).

On the other hand, while the field study is seldom able to manipulate any variables, or to manipulate them at many levels, the manipulations which sometimes can be achieved in field settings are often very powerful. Partly, this power comes from the fact that manipulations of conditions in a field study—whether due to "natural" causes or to experimental plan—affect the very lives of the participants in the study. Manipulations in the laboratory, on the other hand, are often relatively weak, both for ethical reasons and because of the inherent artificiality of the motivational conditions under which participants are operating.

One of the special advantages of the computer simulation lies in the facility which it provides for systematic manipulation of many variables at each of many values. In fact, the computer simulation can generate combinations of conditions which do not exist in the real world, but whose effects may be of vital importance for theoretical development. For example, a computer simulation might be developed to represent an organization whose "human components" perform with perfect efficiency and rationality—a situation not found in nature —to study upper limit conditions for performance of that organization. (Sometimes, computer simulations seem to build such assumptions about human perfection into their models, without recognizing that they are dealing with hypothetical upper limits.)

Treatment Z: Uncontrolled Variables

The uncontrolled and unmeasured operation of a variable (Treatment Z) generates "noise" within a study design. All variables which are neither controlled, manipulated, nor measured are, necessarily, noise-producing variables. The "use" of Treatment Z in a study is always more or less unwitting, either as a result of lack of knowledge about the phenomena being studied or as a result of lack of knowledge about appropriate scientific procedures.

By their very nature, field studies are likely to contain variables handled by Treatment Z (i.e., variables which have been ignored), because field study situations preclude much use of control (W) and manipulation (X), and are likely to contain more variables than can be measured effectively (Y). The major advantage of laboratory studies is their ability to minimize uncontrolled variables (i.e., minimize use of Treatment Z). They do so by applying Treatments W and X, and sometimes Y, to variables which might have received Treatment Z in a field setting. Experimental simulations also share this advantage with the laboratory setting, but to a lesser degree because of the greater complexity and the continuity-of-situation which they contain. Computer simulations essentially eliminate Treatment Z. They have no "noise."[46]

Treatment Y: A Necessary Condition for Obtaining Research Information

The number of variables handled by Treatment Y does not necessarily increase or decrease as we proceed along the continuum of methods from field studies to the laboratory situation. However, the precision with which variables can be measured tends to increase. Precision of measurement is used here to refer both to sensitivity (the number of values of a variable which can be distinguished) and to reliability (the stability of results from independent measures) of the measurement process.

Treatment Y does not exist in the computer situation, for the same reason that Treatment Z is not a part of that class of research settings. Treatment Y refers to permitting a variable to vary freely and measuring its variation; Treatment Z refers to permitting a variable to vary freely but not measuring it. Since no variable is operating outside the control of the investigator in a "closed model" such as a computer simulation, neither Treatment Y nor Treatment Z are possible within it. Even the "output" variables of a computer simulation do not vary freely, but rather are *wholly determined* by the values and relationships built into the model. Thus, even though the complexity of the model and the stochastic nature of some of the variables in it may prevent us from clearly specifying the output of its "operation" in advance, that output is nevertheless determined fully, albeit in a complex manner.

Hence, while the computer simulation entirely eliminates "noise" because it does not permit Treatment Z, it also entirely eliminates *information,* in the sense in which that term is here defined, because it does not permit Treatment Y. Returning to our earlier definition, we can gain research information when and only when something that is free to happen does not happen. That condition is never met by a computer simulation or any logically closed formal model.

Since the presence of Treatment Y is a necessary condition for obtaining research information, maximizing its use would seem to be an unqualified desideratum. However, such a generalization could lead to substantial inefficiency in the collection of empirical data. For example, there may be a particular value of a variable which seldom occurs in nature but which is of key theoretical significance. To obtain information on how that value affects other variables by use of an "all-Treatment *Y*" approach might be prohibitively costly. We would need to obtain a rather large sample of data for all frequently occurring values in order to obtain even a meager sample of cases which include the value of particular concern. The substitution of Treatment *X* in such a situation greatly increases efficiency by controlling the rate at which we sample values of (independent) variables. It permits us to substitute *systematic* for *representative* sampling, hence to provide an adequate amount of data for all values of concern within a minimum total amount of data.

Comprehensiveness, Efficiency, and Effectiveness

Comparisons of the research methods in terms of their comprehensiveness, efficiency, and effectiveness are implicit in the foregoing discussion. Any procedure which reduces the number of combinations of values of variables which can occur in the study situation reduces the comprehensiveness of that study. Use of Treatment *W*, and use of Treatment *X* so that only a small number of values of a variable occur during the study, both lead to a reduction of information potential and hence to a reduction of comprehensiveness. Since the use of both *W* and *X* increases as we move from field study to experimental simulation to laboratory study, comprehensiveness decreases at the same time. Generally, comprehensiveness decreases still further in the computer simulations because of the extensive use of Treatment *W* (often in the form of simplifying assumptions designed to make the model feasible for computer programming). But it is *possible* for a computer simulation to offset the reduction of comprehensiveness somewhat by systematically "playing" many values of many variables (i.e., using Treatment *X* rather than Treatment *W*).

At the same time, permitting a variable to go unmeasured and uncontrolled (Treatment *Z*) introduces noise into the design, which will tend to confound information from other variables, and hence reduce the efficiency of the study. Since the use of Treatment *Z* decreases as we move from the field study to other settings, it follows that field studies are generally less efficient than experimental simulations, which in turn are less efficient than laboratory experiments. Computer simulations eliminate noise in the present sense of the term, but they do so in a manner which also eliminates information. Hence, no meaningful statement of efficiency, in the present sense, can be made about the computer simulation.

Thus, within the framework of the present set of concepts, field studies are relatively comprehensive but inefficient. As study designs they retain almost all of the potential information which exists in the real life situation, but they also contain much noise which reduces the effective information yield. Laboratory experiments, on the other hand, are relatively efficient but low in comprehensiveness. They minimize noise, and hence convert much of the potential information in the study design into information yield. But they do so by restricting the information potential of the study design far below the information potential of the real-world situation to which the study is related. Experimental simulations seem to lie between field studies and laboratory experiments in both comprehensiveness and efficiency. Computer simulations are often relatively low in comprehensiveness, while the concept of efficiency does not apply since they yield no research information in the present use of that term.

We might summarize these comparisons by commenting that field studies may learn a little about a lot, whereas laboratory experiments may learn a lot about a little. In the same vein, computer simulations may learn "everything" about nothing.

But we have not yet commented on the relative *effectiveness* of these four classes of methods. Previously, we defined effectiveness of a research setting such that a loss in *either* scope or efficiency constitutes a loss in effectiveness. No over-all comparison of these four classses of methods in terms of their relative effectiveness can be made from the present context, since methods high in efficiency tend to be low in comprehensiveness and *vice versa*.

It might be argued that experimental simulations provide the most effective setting since they offer an optimal balance of scope and efficiency. To make such a conclusion, however, we would need to be able to formulate the metric properties of our continuum of methods, and accurately place the four classes of methods along that continuum; and this we clearly cannnot do with our present "weak" model. Thus, we cannot reasonably conclude that experimental simulations are inherently more effective research settings than other methods. However, they do seem to provide a research context which lets us avoid an extreme loss of *either* scope or efficiency.

Ultimately, effectiveness depends in a large measure on the specific research procedures which we use in a given case and the rigor with which we apply them. Hence, we can assess the relative effectiveness of specific studies, rather than of classes of study settings, because studies using any of the four types of settings can be executed well or poorly in terms of the rigor of procedures. However, the type of study setting used does place *limits* on the comprehensiveness and efficiency of *any* study done in that kind of setting, hence, effectiveness of a study is not entirely independent of the type of research setting by means of which it is done.

Implications for Programmatic Research

It should be pointed out that use of the different classes of research settings imply different levels of prior knowledge about the problem to be studied. The investigator needs to know a lot more (or assume he knows a lot more) about the phenomena he is studying in order to work with the methods at the laboratory and computer end of the continuum. As we proceed down the continuum from field studies to laboratory and computer studies, our results become more and more a function of the structure which we impose on the situation (by our Treatment W and Treatment X operations). Consequently, the empirical "truth" of the results which we obtain (as they apply to the real-life phenomena which we are studying) becomes more and more dependent upon the empirical "truth" of the structure which we have imposed.

On the field study end of the continuum, however, the investigator needs to know (or assume) less about the phenomena before he starts. He imposes less of a structure or a theory upon the situation. However, it should never be assumed that the field investigator does not also impose some theory as he selects and measures variables. Furthermore, although in one sense the data from the field study is necessarily "true," the investigator needs to know (or assume) a lot about what was and was not operating in his field situation in order for his *interpretations* to be "true." Hence, the field study investigator imposes a "strong" structure *after,* rather than before, he collects his data.

Obviously, then, the choice of methods along this continuum is not to be done in a haphazard way, on the basis of personal preference, or on the basis of mere expedience. We might view the continuum of methods as a two-way street.[47] If we are starting research on a relatively unexplored phenomenon, it would seem to be best to start far over at the field study end of the continuum. As we learn more about the problem, we can then work with methods further along the continuum, with which we can gain more precise information. Then, having explored the problem with precision and in depth, and perhaps having formulated and thoroughly manipulated a formal model, we can return toward the field study end of the street to find out how closely our representations fit the phenomena of the real world. This "path" of programmatic research is illustrated in Fig. 1.

This is, of course, an idealized description of what everyone knows to be the best way to do programmatic research. What is not specified here, and perhaps cannot be answered in the general case, is how to allocate time and effort among the various classes of methods, both on the "way down" and on the "way back" on this two-way street. In any actual case, for example, choice of methods must be determined on the basis of available resources, as well as on the basis of our present stage of knowledge about the problem. Methods differ considerably in the cost of running a given number of "cases." The more artificial and more abstract methods of the laboratory and computer generally have a far lower cost per case.

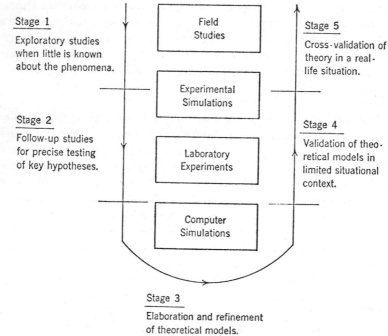

FIGURE 1. DIAGRAM OF A FIVE-STAGE LOGICAL PATH
FOR PROGRAMMATIC RESEARCH

But the ever present need to compromise our idealized research plans on pragmatic grounds does not in any way lessen the need for a full and careful reckoning of the advantages and limitations of methodological alternatives. Only by such a reckoning of the relative information which can be derived from different approaches to a given problem can we possibly be in a position to know how "costly" a given compromise would be. It must be recognized, of course, that the present formulation of a "theory of method" for the study of organizations is only a first step toward that aim. A much more thorough and precise formulation will be needed before we can truly "calculate" the relative losses and gains to be achieved by the choice of one approach over another. Still, it is hoped that this partial and tentative formulation may take us closer to the point where our choices of method for organization research can be done more often in a rational and efficient manner.

NOTES AND REFERENCES

1. Mesarović, M. D., Sanders, J. L., and Sprague, C. F. An Axiomatic Approach to Organizations from a General Systems Viewpoint. In Cooper, W. W., Leavitt, H. J., and Shelly, M. W. II New Perspectives in Organization Research. New York: John Wiley, 1964.
2. Bass, B. M. Production Organization Exercise: An Application of Experimental Techniques to Business Games. In Cooper, W. W., Leavitt, H. J., and Shelly, M. W. II New Perspectives in Organization Research. New York: John Wiley, 1964.
3. Seashore, S. E. and Bowers, D. G. Communications and Decision Processes as Determinants of Organizational Effectiveness, AFOSR Contract No. AF49 (638)-1032. Ann Arbor: Univ. of Michigan Institute for Social Research, 1962.
4. Guetzkow, H., Brody, R. A., and Driver, M. J. An Experimental Approach to the n-Country Problem. St. Louis, Mo.: Washington Univ., 1961.
5. Jenson, L. The Postwar Disarmament Negotiations: A Study in American-Soviet Bargaining Behavior. Ann Arbor: Univ. of Michigan, 1962.
6. Cyert, R. M. and March, J. G. The Behavioral Theory of the Firm: A Behavioral Science-Economics Amalgam. In Cooper, W. W., Leavitt, H. J., and Shelly, M. W. II New Perspectives in Organization Research. New York: John Wiley, 1964.
7. Likert, R. New Patterns of Management. New York: McGraw-Hill, 1961.
8. Homans, G. C. The Human Group. New York: Harcourt, Brace, 1950.
9. Bavelas, A. Communication Patterns in Task Oriented Groups. J. Acoustical Soc. Amer. 22: 725-730, 1950.
10. Leavitt, H. J. Some Effects of Certain Communication Patterns on Group Performance. J. Ab. Soc. Psych. 46: 38-50, 1951.
11. Guetzkow, H., and Simon, H. A. The Impact of Certain Communication Nets upon Organization and Performance in Task-Oriented Groups. Man. Science, 1: 233-250, 1955.

12. Merton, R. K. Bureaucratic Structure and Personality. Soc. Forces, 18: 560-568, 1940.

13. Parsons, T. Structure and Process in Modern Society. Glencoe: Free Press, 1960.

14. Whyte, W. F. Human Relations in the Restaurant Industry. New York: Mc-Graw-Hill, 1948.

15. Selznick, P. TVA and the Grass Roots. Berkeley: University of California Press, 1949.

16. For example, Comrey, et al. (17) and Udy (18).

17. Comrey, A. L., Pfiffner, J. M., and Beem, H. P. Factors Influencing Organizational Effectiveness I: The U. S. Forest Survey. Personnel Psych. 5: 307-325, 1952.

18. Udy, S. H., Jr. Administrative Rationality, Social Setting and Organizational Development. In Cooper, W. W., Leavitt, H. J., and Shelly, M. W. II New Perspectives in Organization Research. New York: John Wiley, 1964.

19. Whyte, W. H., Jr. The Organization Man. New York: Simon and Schuster, 1956.

20. Riesman, D. The Lonely Crowd. New Haven: Yale University Press, 1950.

21. Morse, N. C. and Reimer, E. The Experimental Change of a Major Organizational Variable. J. Ab. Soc. Psych. 52: 120-129, 1956.

22. Rome, S. C. and Rome, B. K. The Leviathan Technique for Large-Group Analysis. Santa Monica: System Development Corp., 1960.

23. See, e.g., Bonini (24), Whinston (25), and Mesarovic, Sanders, and Sprague (1).

24. Bonini, C. P. Simulating Organizational Behavior. In Cooper, W. W., Leavitt, H. J., and Shelly, M. W. II New Perspectives in Organization Research. New York: John Wiley, 1964.

25. Whinston, A. Price Guides in Decentralized Organizations. In Cooper, W. W., Leavitt, H. J., and Shelly, M. W. II New Perspectives in Organization Research. New York: John Wiley, 1964.

26. Alger, C. F. The External Bureaucracy in U. S. Foreign Affairs. Admin. Sci. Quart. 7: 50-78, 1962.

27. For example, Pepinski, et al. (28) and Udy (18).

28. Pepinsky, P. N. et al. The Research Team and Its Organizational Environment. Paper presented at AFSDR Conference on Research on Organization Behavior, Athens, Ga., May 1962.

29. Coch, L. and French, J. R. P. Overcoming Resistance to Change. Hum. Relat. 1: 512-532, 1948.

30. Guetzkow, H. Simulation in Social Science. Englewood Cliffs: Prentice-Hall, 1962.

31. In a sense, all laboratory experiments of human behavior, as individuals and as groups, are relevant to the field of organization research. A few of the many laboratory experiments which seem to have made important direct contributions to organization research, besides the communication net studies, include: studies on communication, development of norms, and pressures for conformity in informal groups (32-36); and studies of cohesiveness and group pressures as they affect productivity (37, 38).

32. Back, K. W. Influence through Social Communication. J. Ab. Soc. Psych. 46: 9-23, 1951.

33. Festinger, L., Gerard, H. B., Hymovitch, B., Kelley, H. H., and Raven, B. The Influence Process in the Presence of Extreme Deviates. Hum. Relat. 5: 327-346, 1952.

34. Kelley, H. H. Communication in Experimentally Created Hierarchies. Hum. Relat. 4: 39-56, 1951.

35. Schachter, S. Deviation, Rejection, and Communication. J. Ab. Soc. Psych. 46: 190-207, 1951.

36. Thibaut, J. W. An Experimental Study of the Cohesiveness of Underprivileged Groups. Hum. Relat. 3: 251-278, 1950.

37. Schachter, S., Ellertson, N., McBride, D., and Gregory, D. An Experimental Study of Cohesiveness and Productivity. Hum. Relat. 4: 229-238, 1951.

38. Berkowitz, L. Group Standards, Cohesiveness and Productivity. Hum. Relat. 7: 509-519, 1954.

39. Christie, L. A., et al. Communication and Learning in Task Oriented Groups. Cambridge: Research Laboratory of Electronics, 1952.

40. Shaw, M. E. Communication Patterns in Small Groups. Res. Rev. 11-12, 1955.

41. See Bonini (24) for an example.

42. It is obvious from the prior discussion that the methodologies being considered vary along a continuum rather than in a categorical manner. For example, the "field experiment," which is here classified as a field study, often shades into the experimental simulation class. Similarly, experimental simulations which are highly abstract representations of generic classes of organizations may become nearly indistinguishable from the laboratory experiment. The four-category classification of methods is used for convenience and clarity of presentation.

43. There are several important special cases of Treatment X. One of the more interesting ones, which is widely used under the name of "Monte Carlo technique," is the random selection of a value k_i for a given variable V_j on a given "trial," out of a predetermined probability distribution of values for V_j. Here, although there is some indeterminacy for any given trial, the distribution of values over a series of trials is predictable in advance, the accuracy of the prediction being a function of the number of trials in the series.

44. This formulation assumes that there are a *finite* number of relevant variables in a situation, and that each has a *finite* range and a *finite* number of possible alternative values.

45. This is equivalent to the ratio of "signal" to "signal-plus-noise." It is an expression of the effects of unsystematic confounding of a variable.

46. One might argue that computer simulations contain "noise" because they deliberately introduce random variation by the use of stochastic processes. Such variation is noise of a different sort than meant here. Although it produces indeterminancy for a given trial, the distribution of values for the total set of trials is predictable in advance. As noted previously [see (43)], these "Monte Carlo" procedures are really a special case of Treatment X.

47. To extend the analogy of the "two-way street," our prior discussion of variations within each class of methods [see (27)] suggests that the four classes of methods here defined are *neighborhoods,* rather than specific addresses, along that street. Within each neighborhood, the specific methods range so that some (such as field experiments) are on the borderline between adjacent neighborhoods.

48. McGrath, J. E., Nordlie, P. G., and Vaughan, W. S. A Systematic Framework for Comparison of System Research Methods. Arlington, Va.: Human Sciences Research, Technical Note HSR-59/7, Contract No. Nonr 2525- (00), 1960.

Many of the ideas presented in this chapter were developed in a research program designed to review and integrate research methodology used in studies of complex man-machine systems, sponsored by the Psychological Sciences Division, Office of Naval Research. See McGrath, et al.[48]

11

Factors Relevant to the Validity of Experiments in Social Settings

DONALD T. CAMPBELL

WHAT do we seek to control in experimental designs? What extraneous variables which would otherwise confound our interpretation of the experiment do we wish to rule out? The present paper attempts a specification of the major categories of such extraneous variables and employs these categories in evaluating the validity of standard designs for experimentation in the social sciences.

Validity will be evaluated in terms of two major criteria. First, and as a basic minimum, is what can be called *internal validity:* did in fact the experimental stimulus make some significant difference in this specific instance? The second criterion is that of *external validity, representativeness,* or *generalizability:* to what populations, settings, and variables can this effect be generalized? Both criteria are obviously important although it turns out that they are to some extent incompatible, in that the controls required for internal validity often tend to jeopardize representativeness.

The extraneous variables affecting internal validity will be introduced in the process of analyzing three pre-experimental designs. In the subsequent evaluation of the applicability of three true experimental designs, factors leading to external invalidity will be introduced. The effects of these extraneous variables will be considered at two levels: as simple or main effects, they occur independently of or in addition to the effects of the experimental variable; as interactions, the effects appear in conjunction with the experimental variable. The main effects typically turn out to be relevant to internal validity, the interaction effects to external validity or representativeness.

The following designation for experimental designs will be used: X will represent the exposure of a group to the experimental variable or event, the effects of which are to be measured; O will refer to the process of observation or measurement, which can include watching what people do, listening, recording, interviewing, administering tests, counting lever depressions, etc. The Xs and Os in a given row are applied to the same specific persons. The left to right dimension indicates temporal order. Parallel rows represent equivalent samples of persons unless otherwise specified. The designs will be numbered and named for cross-reference purposes.

Three Pre-experimental Designs and Their Confounded Extraneous Variables

The One-Shot Case Study. As Stouffer [3] has pointed out, much social science research still uses Design 1, in which a single individual or group is studied in detail only once, and in which the observations are attributed to exposure to some prior situation.

$$X \quad O \qquad \text{1. One-Shot Case Study}$$

This design does not merit the title of experiment, and is introduced only to provide a reference point. The very minimum of useful scientific information involves at least one formal comparison and therefore at least two careful observations. [4]

The One-Group Pretest-Posttest Design. This design does provide for one formal comparison of two observations, and is still widely used.

$$O_1 \quad X \quad O_2 \qquad \text{2. One-Group Pretest-Posttest Design}$$

However, in it there are four or five categories of extraneous variables left uncontrolled which thus become rival explanations of any difference between O_1 and O_2, confounded with the possible effect of X.

The first of these is the main effect of *history*. During the time span between O_1 and O_2 many events have occurred in addition to X, and the results might be attributed to these. Thus in Collier's [5] experiment, while his respondents [6] were reading Nazi propaganda materials, France fell, and the obtained attitude changes seemed more likely a result of this event than of the propaganda. [7] By history is meant the specific event series other than X, i.e., the extra-experimental uncontrolled stimuli. Relevant to this variable is the concept of experimental isolation, the employment of experimental settings in which all extraneous stimuli are eliminated. The approximation of such control in much physical and biological research has permitted the satisfactory employment of Design 2. But in social psychology and the other social sciences, if history is confounded with X the results are generally uninterpretable.

The second class of variables confounded with X in Design 2 is here designated as *maturation*. This covers those effects which are systematic with the passage of time, and not, like history, a function of the specific events involved. Thus between O_1 and O_2 the respondents may have grown older, hungrier, tireder, etc., and these may have produced the difference between O_1 and O_2, independently of X. While in the typical brief experiment in the psychology laboratory, maturation is unlikely to be a source of change, it has been a problem in research in child development and can be so in extended experiments in social psychology and education. In the form of "spontaneous remission" and the general processes of healing it becomes an important variable to control in medical research, psychotherapy, and social remediation.

There is a third source of variance that could explain the difference between O_1 and O_2 without a recourse to the effect of X. This is the effect of *testing* itself. It is often true that persons taking a test for the second time make scores systematically different from those taking the test for the first time. This is indeed the case for intelligence tests, where a second mean may be expected to run as much as five IQ points higher than the first one. This possibility makes important a distinction between *reactive* measures and *nonreactive* measures. A reactive measure is one which modifies the phenomenon under study, which changes the very thing that one is trying to measure. In general, any measurement procedure which makes the subject self-conscious or aware of the fact of the experiment can be suspected of being a reactive measurement. Whenever the measurement process is *not* a part of the normal environment it is probably reactive. Whenever measurement exercises the process under study, it is almost certainly reactive. Measurement of a person's height is relatively nonreactive. However, measurement of weight, introduced into an experimental design involving adult American women, would turn out to be reactive in that the process of measuring would stimulate weight reduction. A photograph of a crowd taken in secret from a second story window would be nonreactive, but a news photograph of the same scene might very well be reactive, in that the presence of the photographer would modify the behavior of people seeing themselves being photographed. In a factory, production records introduced for the purpose of an experiment would be reactive, but if such records were a regular part of the operating environment they would be nonreactive. An English anthropologist may be nonreactive as a participant-observer at an English wedding, but might be a highly reactive measuring instrument at a Dobu nuptials. Some measures are so extremely reactive that their use in a pretest-posttest design is not usually considered. In this class would be tests involving surprise, deception, rapid adaptation, or stress. Evidence is amply present that tests of learning and memory are highly reactive.[8,9] In the field of opinion and attitude research our well-developed interview and attitude test techniques must be rated as reactive, as shown, for example, by Crespi's[10] evidence.

Even within the personality and attitude test domain, it may be found that tests differ in the degree to which they are reactive. For some purposes, tests involving voluntary self-description may turn out to be more reactive (especially at the interaction level to be discussed below) than are devices which focus the respondent upon describing the external world, or give him less latitude in describing himself, e.g.,[11]. It seems likely that, apart from considerations of validity, the Rorschach test is less reactive than the TAT or MMPI. Where the reactive nature of the testing process results from the focusing of attention on the experimental variable, it may be reduced by imbedding the relevant content in a comprehensive array of topics, as has regularly been done in Hovland's attitude change studies.[12] It seems likely that with attention to the problem, observational and measurement techniques can be developed which are much less reactive than those now in use.

Instrument decay provides a fourth uncontrolled source of variance which could produce an O_1–O_2 difference that might be mistaken for the effect of X. This variable can be exemplified by the fatiguing of a spring scales, or the condensation of water vapor in a cloud chamber. For psychology and the social sciences it becomes a particularly acute problem when human beings are used as a part of the measuring apparatus, as judges, observers, raters, coders, etc. Thus O_1 and O_2 may differ because the raters have become more experienced, more fatigued, have acquired a different adaptation level, or have learned about the purpose of the experiment, etc. However infelicitously, this term will be used to typify those problems introduced when shifts in measurement conditions are confounded with the effect of X, including such crudities as having a different observer at O_1 and O_2, or using a different interviewer or coder. Where the use of different interviewers, observers, or experimenters is unavoidable, but where they are used in large numbers, a sampling equivalence of interviewers is required, with the relevant N being the N of interviewers, not interviewees, except as refined through cluster sampling considerations.[13]

A possible fifth extraneous factor deserves mention. This is statistical *regression*. When, in Design 2, the group under investigation has been selected for its extremity on O_1, O_1–O_2 shifts toward the mean will occur which are due to random imperfections of the measuring instrument or random instability within the population, as reflected in the test-retest reliability. In general, regression operates like maturation in that the effects increase systematically with the O_1–O_2 time interval. McNemar[14] has demonstrated the profound mistakes in interpretation which failure to control this factor can introduce in remedial research.

The Static Group Comparison. The third pre-experimental design is the Static Group Comparison.

$$\begin{array}{cc} X & O_1 \\ \hline & O_2 \end{array}$$ 3. The Static Group Comparison

In this design, there is a comparison of a group which has experienced X with a group which has not, for the purpose of establishing the effect of X. In contrast with Design 6, there is in this design no means of certifying that the groups were equivalent at some prior time. (The absence of sampling equivalence of groups is symbolized by the row of dashes.) This design has its most typical occurrence in the social sciences, and both its prevalence and its weakness have been well indicated by Stouffer.[15] It will be recognized as one form of the correlational study. It is introduced here to complete the list of confounding factors. If the Os differ, this difference could have come about through biased *selection* or recruitment of the persons making up the groups; i.e., they might have differed anyway without the effect of X. Frequently, exposure to X (e.g., some mass communication) has been voluntary and the two groups have an inevitable systematic difference on the factors determining the choice involved, a difference which no amount of matching can remove.

A second variable confounded with the effect of X in this design can be called experimental *mortality*. Even if the groups were equivalent at some prior time, O_1 and O_2 may differ now not because individual members have changed, but because a biased subset of members have dropped out. This is a typical problem in making inferences from comparisons of the attitudes of college freshmen and college seniors, for example.

True Experimental Designs

The Pretest-Posttest Control Group Design. One or another of the above considerations led psychologists between 1900 and 1925[16,17] to expand Design 2 by the addition of a control group, resulting in Design 4.

$$\begin{array}{ccc} O_1 & X & O_2 \\ O_3 & & O_4 \end{array}$$ 4. Pretest-Posttest Control Group Design

Because this design so neatly controls for the main effects of history, maturation, testing, instrument decay, regression, selection, and mortality, these separate sources of variance are not usually made explicit. It seems well to state briefly the relationship of the design to each of these confounding factors, with particular attention to the application of the design in social settings.

If the differences between O_1 and O_2 were due to intervening historical events, then they should also show up in the O_3–O_4 comparison. Note, however, several complications in achieving this control. If respondents are run in groups, and if there is only one experimental session and one control session, then there is no control over the unique internal histories of the groups. The O_1–O_2 difference, even if not appearing in O_3–O_4, may be due to a chance distracting factor appearing in one or the other group. Such a design, while controlling for the shared history or event series, still confounds X with the unique session history. Second, the design implies a simultaneity of O_1 with O_3 and O_2 with O_4 which is usually impossible. If one were to try to achieve simultaneity by using two experimenters, one working with the experimental respondents, the other with the controls, this would confound experimenter differences with X (introducing one type of instrument decay). These considerations make it usually imperative that, for a true experiment, the experimental and control groups be tested and exposed individually or in small subgroups, and that sessions of both types be temporally and spatially intermixed.

As to the other factors: if maturation or testing contributed an O_1–O_2 difference, this should appear equally in the O_3–O_4 comparison, and these variables are thus controlled for their main effects. To make sure the design controls for instrument decay, the same individual or small-session approximation to simultaneity needed for history is required. The occasional practice of running the experimental group and control group at different times is thus ruled out on this ground as well as that of history. Otherwise the observers may have become more experienced, more hurried, more careless, the maze more redolent with irrelevant cues, the lever-tension and friction diminished, etc. Only when groups are effectively simultaneous do these factors affect experimental and control groups alike. Where more than one experimenter or observer is used, counter-balancing experimenter, time, and group is recommended. The balanced Latin square is frequently useful for this purpose.[18]

While regression is controlled in the design as a whole, frequently secondary analyses of effects are made for extreme pretest scorers in the experimental group. To provide a control for effects of regression, a parallel analysis of extremes should also be made for the control group.

Selection is of course handled by the sampling equivalence ensured through the randomization employed in assigning persons to groups, perhaps supplemented by, but not supplanted by, matching procedures. Where the experimental and control groups do not have this sort of equivalence, one has a compromise design rather than a true experiment. Furthermore, the O_1-O_3 comparison provides a check on possible sampling differences.

The design also makes possible the examination of experimental mortality, which becomes a real problem for experiments extended over weeks or months. If the experimental and control groups do not differ in the number of lost cases nor in their pretest scores, the experiment can be judged internally valid on this point, although mortality reduces the generalizability of effects to the original population from which the groups were selected.

For these reasons, the Pretest-Posttest Control Group Design has been the ideal in the social sciences for some thirty years. Recently, however, a serious and avoidable imperfection in it has been noted, perhaps first by Schanck and Goodman.[19] Solomon[20] has expressed the point as an *interaction* effect of testing. In the terminology of analysis of variance, the effects of history, maturation, and testing, as described so far, are all *main* effects, manifesting themselves in mean differences independently of the presence of other variables. They are effects that could be added on to other effects, including the effect of the experimental variable. In contrast, interaction effects represent a joint effect, specific to the concomitance of two or more conditions, and may occur even when no main effects are present. Applied to the testing variable, the interaction effect might involve not a shift due solely or directly to the measurement process, but rather a sensitization of respondents to the experimental variable so that when X was preceded by O there would be a change, whereas both X and O would be without effect if occurring alone. In terms of the two types of validity, Design 4 is internally valid, offering an adequate basis for generalization to other sampling-equivalent *pretested* groups. But it has a serious and systematic weakness in representativeness in that it offers, strictly speaking, no basis for generalization to the *unpretested* population. And it is usually the *unpretested* larger universe from which these samples were taken to which one wants to generalize.

A concrete example will help make this clearer. In the NORC study of a United Nations information campaign,[21] two equivalent samples, of a thousand each, were drawn from the city's population. One of these samples was interviewed, following which the city of Cincinnati was subjected to an intensive publicity campaign using all the mass media of communication. This included special features in the newspapers and on the radio, bus cards, public lectures, etc. At the end of two months, the second sample of 1,000 was interviewed and the results compared with the first 1,000. There were no differences between the two groups except that the second group was somewhat more pessimistic about the likelihood of Russia's cooperating for world peace, a result which was attributed to history rather than to the publicity campaign. The second sample was no better informed about the United Nations nor had it noticed in particular the publicity campaign which had been going on. In connection with a program of research on panels and the reinterview problem, Paul Lazarsfeld and the Bureau of Applied Social Research arranged to have the initial sample reinterviewed at the same time as the second sample was interviewed, after the publicity campaign. This reinterviewed group showed significant attitude changes, a high degree of awareness of the campaign and important increases in information. The inference in this case is unmistakably that the initial interview had sensitized the persons interviewed to the topic of the United Nations, had raised in them a focus of awareness which made the subsequent publicity campaign effective for them but for them only. This study and other studies clearly document the possibility of interaction effects which seriously limit our capacity to generalize from the pretested experimental group to the unpretested general population. Hovland[22] reports a general finding which is of the opposite nature but is, nonetheless, an indication of an interactive effect. In his Army studies the initial pretest served to reduce the effects of the experimental variable, presumably by creating a commitment to a given position. Crespi's[23] findings support this expectation. Solomon[24] reports two studies with school children in which a spelling pretest reduced the effects of a training period. But whatever the direction of the effect, this flaw in the Pretest-Posttest Control Group Design is serious for the purposes of the social scientist.

   The Solomon Four-Group Design. It is Solomon's[25] suggestion to control this problem by adding to the traditional two-group experiment two unpretested groups as indicated in Design 5.

$$O_1 \quad X \quad O_2$$
$$O_3 \qquad O_4 \qquad \text{5. Solomon Four-Group Design}$$
$$X \quad O_5$$
$$O_6$$

This Solomon Four-Group Design enables one both to control and measure both the main and interaction effects of testing and the main effects of a composite of maturation and history. It has become the new ideal design for social scientists. A word needs to be said about the appropriate statistical analysis. In Design 4, an efficient single test embodying the four measurements is achieved through computing for each individual a pretest-posttest difference score which is then used for comparing by t test the experimental and control groups. Extension of this mode of analysis to the Solomon Four-Group Design introduces an inelegant awkwardness to the otherwise elegant procedure. It involves assuming as a pretest score for the unpretested groups the mean value of the pretest from the first two groups. This restricts the effective degrees of freedom, violates assumptions of independence, and leaves one without a legitimate base for testing the significance of main effects and interaction. An alternative analysis is available which avoids the assumed pretest scores. Note that the four posttests form a simple two-by-two analysis of variance design:

	No X	X
Pretested	O_4	O_2
Unpretested	O_6	O_5

The column means represent the main effect of X, the row means the main effect of pretesting, and the interaction term the interaction of pretesting and X. (By use of a t test the combined main effects of maturation and history can be tested through comparing O_6 with O_1 and O_3.)

The Posttest-Only Control Group Design. While the statistical procedures of analysis of variance introduced by Fisher[26] are dominant in psychology and the other social sciences today, it is little noted in our discussions of experimental arrangements that Fisher's typical agricultural experiment involves no pretest: equivalent plots of ground receive different experimental treatments and the subsequent yields are measured.[27] Applied to a social experiment as in testing the influence of a motion picture upon attitudes, two randomly assigned audiences would be selected, one exposed to the movie, and the attitudes of each measured subsequently for the first time.

$A \quad X \quad O_1$ 6. Posttest-Only Control Group Design
$A \qquad O_2$

In this design the symbol A had been added, to indicate that at a specific time prior to X the groups were made equivalent by a random

sampling *assignment*. A is the point of selection, the point of allocation of individuals to groups. It is the existence of this process that
distinguishes Design 6 from Design 3, the Static Group Comparison. Design 6 is not a static cross-sectional comparison, but instead
truly involves control and observation extended in time. The sampling
procedures employed assure us that at time A the groups were equal,
even if not measured. A provides a point of prior equality just as does
the pretest. A point A is, of course, involved in all true experiments,
and should perhaps be indicated in Designs 4 and 5. It is essential that
A be regarded as a specific point in time, for groups change as a function of time since A, through experimental mortality. Thus in a public
opinion survey situation employing probability sampling from lists of
residents, the longer the time since A, the more the sample under-
represents the transient segments of society, the newer dwelling units,
etc. When experimental groups are being drawn from a self-selected
extreme population, such as applicants for psychotherapy, time since
A introduces maturation (spontaneous remission) and regression factors. In Design 6 these effects would be confounded with the effect of
X if the As as well as the Os were not contemporaneous for experimental and control groups.

Like Design 4, this design controls for the effects of maturation and
history through the practical simultaneity of both the As and the Os.
In superiority over Design 4, no main or interaction effects of pre-
testing are involved. It is this feature that recommends it in particular.
While it controls for the main and interaction effects of pretesting as
well as does Design 5, the Solomon Four-Group Design, it does not
measure these effects, nor the main effect of history-maturation. It can
be noted that Design 6 can be considered as the two unpretested
"control" groups from the Solomon Design, and that Solomon's two
traditional pretested groups have in this sense the sole purpose of
measuring the effects of pretesting and history-maturation, a purpose
irrelevant to the main aim of studying the effect of X.[29] However,
under normal conditions of not quite perfect sampling control, the
four-group design provides in addition greater assurance against mistakenly attributing to X effects which are not due it, inasmuch as the
effect of X is documented in three different fashions (O_1 vs. O_2, O_2 vs.
O_4, and O_5 vs. O_6). But, short of the four-group design, Design 6 is
often to be preferred to Design 4, and is a fully valid experimental
design.

Design 6 has indeed been used in the social sciences, perhaps first of
all in the classic experiment by Gosnell, *Getting Out the Vote*.[30]

Schanck and Goodman,[31] Hovland[32] and others[33-37] have also employed it. But, in spite of its manifest advantages of simplicity and control, it is far from being a popular design in social research and indeed is usually relegated to an inferior position in discussions of experimental designs if mentioned at all, e.g.,[38-40]. Why is this the case?

In the first place, it is often confused with Design 3. Even where Ss have been carefully assigned to experimental and control groups, one is apt to have an uneasiness about the design because one "doesn't know what the subjects were like before." This objection must be rejected, as our standard tests of significance are designed precisely to evaluate the likelihood of differences occurring by chance in such sample selection. It is true, however, that this design is particularly vulnerable to selection bias and where random assignment is not possible it remains suspect. Where naturally aggregated units, such as classes, are employed intact, these should be used in large numbers and assigned at random to the experimental and control conditions; cluster sampling statistics[41] should be used to determine the error term. If but one or two intact classrooms are available for each experimental treatment, Design 4 should certainly be used in preference.

A second objection to Design 6, in comparison with Design 4, is that it often has less precision. The difference scores of Design 4 are less variable than the posttest scores of Design 6 if there is a pretest-posttest correlation above .50,[42] and hence for test-retest correlations above that level a smaller mean difference would be statistically significant for Design 4 than for Design 6, for a constant number of cases. This advantage to Design 4 may often be more than dissipated by the costs and loss in experimental efficiency resulting from the requirement of two testing sessions, over and above the considerations of representativeness.

Design 4 has a particular advantage over Design 6 if experimental mortality is high. In Design 4, one can examine the pretest scores of lost cases in both experimental and control groups and check on their comparability. In the absence of this in Design 6, the possibility is opened for a mean difference resulting from differential mortality rather than from individual change, if there is a substantial loss of cases.

A final objection comes from those who wish to study the relationship of pretest attitudes to kind and amount of change. This is a valid objection, and where this is the interest, Design 4 or 5 should be used, with parallel analysis of experimental and control groups. Another common type of individual difference study involves classifying persons in terms of amount of change and finding associated characteristics such as sex, age, education, etc. While unavailable in this form in Design 6, essentially the same correlational information can be obtained by subdividing both experimental and control groups in terms of the associated characteristics, and examining the experimental-control difference for such subtypes.

For Design 6, the Posttest-Only Control Group Design, there is a class of social settings in which it is optimally feasible, settings which should be more used than they now are. Whenever the social contact represented by X is made to single individuals or to small groups, and where the response to that stimulus can be identified in terms of individuals or type of X, Design 6 can be applied. Direct mail and door-to-door contacts represent such settings. The alternation of several appeals from door-to-door in a fund-raising campaign can be organized as a true experiment without increasing the cost of the solicitation. Experimental variation of persuasive materials in a direct-mail sales campaign can provide a better experimental laboratory for the study of mass communication and persuasion than is available in any university. The well-established, if little-used, split-run technique in comparing alternative magazine ads is a true experiment of this type, usually limited to coupon returns rather than sales because of the problem of identifying response with stimulus type.[43] The split-ballot technique[44] long used in public opinion polls to compare different question wordings or question sequences provides an excellent example which can obviously be extended to other topics, e.g.,[45]. By and large these laboratories have not yet been used to study social science theories, but they are directly relevant to hypotheses about social persuasion.

Multiple X designs. In presenting the above designs, X has been opposed to No-X, as is traditional in discussions of experimental design in psychology. But while this may be a legitimate description of the stimulus-isolated physical science laboratory, it can only be a convenient shorthand in the social sciences, for any No-X period will not be empty of potentially change-inducing stimuli. The experience of the control group might better be categorized as another type of X, a control experience, an X_C instead of No-X. It is also typical of advance in science that we are soon no longer interested in the qualitative fact of effect or no-effect, but want to specify degree of effect for varying degrees of X. These considerations lead into designs in which multiple groups are used, each with a different X_1, X_2, X_3, X_n, or in multiple factorial design, as X_{1a}, X_{1b}, X_{2a}, X_{2b}, etc. Applied to Designs 4 and 6, this introduces one additional group for each additional X. Applied to 5, The Solomon Four-Group Design, two additional groups (one pre-tested, one not, both receiving X_n) would be added for each variant on X.

In many experiments, X_1, X_2, X_3, and X_n are all given to the same group, differing groups receiving the Xs in different orders. Where the problem under study centers around the effects of order or combination, such counterbalanced multiple X arrangements are, of course, essential. Studies of transfer in learning are a case in point.[46] But where one wishes to generalize to the effect of each X as occurring in isolation, such designs are not recommended because of the sizable interactions among Xs, as repeatedly demonstrated in learning studies under such labels as proactive inhibition and learning sets. The use of counter-balanced sets of multiple Xs to achieve experimental equation, where natural groups not randomly assembled have to be used, will be discussed in a subsequent paper on compromise designs.

Testing for effects extended in time. The researches of Hovland and his associates[47, 48] have indicated repeatedly that the longer range effects of persuasive Xs may be qualitatively as well as quantitatively different from immediate effects. These results emphasize the importance of designing experiments to measure the effect of X at extended periods of time. As the misleading early research on reminiscence and on the consolidation of the memory trace indicate,[49] repeated measurement of the same persons cannot be trusted to do this if a reactive measurement process is involved. Thus, for Designs 4 and 6, two separate groups must be added for each posttest period. The additional control group cannot be omitted, or the effects of intervening history, maturation, instrument decay, regression, and mortality are confounded with the delayed effects of X. To follow fully the logic of Design 5, four additional groups are required for each posttest period.

True experiments in which O is not under E's control. It seems well to call the attention of the social scientist to one class of true experiments which are possible without the full experimental control over both the "when" and "to whom" of both X and O. As far as this analysis has been able to go, no such true experiments are possible without the ability to control X, to withhold it from carefully randomly selected respondents while presenting it to others. But control over O does not seem so indispensable. Consider the following design.

A X O_1
A O_2 6. Posttest Only Design, where O cannot be withheld
     (O) from any respondent
     (O)
     (O)

The parenthetical Os are inserted to indicate that the studied groups, experimental and control, have been selected from a larger universe all of which will get O anyway. An election provides such an O, and using "whether voted" rather than "how voted," this was Gosnell's design.[50] Equated groups were selected at time A, and the experimental group subjected to persuasive materials designed to get out the vote. Using precincts rather than persons as the basic sampling unit, similar studies can be made on the content of the voting.[51] Essential to this design is the ability to create specified randomly equated groups, the ability to expose one of these groups to X while withholding it (or providing X_2) from the other group, and the ability to identify the performance of each individual or unit in the subsequent O. Since such measures are natural parts of the environment to which one wishes to generalize, they are not reactive, and Design 4, the Pretest-Posttest Control Group Design, is feasible if O has a predictable periodicity to it. With the precinct as a unit, this was the design of Hartmann's classic study of emotional vs. rational appeals in a public election.[52] Note that 5, the Solomon Four-Group Design, is not available, as it requires the ability to withhold O experimentally, as well as X.

Further Problems of Representativeness

The interaction effect of testing, affecting the external validity or representativeness of the experiment, was treated extensively in the previous section, inasmuch as it was involved in the comparison of alternative designs. The present section deals with the effects upon representativeness of other variables which, while equally serious, can apply to any of the experimental designs.

The interaction effects of selection. Even though the true experiments control selection and mortality for internal validity purposes, these factors have, in addition, an important bearing on representativeness. There is always the possibility that the obtained effects are specific to the experimental population and do not hold true for the populations to which one wants to generalize. Defining the universe of reference in advance and selecting the experimental and control groups from this at random would guarantee representativeness if it were ever achieved in practice. But inevitably not all those so designated are actually eligible for selection by any contact procedure. Our best survey sampling techniques, for example, can designate for potential contact only those available through residences. And, even of those so designated, up to 19 per cent are not contactable for an interview in their own homes even with five callbacks.[53] It seems legitimate to assume that the more effort and time required of the respondent, the larger the loss through nonavailability and noncooperation. If one were to try to assemble experimental groups away from their own homes it seems reasonable to estimate a 50 per cent selection loss. If, still trying to extrapolate to the general public, one further limits oneself to docile preassembled groups, as in schools, military units, studio audiences, etc., the proportion of the universe systematically excluded through the sampling process must approach 90 per cent or more. Many of the selection factors involved are indubitably highly systematic. Under these extreme selection losses, it seems reasonable to suspect that the experimental groups might show reactions not characteristic of the general population. This point seems worth stressing lest we unwarrantedly assume that the selection loss for experiments is comparable to that found for survey interviews in the home at the respondent's convenience. Furthermore, it seems plausible that the greater the cooperation required, the more the respondent has to deviate from the normal course of daily events, the greater will be the possibility of nonrepresentative reactions. By and large, Design 6 might be expected to require less cooperation than Design 4 or 5, especially in the natural individual contact setting. The interactive effects of experimental mortality are of similar nature. Note that, on these grounds, the longer the experiment is extended in time the more respondents are lost and the less representative are the groups of the original universe.

Reactive arrangements. In any of the experimental designs, the respondents can become aware that they are participating in an experiment, and this awareness can have an interactive effect, in creating reactions to X which would not occur had X been encountered without this "I'm a guinea pig" attitude. Lazarsfeld,[54] Kerr,[55] and Rosenthal and Frank,[56] all have provided valuable discussions of this problem. Such effects limit generalizations to respondents having this awareness, and preclude generalization to the population encountering X with non-experimental attitudes. The direction of the effect may be one of negativism, such as an unwillingness to admit to any persuasion or change. This would be comparable to the absence of any immediate effect from discredited communicators, as found by Hovland.[57] The result is probably more often a cooperative responsiveness, in which the respondent accepts the experimenter's expectations and provides pseudoconfirmation. Particularly is this positive response likely when the respondents are self-selected seekers after the cure that X may offer. The Hawthorne studies[58] illustrate such sympathetic changes due to awareness of experimentation rather than to the specific nature of X. In some settings it is possible to disguise the experimental purpose by providing plausible façades in which X appears as an incidental part of the background, e.g.,[59-61]. We can also make more extensive use of experiments taking place in the intact social situation, in which the respondent is not aware of the experimentation at all.

The discussion of the effects of selection on representativeness has argued against employing intact natural preassembled groups, but the issue of conspicuousness of arrangements argues for such use. The machinery of breaking up natural groups such as departments, squads, and classrooms into randomly assigned experimental and control groups is a source of reaction which can often be avoided by the use of preassembled groups, particularly in educational settings. Of course, as has been indicated, this requires the use of large numbers of such groups under both experimental and control conditions.

The problem of reactive arrangements is distributed over all features of the experiment which can draw the attention of the respondent to the fact of experimentation and its purposes. The conspicuous or reactive pretest is particularly vulnerable, inasmuch as it signals the topics and purposes of the experimenter. For communications of obviously persuasive aim, the experimenter's topical intent is signaled by the X itself, if the communication does not seem a part of the natural environment. Even for the posttest-only groups, the occurrence of the posttest may create a reactive effect. The respondent may say to himself, "Aha, now I see why we got that movie." This consideration justifies the practice of disguising the connection between O and X even for Design 6, as through having different experimental personnel involved, using different façades, separating the settings and times, and embedding the X-relevant content of O among a disguising variety of other topics.[62]

Generalizing to other Xs. After the internal validity of an experiment has been established, after a dependable effect of X upon O has been found, the next step is to establish the limits and relevant dimensions of generalization not only in terms of populations and settings but also in terms of categories and aspects of X. The actual X in any one experiment is a specific combination of stimuli, all confounded for interpretative purposes, and only some relevant to the experimenter's intent and theory. Subsequent experimentation should be designed to purify X, to discover that aspect of the original conglomerate X which is responsible for the effect. As Brunswik[63] has emphasized, the representative sampling of Xs is as relevant a problem in linking experiment to theory as is the sampling of respondents. To define a category of Xs along some dimension, and then to sample Xs for experimental purposes from the full range of stimuli meeting the specification while other aspects of each specific stimulus complex are varied, serves to untie or unconfound the defined dimension from specific others, lending assurance of theoretical relevance.

In a sense, the placebo problem can be understood in these terms. The experiment without the placebo has clearly demonstrated that some aspect of the total X stimulus complex has had an effect; the placebo experiment serves to break up the complex X into the suggestive connotation of pill-taking and the specific pharmacological properties of the drug—separating two aspects of the X previously confounded. Subsequent studies may discover with similar logic which chemical fragment of the complex natural herb is most essential. Still more clearly, the sham operation illustrates the process of X purification, ruling out general effects of surgical shock so that the specific effects of loss of glandular or neural tissue may be isolated. As these parallels suggest, once recurrent unwanted aspects of complex Xs have been discovered for a given field, control groups especially designed to eliminate these effects can be regularly employed.

Generalizing to other Os. In parallel form, the scientist in practice uses a complex measurement procedure which needs to be refined in subsequent experimentation. Again, this is best done by employing multiple Os all having in common the theoretically relevant attribute but varying widely in their irrelevant specificities. For Os this process can be introduced into the initial experiment by employing multiple measures. A major practical reason for not doing so is that it is so frequently a frustrating experience, lending hesitancy, indecision, and a feeling of failure to studies that would have been interpreted with confidence had but a single response measure been employed.

Transition experiments. The two previous paragraphs have argued against the *exact* replication of experimental apparatus and measurement procedures on the grounds that this continues the confounding

of theory-relevant aspects of X and O with specific artifacts of unknown influence. On the other hand, the confusion in our literature
generated by the heterogeneity of results from studies all on what is
nominally the "same" problem but varying in implementation, is leading some to call for exact replication of initial procedures in subsequent research on a topic. Certainly no science can emerge without
dependably repeatable experiments. A suggested resolution is the *transition experiment,* in which the need for varying the theory-indepen-
dent aspects of X and O is met in the form of a multiple X, multiple
O design, one segment of which is an "exact" replication of the original experiment, exact at least in those major features which are normally reported in experimental writings.

Internal vs. external validity. If one is in a situation where either
internal validity or representativeness must be sacrificed, which should
it be? The answer is clear. Internal validity is the prior and indispensable consideration. The optimal design is, of course, one having both
internal and external validity. Insofar as such settings are available,
they should be exploited, without embarrassment from the apparent
opportunistic warping of the content of studies by the availability of
laboratory techniques. In this sense, a science is as opportunistic as a
bacteria culture and grows only where growth is possible. One basic
necessity for such growth is the machinery for selecting among alternative hypotheses, no matter how limited those hypotheses may have to be.

Summary

In analyzing the extraneous variables which experimental designs
for social settings seek to control, seven categories have been distinguished: history, maturation, testing, instrument decay, regression, selection, and mortality. In general, the simple or main effects of these
variables jeopardize the internal validity of the experiment and are
adequately controlled in standard experimental designs. The interactive effects of these variables and of experimental arrangements affect
the external validity or generalizability of experimental results. Standard experimental designs vary in their susceptibility to these interactive effects. Stress is also placed upon the differences among measuring
instruments and arrangements in the extent to which they create unwanted interactions. The value for social science purposes of the Posttest-Only Control Group Design is emphasized.

NOTES AND REFERENCES
1. Stouffer, S. A. Measurement in Sociology. Am. Soc. Rev. 18: 591-597, 1953.

2. Underwood, B. J. Psychological Research. New York: Appleton-Century-Crofts, 1957a.

3. Stouffer, S. A. Some Observations of Study Design. Am. J. Sociol. 55: 355-361, 1949-50.

4. Boring, E. G. The Nature and History of Experimental Control. Am. J. Psychol. 67: 573-589, 1954.

5. Collier, R. M. The Effect of Propaganda upon Attitude Following a Critical Examination of the Propaganda Itself. J. Soc. Psychol. 20: 3-17, 1944.

6. In line with the central focus on social psychology and the social sciences, the term *respondent* is employed in place of the terms *subject, patient,* or *client.*

7. Collier actually used a more adequate design than this, an approximation to Design 4.

8. Underwood, B. J. Interference and Forgetting. Psychol. Rev. 64: 49-60, 1957b.

9. Underwood, 1957a, op. cit.

10. Crespi, L. P. The Interview Effect in Polling. Publ. Opin. Quart. 12: 99-111, 1948.

11. Campbell, D. T. The Indirect Assessment of Social Attitudes. Psychol. Bull. 47: 15-38, 1950.

12. Hovland, C. E., Janis, I. L., and Kelley, H. H. Communication and Persuasion. New Haven: Yale University Press, 1953.

13. Kish, L. Selection of the Sample. In Festinger, L., and Katz, D. (Eds.) Research Methods in the Behavioral Sciences. New York: Dryden Press, 1953, pp. 175-239.

14. McNemar, Q. A Critical Examination of the University of Iowa Studies of Environmental Influences upon the I.Q. Psychol. Bull. 37: 63-92, 1940.

15. Stouffer, 1949-50, op. cit.

16. Boring, op. cit.

17. Solomon, R. W. An Extension of Control Group Design. Psychol. Bull. 46: 137-150, 1949.

18. Bugelski, B. R. A Note on Grant's Discussion of the Latin Square Principle in the Design and Analysis of Psychological Experiments. Psychol. Bull. 46: 49-50, 1949.

19. Schanck, R. L., and Goodman, C. Reactions to Propaganda on Both Sides of a Controversial Issue. Publ. Opin. Quart. 3: 107-112, 1939.

20. Solomon, op. cit.

21. Star, S. A., and Hughes, H. M. Report on an Educational Campaign: The Cincinnati Plan for the United Nations. Amer. J. Sociol. 55: 389, 1949-50.

22. Hovland, C. I., Lumsdaine, A. A., and Sheffield, F. D. Experiments on Mass Communication. Princeton: Princeton Univ. Press, 1949.

23. Crespi, op. cit.

24. Solomon, op. cit.

25. Ibid.

26. Fisher, R. A. The Design of Experiments. Edinburgh: Oliver & Boyd, 1935.

27. This is not to imply that the pretest is totally absent from Fisher's designs. He suggests the use of previous year's yields, etc., in covariance analysis. He notes, however, "with annual agricultural crops, knowledge of yields of the experimental area in a previous year under uniform treatment has not been found sufficiently to increase the precision to warrant the adoption of such uniformity trials as a preliminary to projected experiments." (28)

28. Fisher, op. cit., p. 176.

29. Payne, S. L. The Ideal Model for Controlled Experiments. Publ. Opinion Quart. 15: 557-562, 1951.
30. Gosnell, H. F. Getting out the Vote: An Experiment in the Stimulation of Voting. Chicago: Univ. of Chicago Press, 1927.
31. Schanck & Goodman, op. cit.
32. Hovland, Lumsdaine, and Sheffield, op. cit.
33. Annis, A. D., and Meier, N. C. The Induction of Opinion through Suggestion by Means of Planted Content. J. Soc. Psychol. 5: 65-81, 1934.
34. Greenberg, A. Matched Samples. J. Marketing, 18: 241-245, 1953-54.
35. Menefee, S. C. An Experimental Study of Strike Propaganda. Soc. Forces, 16: 574-582, 1938.
36. Parrish, J. A., and Campbell, D. T. Measuring Propaganda Effects with Direct and Indirect Attitude Tests. J. Abnorm. Soc. Psychol. 48: 3-9, 1953.
37. Rankin, R. E., and Campbell, D. T. Galvanic Skin Response to Negro and White Experimenters. J. Abnorm. Soc. Psychol. 51: 30-33, 1955.
38. Hovland, Lumsdaine, and Sheffield, op. cit.
39. Jahoda, M., Deutsch, M., and Cook, S. W. Research Methods in Social Relations. New York: Dryden Press, 1951.
40. Stouffer, 1949-50, op. cit.
41. Kish, op. cit.
42. Hovland, Lumsdaine, and Sheffield, op. cit., p. 323.
43. Lucas, D. B. and Britt, S. H. Advertising Psychology and Research. New York: McGraw-Hill, 1950.
44. Cantril, H. Gauging Public Opinion. Princeton: Princeton Univ. Press, 1944.
45. Greenberg, op. cit.
46. Underwood, B. J. Experimental Psychology. New York: Appleton-Century-Crofts, 1949.
47. Hovland, Janis, and Kelley, op. cit.
48. Hovland, Lumsdaine, and Sheffield, op. cit.
49. Underwood, 1957 a, op. cit.
50. Gosnell, op. cit.
51. Campbell, D. T. On the Possibility of Experimenting with the "Bandwagon" Effect. Int. J. Opin. Attitude Res. 5: 251-260, 1951.
52. Hartmann, G. W. A Field Experiment on the Comparative Effectiveness of "Emotional" and "Rational" Political Leaflets 18: 241-245, 1953-54.
53. Williams, R. Probability Sampling in the Field: A Case History. Publ. Opin. Quart. 14: 316-330, 1950.
54. Lazarsfeld, P. F. Training Guide on the Controlled Experiment in Social Research. Dittoed. Columbia Univ., Bureau of Applied Social Research, 1948.
55. Kerr, W. A. Experiments on the Effect of Music on Factory Production. Appl. Psychol. Mon. 1945, No. 5.
56. Rosenthal, D., and Frank, J. O. Psychotherapy and the Placebo Effect. Psychol. Bull. 53: 294-302, 1956.
57. Hovland, Janis, and Kelley, op. cit.
58. Mayo, E. The Human Problems of an Industrial Civilization. New York: Macmillan, 1933.
59. Postman, L., and Bruner, J. S. Perception under Stress. Psychol. Rev. 55: 314-322, 1948.
60. Rankin and Campbell, op. cit.

61. Schanck and Goodman, op. cit.

62. For purposes of completeness, the interaction of X with history and maturation should be mentioned. Both affect the generalizability of results. The interaction effect of history represents the possible specificity of results to a given historical moment, a possibility which increases as problems are more societal, less biological. The interaction of maturation and X would be represented in the specificity of effects to certain maturational levels, fatigue states, etc.

63. Brunswick, E. Perception and the Representative Design of Psychological Experiments. Berkeley: University of California Press, 1956.

A dittoed version of this paper was privately distributed in 1953 under the title "Designs for Social Science Experiments." The author has had the opportunity to benefit from the careful reading and suggestions of L. S. Burwen, J. W. Cotton, C. P. Duncan, D. W. Fiske, C. I. Hovland, L. V. Jones, E. S. Marks, D. C. Pelz, and B. J. Underwood, among others, and wishes to express his appreciation. They have not had the opportunity of seeing the paper in its present form and bear no responsibility for it. The author also wishes to thank S. A. Stouffer[1] and B. J. Underwood[2] for their public encouragement.

12

Evaluating the Quality of Medical Care

AVEDIS DONABEDIAN

Introduction

This paper is an attempt to describe and evaluate current methods for assessing the quality of medical care and to suggest some directions for further study. It is concerned with methods rather than findings, and with an evaluation of methodology in general, rather than a detailed critique of methods in specific studies.

This is not an exhaustive review of the pertinent literature. Certain key studies, of course, have been included. Other papers have been selected only as illustrative examples. Those omitted are not, for that reason, less worthy of note.

This paper deals almost exclusively with the evaluation of the medical care process at the level of physician-patient interaction. It excludes, therefore, processes primarily related to the effective delivery of medical care at the community level. Moreover, this paper is not concerned with the administrative aspects of quality control. Many of the studies reviewed here have arisen out of the urgent need to evaluate and control the quality of care in organized programs of medical care. Nevertheless, these studies will be discussed only in terms of their contribution to methods of assessment and not in terms of their broader social goals. The author has remained, by and large, in the familiar territory of care provided by physicians and has avoided incursions into other types of health care. Also, consideration of the difficult problem of economic efficiency as a measurable dimension of quality has been excluded.

Three general discussions of the evaluation of quality have been very helpful in preparing this review. The first is a classic paper by Mindel Sheps which includes an excellent discussion of methods.[1] A more recent paper by Peterson provides a valuable appraisal of the field.[2] The paper by Lerner and Riedel discusses one recent study of quality and raises several questions of general importance.[3]

Definition of Quality

The assessment of quality must rest on a conceptual and operationalized definition of what the "quality of medical care" means.

Many problems are present at this fundamental level, for the quality of care is a remarkably difficult notion to define. Perhaps the best-known definition is that offered by Lee and Jones[4] in the form of eight "articles of faith," some stated as attributes or properties of the process of care and others as goals or objectives of that process. These "articles" convey vividly the impression that the criteria of quality are nothing more than value judgments that are applied to several aspects, properties, ingredients or dimensions of a process called medical care. As such, the definition of quality may be almost anything anyone wishes it to be, although it is, ordinarily, a reflection of values and goals current in the medical care system and in the larger society of which it is a part.

Few empirical studies delve into what the relevant dimensions and values are at any given time in a given setting. Klein, *et al.*,[5] found that 24 "administrative officials," among them, gave 80 criteria for evaluating "patient care." They conclude that patient care, like morale, cannot be considered as a unitary concept and "... it seems likely that there will never be a single comprehensive criterion by which to measure the quality of patient care."

Which of a multitude of possible dimensions and criteria are selected to define quality will, of course, have profound influence on the approaches and methods one employs in the assessment of medical care.

Approaches to Assessment: What to Assess

The outcome of medical care, in terms of recovery, restoration of function and of survival, has been frequently used as an indicator of the quality of medical care. Examples are studies of perinatal mortality,[6,7] surgical fatality rates[8] and social restoration of patients discharged from psychiatric hospitals.[9]

Many advantages are gained by using outcome as the criterion of quality in medical care. The validity of outcome as a dimension of quality is seldom questioned. Nor does any doubt exist as to the stability and validity of the values of recovery, restoration and survival in most situations and in most cultures, though perhaps not in all. Moreover, outcomes tend to be fairly concrete and, as such, seemingly amenable to more precise measurement.

However, a number of considerations limit the use of outcomes as measures of the quality of care. The first of these is whether the outcome of care is, in fact, the relevant measure. This is because outcomes reflect both the power of medical science to achieve certain results under any given set of conditions, and the degree to which "scientific medicine," as currently conceived, has been applied in the instances under study. But the object may be precisely to separate these two effects. Sometimes a particular outcome may be irrelevant, as when survival is chosen as a criterion of success in a situation which is not fatal but is likely to produce suboptimal health or crippling.[10]

Even in situations where outcomes are relevant, and the relevant outcome has been chosen as a criterion, limitations must be reckoned with. Many factors other than medical care may influence outcome, and precautions must be taken to hold all significant factors other than medical care constant if valid conclusions are to be drawn. In some cases long periods of time, perhaps decades, must elapse before relevant outcomes are manifest. In such cases the results are not available when they are needed for appraisal and the problems of maintaining comparability are greatly magnified. Also, medical technology is not fully effective and the measure of success that can be expected in a particular situation is often not precisely known. For this reason comparative studies of outcome, under controlled situations, must be used.

Although some outcomes are generally unmistakable and easy to measure (death, for example) other outcomes, not so clearly defined, can be difficult to measure. These include patient attitudes and satisfactions, social restoration and physical disability and rehabilitation.[11] Even the face validity that outcomes generally have as criteria of success or failure, is not absolute. One may debate, for example, whether the prolongation of life under certain circumstances is evidence of good medical care. McDermott, et al., have shown that, although fixing a congenitally dislocated hip joint in a given position is considered good medicine for the white man, it can prove crippling for the Navajo Indian who spends much time seated on the floor or in the saddle.[12] Finally, although outcomes might indicate good or bad care in the aggregate, they do not give an insight into the nature and location of the deficiencies or strengths to which the outcome might be attributed.

All these limitations to the use of outcomes as criteria of medical care are presented not to demonstrate that outcomes are inappropriate indicators of quality but to emphasize that they must be used with discrimination. Outcomes, by and large, remain the ultimate validators of the effectiveness and quality of medical care.

Another approach to assessment is to examine the process of care itself rather than its outcomes. This is justified by the assumption that one is interested not in the power of medical technology to achieve results, but in whether what is now known to be "good" medical care has been applied. Judgments are based on considerations such as the appropriateness, completeness and redundancy of information obtained through clinical history, physical examination and diagnostic tests; justification of diagnosis and therapy; technical competence in the performance of diagnostic and therapeutic procedures, including surgery; evidence of preventive management in health and illness; coordination and continuity of care; acceptability of care to the recipient and so on. This approach requires that a great deal of attention be given to specifying the relevant dimensions, values and standards to be used in assessment. The estimates of quality that one obtains are less stable and less final than those that derive from the measurement of outcomes. They may, however, be more relevant to the question at hand: whether medicine is properly practiced.

This discussion of process and outcome may seem to imply a simple separation between means and ends. Perhaps more correctly, one may think of an unbroken chain of antecedent means followed by intermediate ends which are themselves the means to still further ends.[13] Health itself may be a means to a further objective. Several authors have pointed out that this formulation provides a useful approach to evaluation.[14,15] It may be designated as the measurement of procedural end points and included under the general heading of "process" because it rests on similar considerations with respect to values, standards and validation.

A third approach to assessment is to study not the process of care itself, but the settings in which it takes place and the instrumentalities of which it is the product. This may be roughly designated as the assessment of structure, although it may include administrative and related processes that support and direct the provision of care. It is concerned with such things as the adequacy of facilities and equipment; the qualifications of medical staff and their organization; the administrative structure and operations of programs and institutions providing care; fiscal organization and the like.[16,17] The assumption is made that given the proper settings and instrumentalities, good medical care will follow. This approach offers the advantage of dealing, at least in part, with fairly concrete and accessible information. It has the major limitation that the relationship between structure and process or structure and outcome, is often not well established.

Sources and Methods of Obtaining Information

The approach adopted for the appraisal of quality determines, in large measure, the methods used for collecting the requisite information. Since these range the gamut of social science methods, no attempt will be made to describe them all. Four, however, deserve special attention.

Clinical records are the source documents for most studies of the medical care process. In using them one must be aware of their several limitations. Since the private office practice of most physicians is not readily accessible to the researcher, and the records of such practice are generally disappointingly sketchy, the use of records has been restricted to the assessment of care in hospitals, outpatient departments of hospitals and prepaid group practice. Both Peterson[18] and Clute[19] have reported the prevailing inadequacies of recording in general practice. In addition, Clute has pointed out that, in general practice, ". . . the lack of adequate records is not incompatible with practice of a good, or even an excellent quality. . . ." On the other hand, a recent study of the office practice of a sample of members of the New York Society of Internal Medicine[20] suggests that abstracts of office records can be used to obtain reproducible judgments concerning the quality of care. But to generalize from this finding is difficult. It concerns a particular group of physicians more likely to keep good records than the average. Moreover, for one reason or another, the original sample drawn for this study suffered a 61 per cent attrition rate.

Assuming the record to be available and reasonably adequate, two further issues to be settled are the veracity and the completeness of the record. Lembcke[10] has questioned whether key statements in the record can be accepted at face value. He has questioned not only the statements of the physician about the patient and his management, but also the validity of the reports of diagnostic services. The first is verified by seeking in the record, including the nurses' notes, what appears to be the most valid evidence of the true state of affairs. The second is verified by having competent judges re-examine the evidence (films, tracings, slides) upon which diagnostic reports are made. Observer error tends to be a problem under the best of circumstances.[21] But nothing can remove the incredulity from the finding by Lembcke, in one hospital, that the true incidence of uterine hyperplasia was between 5 and 8 per cent rather than 60 to 65 per cent of uterine curettages, as reported by the hospital pathologist. In any case, the implications of verification as part of the assessment of quality must be carefully considered. Errors in diagnostic reports no doubt reflect particularly on the quality of diagnostic service and on the care provided by the hospital, in general. But the physician may be judged to perform well irrespective of whether the data he works with are or are not valid. This is so when the object of interest is the logic that governs the physician's activities rather than the absolute validity of these activities.

Much discussion has centered on the question of the completeness of clinical records and whether, in assessing the quality of care based on what appears in the record, one is rating the record or the care provided. What confuses the issue is that recording is itself a separate and legitimate dimension of the quality of practice, as well as the medium of information for the evaluation of most other dimensions. These two aspects can be separated when an alternative source of information about the process of care is available, such as the direct observation of practice.[18,19] In most instances, however, they are confounded. Rosenfeld[22] handled the problem of separating recording from care by examining the reasons for downrating the quality of care in each patient record examined. He demonstrated that the quality of care was rated down partly because of what could have been poor recording ("presumptive" evidence) and partly for reasons that could not have been a matter of recording ("substantial" evidence). He also found that hospitals tended to rank high or low on both types of errors, showing that these errors were correlated. Since routine recording is more likely to be complete in the wards, comparison of ward and private services in each hospital by type of reason for downrating might have provided further information on this important question. Other investigators have tried to allow for incompleteness in the record by supplementing it with interviews with the attending physician and making appropriate amendments.[23-25] Unfortunately, only one of these studies (length of stay in Michigan hospitals) contains a report of what difference this additional step made. In this study "the additional medical information elicited by means of personal interviews with attending physicians was of sufficient importance in 12.6 per cent of the total number of cases studied to warrant a reclassification of the evaluation of necessity for admission and/or the appropriateness of length of stay."[3,25] When information obtained by interview is used to amend or supplement the patient record, the assumption may have to be made that this additional information has equal or superior validity. Morehead, who has had extensive experience with this method, said, "Many of the surveyors engaged in the present study employed the technique of physician interview in earlier studies without fruitful results.... The surveyor was ... left in the uncomfortable position of having to choose between taking at face value statements that medical care was indeed optimal, or concluding that statements presented were untrue."[26] Even in an earlier study, where supplementation by interview is reported to have been used,[24] verbal information was discarded unless it was further corroborated by the course of action or by concrete evidence.[27]

Another question of method is whether the entire record or abstracted digests of it should be used as a basis for evaluation. The question arises because summaries and abstracts can presumably be prepared by less skilled persons allowing the hard-to-get expert to concentrate on the actual task of evaluation. Abstracting, however, seemingly involves the exercise of judgment as to relevance and importance. For that reason, it has been used as a first step in the evaluation of quality only in those studies that use very specific and detailed standards.[10] Even then, little information is available about how reliable the process of abstracting is, or how valid when compared with a more expert reading of the chart. The study of New York internists, already referred to, demonstrated a high level of agreement between physicians and highly trained non-physicians abstracting the same office record.[20]

While the controversy about the record as a source of information continues, some have attempted to reduce dependence on the physician's recording habits by choosing for evaluation diagnostic categories which are likely to be supported by recorded evidence additional to the physician's own entries.[28] This explains, in part, the frequent use of surgical operations as material for studies of quality.

In general practice, patient records are too inadequate to serve as a basis for evaluation. The alternative is *direct observation* of the physician's activities by a well qualified colleague.[18,19] The major limitation of this method would seem to be the changes likely to occur in the usual practice of the physician who knows he is being observed. This has been countered by assurances that the physician is often unaware of the true purpose of the study, becomes rapidly accustomed to the presence of the observer, and is unable to change confirmed habits of practice. Even if changes do occur, they would tend to result in an overestimate of quality rather than the reverse. These assurances notwithstanding, measuring the effect of observation on practice remains an unsolved problem.   ·

Those who have used the method of direct observation have been aware that the problem of completeness is not obviated. The practicing physician often knows a great deal about the patient from previous contacts with him. Hence the need to select for observation "new" cases and situations that require a thorough examination irrespective of the patient's previous experience. Moreover, not all of the managing physician's activities are explicit. Some dimensions of care, not subject to direct observation, must be excluded from the scheme of assessment. Selective perception by the observer may be an additional problem. The observer is not likely to be first a neutral recorder of events and then a judge of these same events. His knowledge and criteria are likely to influence what he perceives, and thus to introduce a certain distortion into perception.

An indirect method of obtaining information is to study *behaviors* and *opinions* from which inferences may be drawn concerning quality. A *sociometric* approach has been reported by Maloney, *et al.*, which assumes that physicians, in seeking care for themselves and their families, exhibit critical and valid judgments concerning the capacity of their colleagues to provide care of high quality.[29] Such choices were shown to identify classes of physicians presumed to be more highly qualified than others. But both sensitivity and specificity, using as criterion more rigorous estimates of the quality of care, lack validation. Georgopoulos and Mann[30] used what might be called an *autoreputational*[31] approach in assessing the quality of care in selected community hospitals. This grew out of previous studies showing that people are pretty shrewd judges of the "effectiveness" of the organizations in which they work.[32] The hospitals were rated and ranked using opinions concerning the quality of medical care, and other characteristics, held by different categories of managerial, professional and technical persons working in, or connected with, each hospital, as well as by knowledgeable persons in the community. The responses were sufficiently consistent and discriminating to permit the hospitals to be ranked with an apparently satisfactory degree of reliability. This in spite of the generally self-congratulatory nature of the responses that classified the quality of medical care in the hospitals as "very good," "excellent," or "outstanding" in 89 per cent of cases, and "poor" in almost none. The authors provide much evidence that the several opinions, severally held, were intercorrelated to a high degree. But little evidence supports the validity of the judgments by using truly external criteria of the quality of care.

Sampling and Selection

The first issue in sampling is to specify precisely the universe to be sampled, which, in turn, depends on the nature of the generalizations that one wishes to make. Studies of quality are ordinarily con-

cerned with one of three objects: 1. the actual care provided by a
specified category of providers of care; 2. the actual care received by a
specified group of people and 3. the capacity of a specified group of
providers to provide care. In the first two instances representative samples of potential providers or recipients are required, as well as representative samples of care provided or received. In the third instance
a representative sample of providers is needed, but not necessarily a
representative sample of care. A more important aspect is to select, uniformly of course, significant dimensions of care. Perhaps performance
should be studied in certain clinical situations that are particularly
stressful and therefore more revealing of latent capacities or weaknesses
in performance. Hypothetical test situations may even be set up to
assess the capacity to perform in selected dimensions of care.[33-35] The
distinctions made above, and especially those between the assessment of
actual care provided and of the capacity to provide care, are useful in
evaluating the sampling procedures used in the major studies of
quality. By these criteria, some studies belong in one category or another, but some seem to combine features of several in such a way that
generalization becomes difficult. For example, in the first study of the
quality of care received by Teamster families, the findings are meant
to apply only to the management of specific categories of hospitalized
illness in a specified population group.[28] In the second study of this
series, somewhat greater generalizability is achieved by obtaining a
representative sample (exclusive of seasonal variation) of all hospitalized illness in the same population group.[26] Neither study is
meant to provide information about all the care provided by a representative sample of physicians.

The degree of homogeneity in the universe to be sampled is, of
course, a matter of great importance in any scheme of sampling or
selection. The question that must be asked is to what extent the care
provided by a physician maintains a consistent level. Do specific diagnostic categories, levels of difficulty or dimensions of care exist in
which a physician performs better than in others? Can one find, in
fact, an "overall capacity for goodness in medical care,"[18] or is he
dealing with a bundle of fairly disparate strands of performance? One
might, similarly, ask whether the care provided by all subdivisions of
an institution are at about the same level in absolute terms or in relation to performance in comparable institutions. Makover, for example, makes an explicit assumption of homogeneity when he writes, "No
attempt was made to relate the number of records to be studied to the
size of enrollment of the medical groups. The medical care provided

to one or another individual is valid evidence of quality and there should be little or no chance variation which is affected by adjusting the size of the sample."[23] Rosenfeld began his study with the hypothesis "that there is a correspondence in standards of care in the several specialties and for various categories of illness in an institution."[22]

The empirical evidence concerning homogeneity is not extensive. Both the Peterson and Clute studies of general practice[18,19] showed a high degree of correlation between performance of physicians in different components or dimensions of care (history, physical examination, treatment, etc.). Rosenfeld demonstrated that the differences in quality ratings among several diagnoses selected within each area of practice (medicine, surgery and obstetrics-gynecology) were not large. Although the differences among hospitals by area of practice appeared by inspection to be larger, they were not large enough to alter the rankings of the three hospitals studied.

The two studies of care received by Teamster families[26,28] arrived at almost identical proportions of optimal and less than optimal care for the entire populations studied. This must have been coincidental, since the percent of optimal care, in the second study, varied greatly by diagnostic category from 31 per cent for medicine to 100 per cent for ophthalmology (nine cases only). If such variability exists, the "diagnostic mix" of the sample of care must be a matter of considerable importance in assessment. In the two Teamster studies, differences in "diagnostic mix" were thought to have resulted in lower ratings for medicine and higher ratings for obstetrics-gynecology in the second study than in the first. That the same factor may produce effects in two opposite directions is an indication of the complex interactions that the researcher must consider. "The most probable explanation for the ratings in medicine being lower in the present (second) study is the nature of the cases reviewed." The factor responsible is less ability to handle illness "which did not fall into a well recognized pattern." For obstetrics and gynecology the finding of the second study ". . . differed in one major respect from the earlier study where serious questions were raised about the management of far more patients. The earlier study consisted primarily of major abdominal surgery, whereas this randomly selected group contained few such cases and had more patients with minor conditions."[26] In studies such as these, where the care received by total or partial populations is under study, the variations noted stem partly from differences in diagnostic content and partly from institutionalized patterns of practice associated with diagnostic content. For example, all nine cases of eye disease received optimal care because "this is a highly specialized area, where physicians not trained in this field rarely venture to perform procedures."[26]

Sampling and selection influence, and are influenced by, a number of considerations in addition to generalization and homogeneity. The specific dimensions of care that interest one (preventive management or surgical technique, to mention two rather different examples) may dictate the selection of medical care situations for evaluation. The situations chosen are also related to the nature of the criteria and standards used and of the rating and scoring system adopted. Attempts to sample problem situations, rather than traditional diagnoses or operations, can be very difficult, because of the manner in which clinical records are filed and indexed. This is unfortunate, because a review of operations or established diagnoses gives an insight into the bases upon which the diagnosis was made or the operation performed. It leaves unexplored a complementary segment of practice, namely the situations in which a similar diagnosis or treatment may have been indicated but not made or performed.

Measurement Standards

Measurement depends on the development of standards. In the assessment of quality, standards derive from two sources.

Empirical standards are derived from actual practice and are generally used to compare medical care in one setting with that in another, or with statistical averages and ranges obtained from a larger number of similar settings. The Professional Activities Study is based, in part, on this approach.[36]

Empirical standards rest on demonstrably attainable levels of care and, for that reason, enjoy a certain degree of credibility and acceptability. Moreover, without clear normative standards, empirical observations in selected settings must be made to serve the purpose. An interesting example is provided by Furstenberg, *et al.*, who used patterns of prescribing in medical care clinics and outpatient hospitals as the standard to judge private practice.[37]

In using empirical standards one needs some assurance that the clinical material in the settings being compared is similar. The Professional Activities Study makes some allowance for this by reporting patterns of care for hospitals grouped by size. The major shortcoming, however, is that care may appear to be adequate in comparison to that in other situations and yet fall short of what is attainable through the full application of current medical knowledge.

Normative standards derive, in principle, from the sources that legitimately set the standards of knowledge and practice in the dominant medical care system. In practice, they are set by standard textbooks or publications,[10] panels of physicians,[25] highly qualified practitioners who serve as judges[26] or a research staff in consultation with qualified practitioners.[22] Normative standards can be put very high and represent the "best" medical care that can be provided, or they can be set at a more modest level signifying "acceptable" or "adequate" care. In any event, their distinctive characteristic is that they stem from a body of legitimate knowledge and values rather than from specific examples of actual practice. As such, they depend for their validity on the extent of agreement concerning facts and values within the profession or, at least, among its leadership. Where equally legitimate sources differ in their views, judgments concerning quality become correspondingly ambiguous.

The relevance of certain normative standards, developed by one group, to the field of practice of another group, has been questioned. For example, Peterson and Barsamian report that although spermatic fluid examination of the husband should precede surgery for the Stein-Leventhal syndrome, not one instance of such examination was noted, and that this requirement was dropped from the criteria for assessment.[38] Dissatisfaction has also been voiced concerning the application to general practice of standards and criteria elaborated by specialists who practice in academic settings. The major studies of general practice have made allowances for this. Little is known, however, about the strategies of "good" general practice and the extent to which they are similar to, or different from, the strategies of specialized practice in academic settings.

Some researchers have used both types of standards, normative and empirical, in the assessment of care. Rosenfeld used normative standards but included in his design a comparison between university affiliated and community hospitals. "Use of the teaching hospital as a control provides the element of flexibility needed to adjust to the constantly changing scientific basis of the practice of medicine. No written standards, no matter how carefully drawn, would be adequate in five years."[22] Lembcke used experience in the best hospitals to derive a corrective factor that softens the excessive rigidity of his normative standards. This factor, expressed in terms of an acceptable percent of compliance with the standard, was designed to take account of contingencies not foreseen in the standards themselves. It does, however, have the effect of being more realistically permissive as well. This is because the correction factor is likely to be made up partly of acceptable departures from the norm and partly of deviations that might be unacceptable.

Standards can also be differentiated by the extent of their specificity and directiveness. At one extreme the assessing physician may be very simply instructed as follows: "You will use as a yardstick in relation to the quality of care rendered, whether you would have treated this particular patient in this particular fashion during this specific hospital admission."[26] At the other extreme, a virtually water-tight "logic system" may be constructed that specifies all the decision rules that are acceptable to justify diagnosis and treatment.[38,39] Most cases fall somewhere in between.

Highly precise and directive standards are associated with the selection of specific diagnostic categories for assessment. When a representative sample of all the care provided is to be assessed, little more than general guides can be given to the assessor. Lembcke, who has stressed the need for specific criteria, has had to develop a correspondingly detailed diagnostic classification of pelvic surgery, for example.[10] In addition to diagnostic specificity, highly directive standards are associated with the preselection of specific dimensions of care for evaluation. Certain diagnoses, such as surgical operations, lend themselves more readily to this approach. This is evident in Lembcke's attempt to extend his system of audits to nonsurgical diagnoses.[40] The clear, almost rule-of-thumb judgments of adequacy become blurred. The data abstracted under each diagnostic rubric are more like descriptions of patterns of management, with insufficient normative criteria for decisive evaluation. The alternative adopted is comparison with a criterion institution.

Obviously, the more general and nondirective the standards are, the more one must depend on the interpretations and norms of the person entrusted with the actual assessment of care. With greater specificity, the research team is able, collectively, to exercise much greater control over what dimensions of care require emphasis and what the acceptable standards are. A great deal appears in common between the standards used in structured and unstructured situations as shown by the degree of agreement between "intuitive" ratings and directed ratings in the Rosenfeld study,[22] and between the "qualitative" and "quantitative" ratings in the study by Peterson, et al.[18] Indeed, these last two were so similar that they could be used interchangeably.

When standards are not very specific and the assessor must exercise his own judgment in arriving at an evaluation, very expert and careful judges must be used. Lembcke claims that a much more precise and directive system such as his does not require expert judges. "It is said that with a cookbook, anyone who can read can cook. The same is true, and to about the same extent, of the medical audit using objective criteria; anyone who knows enough medical terminology to understand the definitions and criteria can prepare the case abstracts and tables for the medical audit. However, the final acceptance, interpretation and application of the findings must be the responsibility of a physician or group of physicians."[41] The "logic system" developed by Peterson and Barsamian appears well suited for rating by computer, once the basic facts have been assembled, presumably by a record abstractor.[38,39]

The dimensions of care and the values that one uses to judge them are, of course, embodied in the criteria and standards used to assess care.[42] These standards can, therefore, be differentiated by their selectivity and inclusiveness in the choice of dimensions to be assessed. The dimensions selected and the value judgments attached to them constitute the operationalized definition of quality in each study.

The preselection of dimensions makes possible, as already pointed out, the development of precise procedures, standards and criteria. Lembcke[10] has put much stress on the need for selecting a few specific dimensions of care within specified diagnostic categories rather than attempting general evaluations of unspecified dimensions which, he feels, lack precision. He uses dimensions such as the following: confirmation of clinical diagnosis, justification of treatment (including surgery) and completeness of the surgical procedure. Within each dimension, and for each diagnostic category, one or more previously defined activities are often used to characterize performance for that dimension as a whole. Examples are the compatibility of the diagnosis of pancreatitis with serum amylase levels or of liver cirrhosis with biopsy findings, the performance of sensitivity tests prior to antibiotic therapy in acute bronchitis, and the control of blood sugar levels in diabetes.

In addition to the extent to which preselection of dimensions takes place, assessments of quality differ with respect to the number of dimensions used and the exhaustiveness with which performance in each dimension is explored. For example, Peterson, *et al.,*[18] and Rosenfeld[22] use a large number of dimensions. Peterson and Barsamian,[38,39] on the other hand, concentrate on two basic dimensions, justification of diagnosis and of therapy, but require complete proof of justification. A much more simplified approach is illustrated by Huntley, *et al.*,[43] who evaluate outpatient care using two criteria only: the percent of work-ups not including certain routine procedures, and the percent of abnormalities found that were not followed up.

Judgments of quality are incomplete when only a few dimensions are used and decisions about each dimension are made on the basis of partial evidence. Some dimensions, such as preventive care or the psychological and social management of health and illness, are often excluded from the definition of quality and the standards and criteria that make it operational. Examples are the intentional exclusion of psychiatric care from the Peterson study[18] and the planned exclusion of the patient-physician relationship and the attitudes of physicians in studies of the quality of care in the Health Insurance Plan of Greater New York.[27] Rosenfeld[22] made a special point of including the performance of specified screening measures among the criteria of superior care; but care was labeled good in the absence of these measures. In the absence of specific instructions to the judges, the study by Morehead, *et al.*,[26] includes histories of cases, considered to have received optimal care, in which failure of preventive management could have resulted in serious consequences to the patient.

Another characteristic of measurement is the level at which the standard is set. Standards can be so strict that none can comply with them, or so permissive that all are rated "good." For example, in the study of general practice reported by Clute,[19] blood pressure examinations, measurement of body temperature, otoscopy and performance of immunizations did not serve to categorize physicians because all physicians performed them well.

Measurement Scales

The ability to discriminate different levels of performance depends on the scale of measurement used. Many studies of quality use a small number of divisions to classify care, seen as a whole, into categories such as "excellent," "good," "fair" or "poor." A person's relative position in a set can then be further specified by computing the percent of cases in each scale category. Other studies assign scores to performance of specified components of care and cumulate these to obtain a numerical index usually ranging from 0-100. These practices raise questions relative to scales of measurement and legitimate operations on these scales. Some of these are described below.

Those who adhere to the first practice point out that any greater degree of precision is not possible with present methods. Some have even reduced the categories to only two: optimal and less than optimal. Clute[19] uses three, of which the middle one is acknowledged to be doubtful or indeterminate. Also, medical care has an all-or-none aspect that the usual numerical scores do not reflect. Care can be good in many of its parts and be disastrously inadequate in the aggregate due to a vital error in one component. This is, of course, less often a problem if it is demonstrated that performance on different components of care is highly intercorrelated.

Those who have used numerical scores have pointed out much loss of information in the use of overall judgments,[38] and that numerical scores, cumulated from specified subscores, give a picture not only of the whole but also of the evaluation of individual parts. Rosenfeld[22] has handled this problem by using a system of assigning qualitative scores to component parts of care and an overall qualitative score based on arbitrary rules of combination that allow for the all-or-none attribute of the quality of medical care. As already pointed out, a high degree of agreement was found between intuitive and structured ratings in the Rosenfeld study[22] and between qualitative and quantitative ratings in the study by Peterson, *et al.*[18]

A major problem, yet unsolved, in the construction of numerical scores, is the manner in which the different components are to be weighted in the process of arriving at the total. At present this is an arbitrary matter. Peterson, *et al.*,[18] for example, arrive at the following scale: clinical history 30, physical examination 34, use of laboratory aids 26, therapy 9, preventive medicine 6, clinical records 2, total 107. Daily and Morehead[24] assign different weights as follows: records 30, diagnostic work-up 40, treatment and follow-up 30, total 100. Peterson, *et al.*, say: "Greatest importance is attached to the process of arriving at a diagnosis since, without a diagnosis, therapy cannot be rational. Furthermore, therapy is in the process of constant change, while the form of history and physical examination has changed very little over the years."[18] Daily and Morehead offer no justification for their weightings, but equally persuasive arguments could probably be made on their behalf. The problem of seeking external confirmation remains.[11]

The problem of weights is related to the more general problem of value of items of information or of procedures in the medical care process. Rimoldi, *et al.*,[34] used the frequency with which specified items of information were used in the solution of a test problem as a measure of the value of that item. Williamson had experts classify specified procedures, in a specified diagnostic test setting, on a scale ranging from "very helpful" to "very harmful." Individual performance in the test was then rated using quantitative indices of "efficiency," "proficiency" and overall "competence," depending on the frequency and nature of the procedures used.[35]

A problem in the interpretation of numerical scores is the meaning of the numerical interval between points on the scale. Numerical scores derived for the assessment of quality are not likely to have the property of equal intervals. They should not be used as if they had.

Reliability

The reliability of assessments is a major consideration in studies of quality, where so much depends on judgment even when the directive types of standards are used. Several studies have given some attention to agreement between judges. The impression gained is that this is considered to be at an acceptable level. Peterson, et al.,[18] on the basis of 14 observer revisits, judged agreement to be sufficiently high to permit all the observations to be pooled together after adjustment for observer bias in one of the six major divisions of care. In the study by Daily and Morehead, "several cross-checks were made between the two interviewing internists by having them interview the same physicians. The differences in the scores of the family physicians based on these separate ratings did not exceed 7 per cent."[24] Rosenfeld[22] paid considerable attention to testing reliability, and devised mathematical indices of "agreement" and "dispersion" to measure it. These indicate a fair amount of agreement, but a precise evaluation is difficult since no other investigator is known to have used these same measures. Morehead, et al.,[26] in the second study of medical care received by Teamster families, report initial agreement between two judges in assigning care to one of two classes in 78 per cent of cases. This was raised to 92 per cent following reevaluation of disagreements by the two judges.

By contrast to between-judge reliability, very little has been reported about the reliability of repeated judgments of quality made by the same person. To test within-observer variation, Peterson, et al.,[18] asked each of two observers to revisit four of his own previously visited physicians. The level of agreement was lower within observers than between observers, partly because revisits lasted a shorter period of time and related, therefore, to a smaller sample of practice.

The major mechanism for achieving higher levels of reliability is the detailed specification of criteria, standards and procedures used for the assessment of care. Striving for reproducibility was, in fact, a major impetus in the development of the more rigorous rating systems by Lembcke, and by Peterson and Barsamian. Unfortunately, no comparative studies of reliability exist using highly directive versus non-directive methods of assessment. Rosenfeld's raw data might permit a comparison of reliability of "intuitive" judgments and the reliability of structured judgments by the same two assessors. Unreported data by Morehead, *et al.*,[26] could be analyzed in the same way as those of Rosenfeld[22] to give useful information about the relationship between degree of reliability and method of assessment. The partial data that have been published suggest that the post-review reliability achieved by Morehead, *et al.*, using the most non-directive of approaches, is quite comparable with that achieved by Rosenfeld who used a much more directive technique.

Morehead, *et al.*, raised the important question of whether the reliability obtained through the detailed specification of standards and criteria may not be gained at the cost of reduced validity. "Frequently, such criteria force into a rigid framework similar actions or factors which may not be appropriate in a given situation due to the infinite variations in the reaction of the human body to illness.... The study group rejects the assumption that such criteria are necessary to evaluate the quality of medical care. It is their unanimous opinion that it is as important for the surveyors to have flexibility in the judgment of an individual case as it is for a competent physician when confronting a clinical problem in a given patient."[26]

The reasons for disagreement between judges throw some light on the problems of evaluation and the prospects of achieving greater reliability. Rosenfeld found that "almost half the differences were attributable to situations not covered adequately by standards, or in which the standards were ambiguous. In another quarter differences developed around questions of fact, because one consultant missed a significant item of information in the record. It would therefore appear that with revised standards, and improved methods of orienting consultants, a substantially higher degree of agreement could be achieved."[22] Less than a quarter of the disagreements contain differences of opinion with regard to the requirements of management. This is a function of ambiguity in the medical care system and sets an upper limit of reproducibility. Morehead, *et al.*, report that in about half the cases of initial disagreement "there was agreement on the most serious aspect of the patient's care, but one surveyor later agreed that he had not taken into account corollary aspects of patient care."[26] Other reasons for disagreement were difficulty in adhering to the rating categories or failure to note all the facts. Of the small number of unresolved disagreements (8 per cent of all admissions and 36 per cent of initial disagreements) more than half were due to honest differences of opinion regarding the clinical handling of the problem. The remainder arose out of differences in interpreting inadequate records, or the technical problems of where to assess unsatisfactory care in a series of admissions.[27]

A final aspect of reliability is the occasional breakdown in the performance of an assessor, as so dramatically demonstrated in the Rosenfeld study.[22] The question of what the investigator does when a well defined segment of his results are so completely aberrant will be raised here without any attempt to provide an answer.

Bias

When several observers or judges describe and evaluate the process of medical care, one of them may consistently employ more rigid standards than another, or interpret predetermined standards more strictly. Peterson, et al.,[18] discovered that one of their observers generally awarded higher ratings than the other in the assessment of performance of physical examination, but not in the other areas of care. Rosenfeld[22] showed that, of two assessors, one regularly awarded lower ratings to the same cases assessed by both. An examination of individual cases of disagreement in the study by Morehead, et al.,[26] reveals that, in the medical category, the same assessor rated the care at a lower level in 11 out of 12 instances of disagreement. For surgical cases, one surveyor rated the care lower than the other in all eight instances of disagreement. The impression is gained from examining reasons for disagreement on medical cases that one of the judges had a special interest in cardiology and was more demanding of clarity and certainty in the management of cardiac cases.

The clear indication of these findings is that bias must be accepted as the rule rather than the exception, and that studies of quality must be designed with this in mind. In the Rosenfeld study,[22] for example, either of the two raters used for each area of practice would have ranked the several hospitals in the same order, even though one was consistently more generous than the other. The Clute study of general practice in Canada,[19] on the other hand, has been criticized for comparing the quality of care in two geographic areas even though different observers examined the care in the two areas in question.[45] The author was aware of this problem and devised methods for comparing the performance of the observers in the two geographic areas, but the basic weakness remains.

Predetermined order or regularity in the process of study may be associated with bias. Therefore, some carefully planned procedures may have to be introduced into the research design for randomization. The study by Peterson, *et al.,*[18] appears to be one of the few to have paid attention to this factor. Another important source of bias is knowledge, by the assessor, of the identity of the physician who provided the care or of the hospital in which care was given. The question of removing identifying features from charts under review has been raised,[3] but little is known about the feasibility of this procedure and its effects on the ratings assigned. Still another type of bias may result from parochial standards and criteria of practice that may develop in and around certain institutions or "schools" of medical practice. To the extent that this is true, or suspected to be true, appropriate precautions need to be taken in the recruitment and allocation of judges.

Validity

The effectiveness of care as has been stated, in achieving or producing health and satisfaction, as defined for its individual members by a particular society or subculture, is the ultimate validator of the quality of care. The validity of all other phenomena as indicators of quality depends, ultimately, on the relationship between these phenomena and the achievement of health and satisfaction. Nevertheless, conformity of practice to accepted standards has a kind of conditional or interim validity which may be more relevant to the purposes of assessment in specific instances.

The validation of the details of medical practice by their effect on health is the particular concern of the clinical sciences. In the clinical literature one seeks data on whether penicillin promotes recovery in certain types of pneumonia, anticoagulants in coronary thrombosis, or corticosteroids in rheumatic carditis; what certain tests indicate about the function of the liver; and whether simple or radical mastectomy is the more life-prolonging procedure in given types of breast cancer. From the general body of knowledge concerning such relationships arise the standards of practice, more or less fully validated, by which the medical care process is ordinarily judged.

Intermediate, or procedural, end points often represent larger bundles of care. Their relationship to outcome has attracted the attention of both the clinical investigator and the student of medical care organization. Some examples of the latter are studies of relationships between prenatal care and the health of mothers and infants[46,47] and the relationship between multiple screening examinations and subsequent health.[48] An interesting example of the study of the relationship between one procedural end point and another is the attempt to demonstrate a positive relationship between the performance of rectal and vaginal examinations by the physician, and the pathological confirmation of appendicitis in primary appendectomies, as reported by the Professional Activities Study.[49]

Many studies reviewed[18,19,23,26,28] attempt to study the relationship between structural properties and the assessment of the process of care. Several of these studies have shown, for example, a relationship between the training and qualifications of physicians and the quality of care they provide. The relationship is, however, a complex one, and is influenced by the type of training, its duration and the type of hospital within which it was obtained. The two studies of general practice[18,19] have shown additional positive relationships between quality and better office facilities for practice, the presence or availability of laboratory equipment, and the institution of an appointment system. No relationship was shown between quality and membership of professional associations, the income of the physician or the presence of x-ray equipment in the office. The two studies do not agree fully on the nature of the relationship between quality of practice and whether the physician obtained his training in a teaching hospital or not, the number of hours worked or the nature of the physician's hospital affiliation. Hospital accreditation, presumably a mark of quality conferred mainly for compliance with a wide range of organizational standards, does not appear, in and of itself, to be related to the quality of care, at least in New York City.[26]

Although structure and process are no doubt related, the few examples cited above indicate clearly the complexity and ambiguity of these relationships. This is the result partly of the many factors involved, and partly of the poorly understood interactions among these factors. For example, one could reasonably propose, based on several findings[26,38] that both hospital factors and physician factors influence the quality of care rendered in the hospital, but that differences between physicians are obliterated in the best and worst hospital and express themselves, in varying degrees, in hospitals of intermediate quality.

An approach particularly favored by students of medical care organization is to examine relations between structure and outcome without reference to the complex processes that tie them together. Some examples of such studies have been cited already.[6-9] Others include studies of the effects of reorganizing the outpatient clinic on health status,[50] the effects of intensive hospital care on recovery,[51] the effects of home care on survival[52] and the effect of a rehabilitation program on the physical status of nursing home patients.[53,54] The lack of relationship to outcome in the latter two studies suggests that current opinions about how care should be set up are sometimes less than well established.

This brief review indicates the kinds of evidence pertaining to the validity of the various approaches to the evaluation of quality of care. Clearly, the relationships between process and outcome, and between structure and both process and outcome, are not fully understood. With regard to this, the requirements of validation are best expressed by the concept, already referred to, of a chain of events in which each event is an end to the one that comes before it and a necessary condition to the one that follows. This indicates that the means-end relationship between each adjacent pair requires validation in any chain of hypothetical or real events.[55] This is, of course, a laborious process. More commonly, as has been shown, the intervening links are ignored. The result is that causal inferences become attenuated in proportion to the distance separating the two events on the chain.

Unfortunately, very little information is available on actual assessments of quality using more than one method of evaluation concurrently. Makover has studied specifically the relationships between multifactorial assessments of structure and of process in the same medical groups. "It was found that the medical groups that achieved higher quality ratings by the method used in this study were those that, in general, adhered more closely to HIP's Minimum Medical Standards. However, the exceptions were sufficiently marked, both in number and degree, to induce one to question the reliability[56] of one or the other rating method when applied to any one medical group. It would seem that further comparison of these two methods of rating is clearly indicated."[23]

Indices of Medical Care

Since a multidimensional assessment of medical care is a costly and laborious undertaking, the search continues for discrete, readily measurable data that can provide information about the quality of medical care. The data used may be about aspects of structure, process or outcome. The chief requirement is that they be easily, sometimes routinely, measurable and be reasonably valid. Among the studies of quality using this approach are those of the Professional Activities Study,[36] Ciocco, *et al.*,[57] and Furstenberg, *et al.*[37]

Such indices have the advantage of convenience; but the inferences that are drawn from them may be of doubtful validity. Myers has pointed out the many limitations of the traditional indices of the quality of hospital care, including rates of total and postoperative mortality, complications, postoperative infection, Caesarian section, consultation and removal of normal tissue at operation.[58] The accuracy and completeness of the basic information may be open to question. More important still, serious questions may be raised about what each index means since so many factors are involved in producing the phenomenon which it measures. Eislee has pointed out, on the other hand, that at least certain indices can be helpful, if used with care.[36]

The search for easy ways to measure a highly complex phenomenon such as medical care may be pursuing a will-o'-the-wisp. The use of simple indices in lieu of more complex measures may be justified by demonstrating high correlations among them.[1] But, in the absence of demonstrated causal links, this may be an unsure foundation upon which to build. On the other hand, each index can be a measure of a dimension or ingredient of care. Judiciously selected multiple indices may, therefore, constitute the equivalent of borings in a geological survey which yield sufficient information about the parts to permit reconstruction of the whole. The validity of inferences about the whole will depend, of course, on the extent of internal continuities in the individual or institutional practice of medicine.

Some Problems of Assessing Ambulatory Care

Some of the special difficulties in assessing the quality of ambulatory care have already been mentioned. These include the paucity of recorded information, and the prior knowledge, by the managing physician, of the patient's medical and social history. The first of these problems has led to the use of trained observers and the second to the observation of cases for which prior knowledge is not a factor in current management. The degree of relevance to general practice of standards and strategies of care developed by hospital centered and academically oriented physicians has also been questioned.

Another problem is the difficulty of defining the segment of care that may be properly the object of evaluation in ambulatory care. For hospital care, a single admission is usually the appropriate unit.[59] In office or clinic practice, a sequence of care may cover an indeterminate number of visits so that the identification of the appropriate unit is open to question. Usually the answer has been to choose an arbitrary time period to define the relevant episode of care. Ciocco, *et al.,*[57] defined this as the first visit plus 14 days of follow-up. Huntley, *et al.,*[43] use a four-week period after the initial work-up.

Conclusions and Proposals

This review has attempted to give an impression of the various approaches and methods that have been used for evaluating the quality of medical care, and to point out certain issues and problems that these approaches and methods bring up for consideration.

The methods used may easily be said to have been of doubtful value and more frequently lacking in rigor and precision. But how precise do estimates of quality have to be? At least the better methods have been adequate for the administrative and social policy purposes that have brought them into being. The search for perfection should not blind one to the fact that present techniques of evaluating quality, crude as they are, have revealed a range of quality from outstanding to deplorable. Tools are now available for making broad judgments of this kind with considerable assurance. This degree of assurance is supported by findings, already referred to, that suggest acceptable levels of homogeneity in individual practice and of reproducibility of qualitative judgments based on a minimally structured approach to evaluation. This is not to say that a great deal does not remain to be accomplished in developing the greater precision necessary for certain other purposes.

One might begin a catalogue of needed refinements by considering the nature of the information which is the basis for judgments of quality. More must be known about the effect of the observer on the practice being observed, as well as about the process of observation itself—its reliability and validity. Comparisons need to be made between direct observation and recorded information both with and without supplementation by interview with the managing physician. Recording agreement or disagreement is not sufficient. More detailed study is needed of the nature of, and reasons for, discrepancy in various settings. Similarly, using abstracts of records needs to be tested against using the records themselves.

The process of evaluation itself requires much further study. A great deal of effort goes into the development of criteria and standards which are presumed to lend stability and uniformity to judgments of quality; and yet this presumed effect has not been empirically demonstrated. How far explicit standardization must go before appreciable gains in reliability are realized is not known. One must also consider whether, with increasing standardization, so much loss of the ability to account for unforeseen elements in the clinical situation occurs that one obtains reliability at the cost of validity. Assessments of the same set of records using progressively more structured standards and criteria should yield valuable information on these points. The contention that less well trained assessors using exhaustive criteria can come up with reliable and valid judgments can also be tested in this way.

Attention has already been drawn, in the body of the review, to the little that is known about reliability and bias when two or more judges are compared, and about the reliability of repeated judgments of the same items of care by the same assessor. Similarly, very little is known about the effects on reliability and validity, of certain characteristics of judges including experience, areas of special interest and personality factors. Much may be learned concerning these and related matters by making explicit the process of judging and subjecting it to careful study. This should reveal the dimensions and values used by the various judges and show how differences are resolved when two or more judges discuss their points of view. Some doubt now exists about the validity of group reconciliations in which one point of view may dominate, not necessarily because it is more valid.[1] The effect of masking the identity of the hospital or the physician providing care can be studied in the same way. What is proposed here is not only to demonstrate differences or similarities in overall judgments, but to attempt, by making explicit the thought processes of the judges, to determine how the differences and similarities arise, and how differences are resolved.

In addition to defects in method, most studies of quality suffer from having adopted too narrow a definition of quality. In general, they concern themselves with the technical management of illness and pay little attention to prevention, rehabilitation, coordination and continuity of care, or handling the patient-physician relationship. Presumably, the reason for this is that the technical requirements of management are more widely recognized and better standardized. Therefore, more complete conceptual and empirical exploration of the definition of quality is needed.

What is meant by "conceptual exploration" may be illustrated by considering the dimension of efficiency which is often ignored in studies of quality. Two types of efficiency might be distinguished: logical and economic. Logical efficiency concerns the use of information to arrive at decisions. Here the issue might be whether the information obtained by the physician is relevant or irrelevant to the clinical business to be transacted. If relevant, one might consider the degree of replication or duplication in information obtained and the extent to which it exceeds the requirements of decision making in a given situation. If parsimony is a value in medical care, the identification of redundancy becomes an element in the evaluation of care.

Economic efficiency deals with the relationships between inputs and outputs and asks whether a given output is produced at least cost. It is, of course, influenced by logical efficiency, since the accumulation of unnecessary or unused information is a costly procedure which yields no benefit. Typically it goes beyond the individual and is concerned with the social product of medical care effort. It considers the possibility that the "best" medical care for the individual may not be the "best" for the community. Peterson, *et al.*, cite an example that epitomizes the issue. "Two physicians had delegated supervision of routine prenatal visits to office nurses, and the doctor saw the patient only if she had specific complaints."[18] In one sense, this may have been less than the best care for each expectant mother. In another sense, it may have been brilliant strategy in terms of making available to the largest number of women the combined skills of a medical care team. Cordero, in a thought provoking paper, has documented the thesis that, when resources are limited, optimal medical care for the community may require less than "the best" care for its individual members.[60]

In addition to conceptual exploration of the meaning of quality, in terms of dimensions of care and the values attached to them, empirical studies are needed of what are the prevailing dimensions and values in relevant population groups.[5] Little is known, for example, about how physicians define quality, nor is the relationship known between the physician's practice and his own definition of quality. This is an area of research significant to medical education as well as quality. Empirical studies of the medical care process should also contribute greatly to the identification of dimensions and values to be incorporated into the definition of quality.

A review of the studies of quality shows a certain discouraging repetitiousness in basic concepts, approaches and methods. Further substantive progress, beyond refinements in methodology, is likely to come from a program of research in the medical care process itself rather than from frontal attacks on the problem of quality. This is believed to be so because, before one can make judgments about quality, one needs to understand how patients and physicians interact and how physicians function in the process of providing care. Once the elements of process and their interrelationships are understood, one can attach value judgments to them in terms of their contributions to intermediate and ultimate goals. Assume, for example, that authoritarianism-permissiveness is one dimension of the patient-physician relationship. An empirical study may show that physicians are in fact differentiated by this attribute. One might then ask whether authoritarianism or permissiveness should be the criterion of quality. The answer could be derived from the general values of society that may endorse one or the other as the more desirable attribute in social interactions. This is one form of quality judgment, and is perfectly valid, provided its rationale and bases are explicit. The study of the medical care process itself may however offer an alternative, and more pragmatic, approach. Assume, for the time being, that compliance with the recommendations of the physician is a goal and value in the medical care system. The value of authoritarianism or permissiveness can be determined, in part, by its contribution to compliance. Compliance is itself subject to validation by the higher order criterion of health outcomes. The true state of affairs is likely to be more complex than the hypothetical example given. The criterion of quality may prove to be congruence with patient expectations, or a more complex adaptation to specific clinical and social situations, rather than authoritarianism or permissiveness as a predominant mode. Also, certain goals in the medical care process may not be compatible with other goals, and one may not speak of quality in global terms but of quality in specified dimensions and for specified purposes. Assessments of quality will not, therefore, result in a summary judgment but in a complex profile, as Sheps has suggested.[1]

A large portion of research in the medical care process will, of course, deal with the manner in which physicians gather clinically relevant information, and arrive at diagnostic and therapeutic decisions. This is not the place to present a conceptual framework for research in this portion of the medical care process. Certain specific studies may, however, be mentioned and some directions for further research indicated.

Research on information gathering includes studies of the perception and interpretation of physical signs.[61,62] Evans and Bybee have shown, for example, that in interpreting heart sounds errors of perception (of rhythm and timing) occurred along with additional errors of interpretation of what was perceived. Faulty diagnosis, as judged by comparison with a criterion, was the result of these two errors.[62] This points to the need for including, in estimates of quality, information about the reliability and validity of the sensory data upon which management, in part, rests.

The work of Peterson and Barsamian[38,39] represents the nearest approach to a rigorous evaluation of diagnostic and therapeutic decision making. As such, it is possibly the most significant recent advance in the methods of quality assessment. But this method is based on record reviews and is almost exclusively preoccupied with the justification of diagnosis and therapy. As a result, many important dimensions of care are not included in the evaluation. Some of these are considerations of efficiency, and of styles and strategies in problem solving.

Styles and strategies in problem solving can be studied through actual observation of practice, as was done so effectively by Peterson, *et al.,* in their study of general practice.[18] A great deal that remains unobserved can be made explicit by asking the physician to say aloud what he is doing and why. This method of *réflexion parlée* has been used in studies of problem solving even though it may, in itself, alter behavior.[63] Another approach is to set up test situations, such as those used by Rimoldi, *et al.,*[34] and by Williamson,[35] to observe the decision making process. Although such test situations have certain limitations arising out of their artificiality,[64] the greater simplicity and control that they provide can be very helpful.

At first sight, the student of medical care might expect to be helped by knowledge and skill developed in the general field of research in problem solving. Unfortunately, no well developed theoretical base is available which can be exploited readily in studies of medical care. Some of the empirical studies in problem solving might, however, suggest methods and ideas applicable to medical care situations.[63-67] Some of the studies of "troubleshooting" in electronic equipment, in particular, show intriguing similarities to the process of medical diagnosis and treatment. These and similar studies have identified behavioral characteristics that might be used to categorize styles in clinical management. They include amount of information collected, rate of seeking information, value of items of information sought as modified by place in a sequence and by interaction with other items of information, several types of redundancy, stereotypy, search patterns in relation to the part known to be defective, tendencies to act prior to amassing sufficient information or to seek information beyond the point of reasonable assurance about the solution, "error distance" and degrees of success in achieving a solution, and so on.

Decision making theory may also offer conceptual tools of research in the medical care process. Ledley and Lusted,[68,69] among others, have attempted to apply models based on conditional probabilities to the process of diagnosis and therapy. Peterson and Barsamian[38,39] decided against using probabilities in their logic systems for the very good reason that the necessary data (the independent probabilities of diseases and of symptoms, and the probabilities of specified symptoms in specified diseases) were not available. But Edwards, et al.,[70] point out that one can still test efficiency in decision making by substituting subjective probabilities (those of the decision maker himself or of selected experts) for the statistical data one would prefer to have.

A basic question that has arisen frequently in this review is the degree to which performance in medical care is a homogeneous or heterogeneous phenomenon. This was seen, for example, to be relevant to sampling, the use of indices in place of multidimensional measurements, and the construction of scales that purport to judge total performance. When this question is raised with respect to individual physicians, the object of study is the integration of various kinds of knowledge and of skills in the personality and behavior of the physician. When it is raised with respect to institutions and social systems the factors are completely different. Here one is concerned with the formal and informal mechanisms for organizing, influencing and directing human effort in general, and the practice of medicine in particular. Research in all these areas is expected to contribute to greater sophistication in the measurement of quality.

Some of the conventions accepted in this review are, in themselves, obstacles to more meaningful study of quality. Physicians' services are not, in the real world, separated from the services of other health professionals, nor from the services of a variety of supportive personnel. The separation of hospital and ambulatory care is also largely artificial. The units of care which are the proper objects of study include the contributions of many persons during a sequence which may include care in a variety of settings. The manner in which these sequences are defined and identified has implications for sampling, methods of obtaining information, and standards and criteria of evaluation.

A final comment concerns the frame of mind with which studies of quality are approached. The social imperatives that give rise to assessments of quality have already been referred to. Often associated with these are the zeal and values of the social reformer. Greater neutrality and detachment are needed in studies of quality. More often one needs to ask, "What goes on here?" rather than, "What is wrong; and how can it be made better?" This does not mean that the researcher disowns his own values or social objectives. It does mean, however, that the distinction between values, and elements of structure, process or outcome, is recognized and maintained; and that both are subjected to equally critical study. Partly to achieve this kind of orientation, emphasis must be shifted from preoccupation with evaluating quality to concentration on understanding the medical care process itself.

NOTES AND REFERENCES

1. Sheps, M. C. Approaches to the Quality of Hospital Care. Public Illth. Rep. 70: 877-886, 1955.
2. Peterson, O. L. Evaluation of the Quality of Medical Care. N.E.J. Med. 269: 1238-1245, 1963.
3. Lerner, M., and Riedel, D. C. The Teamster Study and the Quality of Medical Care. Inquiry, 1: 69-80, 1964.
4. Lee, R. I., and Jones, L. W. The Fundamentals of Good Medical Care. Chicago: Univ. of Chicago Press, 1933.
5. Klein, M. W.; Malone, M.; Bennis, W. G.; and Berkowitz, N. Problems of Measuring Patient Care in the Out Patient Department. J. Hlth. and Hum. Behav. 2: 138-144, 1961.
6. Kohl, S. G. Perinatal Mortality in New York City: Responsible Factors. Cambridge: Harvard University Press, 1955.
7. Shapiro, S.; Jacobziner, H.; Densen, P. M.; and Weiner, L. Further Observations on Prematurity and Perinatal Mortality in a General Population and in the Population of a Prepaid Group Practice Medical Care Plan. Am. J. Public Hlth. 50: 1304-1317, 1960.
8. Lipworth, L., Lee, J. A. H., and Morris, J. N. Case Fatality in Teaching and Nonteaching Hospitals, 1956-1959. Med. Care, 1: 71-76, 1963.
9. Rice, C. E.; Berger, D. G.; Sewall, L. G.; and Lemkau, P. V. Measuring Social Restoration Performance of Public Psychiatric Hospitals. Public Hlth. Rep. 76: 437-446, 1961.
10. Lembcke, P. A. Medical Auditing by Scientific Methods. J.A.M.A. 162: 646-655, 1956. (Appendices A and B supplied by the author.)
11. Kelman, H. R., and Willner, A. Problems in Measurement and Evaluation of Rehabilitation. Arch. Phys. Med. and Rehab. 43: 172-181, 1962.
12. McDermott, W.; Deuschle, K.; Adair, J.; Fulmer, H.; and Loughlin, B. Introducing Modern Medicine in a Navajo Community. Science, 131: 197-205, 280-287, 1960.
13. Simon, II. A. Administrative Behavior. New York: Macmillan, 1961, pp. 62-66.
14. Hutchison, G. B. Evaluation of Preventive Services. J. Chronic Dis. 11: 497-508, 1960.
15. James, G. Evaluation of Public Health, Report of the Second National Conference on Evaluation in Public Health, Ann Arbor, The University of Michigan, School of Public Health, 1960, pp. 7-17.
16. Weinerman, E. R. Appraisal of Medical Care Programs. Am. J. Public Hlth. 40: 1129-1134, 1950.
17. Goldmann, F., and Graham, E. A. The Quality of Medical Care Provided at

the Labor Health Institute, St. Louis, Missouri. St. Louis: The Labor Health Institute, 1954.

18. Peterson, O. L.; Andrews, L. P.; Spain, R. S.; and Greenberg, B. G. An Analytical Study of North Carolina General Practice: 1953-1954. J. Med. Educ. 31: 1-165, Part 2, 1956.

19. Clute, K. F. The General Practitioner: A Study of Medical Education and Practice in Ontario and Nova Scotia. Toronto: Univ. of Toronto Press, 1963, Chapters 1, 2, 16, 17 and 18.

20. Kroeger, H.; Altman, I.; Clark, D. A.; Johnson, A. C.; and Sheps, C. G. The Office Practice of Internists, I. The Feasibility of Evaluating Quality of Care. J.A.M.A. 193: 371-376, 1965.

21. Kilpatrick, G. S. Observer Error in Medicine. J. Med. Educ. 38: 38-43, 1963. For a useful bibliography on observer error, see Witts, L. J. (Ed.) Medical Surveys and Clinical Trials. London: Oxford University Press, 1959, pp. 39-44.

22. Rosenfeld, L. S. Quality of Medical Care in Hospitals. Am. J. Public Hlth. 47: 856-865, 1957.

23. Makover, H. B. The Quality of Medical Care: Methodological Survey of the Medical Groups Associated with the Health Insurance Plan of New York. Am. J. Public Hlth. 41: 824-832, 1951.

24. Daily, E. F., and Morehead, M. A. A Method of Evaluating and Improving the Quality of Medical Care. Am. J. Public Hlth. 46: 848-854, 1956.

25. Fitzpatrick, T. B., Riedel, D. C., and Payne, B. C. Character and Effectiveness of Hospital Use, in McNerney, W. J. et al. Hospital and Medical Economics. Chicago: Hospital Research and Educational Trust, American Hospital Association, 1962, pp. 495-509.

26. Morehead, M. A., et al. A Study of the Quality of Hospital Care Secured by a Sample of Teamster Family Members in New York City. New York: Columbia University, School of Public Health and Administrative Medicine, 1964.

27. Morehead, M. A. Personal communication.

28. Ehrlich, J., Morehead, M. A., and Trussell, R. E. The Quantity, Quality and Costs of Medical and Hospital Care Secured by a Sample of Teamster Families in the New York Area. New York: Columbia Univ. School of Public Health and Administrative Medicine, 1962.

29. Maloney, M. C., Trussell, R. E., and Elinson, J. Physicians Choose Medical Care: A Sociometric Approach to Quality Appraisal. Am. J. Publ. Hlth. 50: 1678-1686, 1960.

30. Georgopoulos, B. S., and Mann, F. C. The Community General Hospital. New York: Macmillan, 1962.

31. One of the author's students, Mr. Arnold D. Kaluzny, helped the author coin this word.

32. Georgopoulos, B. S., and Tannenbaum, A. S. A Study of Organizational Effectiveness. Am. Sociol. Rev. 22: 534-540, 1957.

33. Evans, L. R., and Bybee, J. R. Evaluation of Student Skills in Physical Diagnosis. J. Med. Educ. 40: 199-204, 1965.

34. Rimoldi, H. J. A., Haley, J. V., and Fogliatto, H. The Test of Diagnostic Skills, Loyola Psychometric Laboratory Publication No. 25. Chicago: Loyola University Press, 1962.

35. Williamson, J. W. Assessing Clinical Judgment. J. Med. Educ. 40: 180-187, 1965.

36. Eislee, C. W., Slee, V. N., and Hoffmann, R. G. Can the Practice of Internal Medicine Be Evaluated? Ann. Int. Med. 44: 144-161, 1956.

37. Furstenberg, F. F.; Taback, M.; Goldberg, H.; and Davis, J. W. Prescribing as an Index to Quality of Medical Care: A Study of the Baltimore City Medical Care Program. Am. J. Public Hlth. 43: 1299-1309, 1953.
38. Peterson, O. L., and Barsamian, E. M. An Application of Logic to a Study of Quality of Surgical Care. Paper read at the Fifth IBM Medical Symposium, Endicott, New York, October 7-11, 1963.
39. Peterson, O. L., and Barsamian, E. M. Diagnostic Performance, in Jacquez, J. A. (Ed.) The Diagnostic Process. Ann Arbor: University of Michigan Press, 1964, pp. 347-362.
40. Lembcke, P. A., and Johnson, O. G. A Medical Audit Report. Los Angeles: University of California, School of Public Health, 1963 (mimeo.).
41. Lembcke, P. A. A Scientific Method for Medical Auditing. Hospitals, 33: 65-71, June 16, 1969; 65-72, July 1, 1959.
42. The dimensionality of the set of variables incorporating these standards remains to be determined.
43. Huntley, R. R.; Steinhauser, R.; White, K. L.; Williams, T. F.; Martin, D. A.; and Pasternack, B. S. The Quality of Medical Care: Techniques and Investigation in the Outpatient Clinic. J. Chronic Dis. 14: 630-642, 1961.
44. Peterson, et al., loc. cit., attempted to get some confirmation of weightings through the procedure of factor analysis. The mathematically sophisticated are referred to their footnote, p. 14-15.
45. Mainland, D. Calibration of the Human Instrument. Notes from a Laboratory of Medical Statistics, Number 81, August 24, 1964 (mimeo).
46. Joint Committee of the Royal College of Obstetricians and Gynecologists and the Population Investigation Committee. Maternity in Great Britain. London: Oxford Univ. Press, 1948.
47. Yankauer, A., Goss, K. G., and Romeo, S. M. An Evaluation of Prenatal Care and its Relationship to Social Class and Social Disorganization. Am. J. Publ. Hlth. 43: 1001-1010, 1953.
48. Wylie, C. M. Participation in a Multiple Screening Clinic with Five Year Follow Up. Publ. Hlth. Rep. 76: 596-602, 1961.
49. Commission on Professional and Hospital Activities. Medical Audit Study Report 5: Primary Appendectomies. Ann Arbor: The Commission on Professional and Hospital Activities, 1957.
50. Simon, A. J. Social Structure of Clinics and Patient Improvement. Admin. Sci. Quart. 4: 197-206, 1959.
51. Lockward, H. J., Lundberg, G. A. F., and Odoroff, M. E. Effect of Intensive Care on Mortality Rate of Patients with Myocardial Infarcts. Publ. Hlth. Rep. 78: 655-661, 1963.
52. Bakst, J. N., and Marra, E. F. Experiences with Home Care for Cardiac Patients. Am. J. Publ. Hlth. 45: 444-450, 1955.
53. Muller, J. N., Tobis, J. S., and Kelman, H. R. The Rehabilitation Potential of Nursing Home Residents. Am. J. Publ. Hlth. 53: 243-247, 1963.
54. These studies also include data on the relationships between structural features and procedural end points. Examples are the effect of clinic structure on the number of outpatient visits,(50) and the effect of a home care program on hospital admissions.(52)
55. Getting, V. A., et al. Research in Evaluation in Public Health Practices. Paper presented at the ninety-second annual meeting, American Public Health Association, New York, October 5, 1964.

56. Assuming the direct evaluation of process to be the criterion, the issue becomes one of the implications of reliability measures for validity.

57. Ciocco, A., Hunt, H., and Altman, I. Statistics on Clinical Services to New Patients in Medical Groups. Publ. Hlth. Rep. 65: 99-115, 1950.

58. Myers, R. S. Hospital Statistics Don't Tell the Truth. Modern Hospital, 83:
53-54, 1954.

59. Even for hospital care the appropriate unit may include care before and after
admission, as well as several hospital admissions.(3)

60. Cordero, A. L. The Determination of Medical Care Needs in Relation to a
Concept of Minimal Adequate Care: An Evaluation of the Curative Outpatient
Services in a Rural Health Center. Med. Care, 2: 95-103, 1964.

61. Butterworth, J. S., and Reppert, E. H. Auscultatory Acumen in the General
Medical Population. J.A.M.A. 174: 32-34, 1960.

62. Evans, L. R., and Bybee, J. R. Evaluation of Student Skills in Physical Diagnosis. J. Med. Educ. 40: 199-204, 1965.

63. Fattu, N. C. Experimental Studies of Problem Solving. J. Med. Educ. 39: 212-
225, 1964.

64. John, E. R. Contributions to the Study of the Problem Solving Process. Psych.
Mon. 71, 1957.

65. Duncan, C. P. Recent Research in Human Problem Solving. Psych. Bull. 56:
397-429, 1959.

66. Fattu, N. A., Mech. E., and Kapos, E. Some Statistical Relationships between
Selected Response Dimensions and Problem Solving Proficiency. Psych. Mon.
68, 1954.

67. Stolurow, L.; Bergum, B.; Hodgson, T.; and Silva, J. The Efficient Course of
Action in "Trouble Shooting" as a Joint Function of Probability and Cost.
Educ. and Psych. Meas. 15: 462-477, 1955.

68. Ledley, R. S., and Lusted, L. B. Reasoning Foundations of Medical Diagnosis.
Science, 130: 9-21, 1959.

69. Lusted, L. B., and Stahl, W. R. Conceptual Models of Diagnosis, in Jacquez,
J. A. (Ed.) The Diagnostic Process. Ann Arbor: Univ. of Michigan Press, 1964,
pp. 157-174.

70. Edwards, W., Lindman, H., and Phillips, L. D. Emerging Technologies for
Making Decisions, in Newcomb, T. M. (Ed.) New Directions in Psychology.
New York: Holt, Rinehart & Winston, 1965, pp. 261-325.

Included among the reviewed authors who read the manuscript and made cor-
rections or comments are Georgopoulos, Makover, Morehead, Peterson, Riedel,
Rosenstock, Rosenfeld, Sheps and Weinerman. The author is especially indebted to
Dr. Mildred A. Morehead and to Professors Basil S. Georgopoulos, Herbert E.
Klarman, and Charles A. Metzner for taking time to make extensive comments.
The official critics, Mr. Sam Shapiro and Dr. Jonas N. Muller, were helpful in
sharpening some of the issues in the assessment of quality. Since the author was
unable to use all the excellent advice he received, he alone is responsible for defects
in this paper.

This review has been supported, in part, by Grant CH-00108 from the Division
of Community Health Services, United States Public Health Service.

13

Evaluation of Program Effectiveness

O. L. DENISTON, I. M. ROSENSTOCK, and V. A. GETTING

A SYSTEMATIC, comprehensive approach is needed to evaluate the effectiveness of programs in public health. Our approach is based on the assumption that all programs in public health can be viewed as consisting of a combination of resources, activities, and objectives of several kinds. We maintain that each program is characterized by one or more program "objectives," which represent the desired end result of program activities, and that each objective implies one or more necessary conditions, termed "sub-objectives," which must be accomplished in order that the program objective may be accomplished. "Activities" are performed to achieve each sub-objective and consequently the program objectives. "Resources" are expended to support the performance of activities. A sharp distinction is made between activities, which imply the performance of work, and objectives, which refer to conditions of people or of the environment deemed desirable. Every program plan, whether written or not, makes three kinds of assumptions: (a) the expenditure of resources as planned will result in the performance of planned activity, (b) each activity, if properly performed, will result in the attainment of the sub-objective with which it is linked, and (c) each sub-objective must necessarily be accomplished before the next one can be achieved and, if all sub-objectives are attained, the program objective will be attained.

In evaluating the effectiveness of programs, specific measures of accomplishment of each sub-objective and the program objectives are set up, and data on attainment of each are collected systematically, following accepted principles of research design. In addition, data are collected on the extent to which each activity is performed as planned and on the extent to which resources are used as planned. Findings from the several sets of data are used to strengthen subsequent program planning.

A second paper will deal with program efficiency, defined as the cost in resources of attaining objectives.

Our logic and methods of evaluating program performance have been and are being applied successfully. An account of a field application, "Report of Evaluation of Agricultural Labor Camp Program, 1966," an unpublished report, is available on request to the Michigan Department of Public Health.

Kinds of Evaluative Questions

The evaluative questions that program directors ask most frequently can be grouped into four categories.

Appropriateness

Questions on appropriateness concern the importance of the specific problems selected for programing and the relative emphasis or priority accorded to each. Program directors are concerned with appropriateness when they ask, "Are our program objectives worthwhile and do they have a higher priority than other possible objectives of this or other programs?"

Adequacy

Ideally, objectives are oriented toward elimination of the problem which gave rise to the program, but various constraints may necessitate reducing the scope of an objective from focus on complete solution of a problem to the more modest scope of reducing a problem by a specific amount or limiting an objective to a portion of a population experiencing the problem rather than trying to reach all those at risk. Questions concerning how much of the entire problem the program is directed toward overcoming refer to the adequacy of program objectives.

Effectiveness

Programs may differ in their effectiveness; that is, in the extent to which pre-established objectives are attained as a result of activity. Effectiveness in attaining objectives is distinct from program appropriateness and adequacy.

Efficiency

Program efficiency is defined as the cost in resources of attaining objectives. The efficiency of a program may be unrelated to its effectiveness, adequacy, and appropriateness.

These four kinds of evaluative questions may be asked before a program begins or at some point after it has been in operation. Applied beforehand, the questions are an evaluation of the planning process.

They can then be phrased as asking whether the proposed program has important objectives, whether it is aimed at overcoming a large proportion of the problem, whether the activities proposed are likely to attain the objectives, and whether the unit cost of attaining objectives is likely to be acceptably low.

When these four questions are asked about an operating program, they constitute an evaluation of performance. The questions then focus on (a) whether the program has in fact been directed toward important problems, (b) how much of the total problem has been controlled, (c) the extent to which the predetermined program objectives have been attained, and (d) the actual costs of attaining objectives.

Our proposed model for evaluation is applicable only to assessing performance of a program and not the planning of a program. Furthermore, the model does not deal with appropriateness. Our model is applicable to adequacy only when all the dimensions of a problem can be specified. We can determine the extent to which a home health care program solved a specified set of problems in a specified sample of a population. But we cannot determine how adequately it solved the entire range of health problems in the whole population unless we are able to identify in advance the total range of health problems in the total population affected. If such information is available, the measurement of program adequacy can be computed simply from the measure of program effectiveness.

Our model is intended to answer two questions: (a) to what extent were objectives attained as the result of activities (program effectiveness) and (b) at what cost (program efficiency)? The model builds upon a number of contributions to program evaluation, especially those of Paul,[1] MacMahon and co-workers,[2] Hutchison,[3] Freeman,[4] and James.[5] If there is anything unique in our model, it is the attempt to be comprehensive, uniform, and consistent in our definitions and logic and in the application of the definitions and logic to health programs.

Model to Evaluate Program Effectiveness

Our model for evaluating effectiveness requires systematic description and measurement of each variable of a program, that is, resources, activities, and objectives. If a variable or portion of a variable cannot be measured, the model cannot be fully applied. However, even partial application of the model will provide information useful to subsequent planning; in addition, it will show the evaluator precisely where additional measurements are needed.

The model is intended primarily for use by program personnel to evaluate certain aspects of their own performance. However, an outside evaluator can also use it. Regardless of who performs the evaluation, it should be remembered that the purpose of evaluation is improvement. Therefore, the evaluation should be endorsed, if not performed, by those who have the authority to make changes.

As a final constraint, the model does not offer a systematic procedure for assessing any unplanned impact of activities, although activities performed for a specific purpose may indeed have side effects. We recommend that program personnel attempt to assess side effects on a subjective, impressionistic basis until a more systematic way of measuring them is developed.

Definition of Terms

The model uses terms that are familiar but have not always been used consistently. First, therefore, these terms will be defined.

Program. An organized response to reduce or eliminate one or more problems. This response includes (a) specification of one or more objectives, (b) selection and performance of one or more activities, and (c) acquisition and use of resources. Although the term "program" probably suggests similar concepts to most health workers, two ambiguities are common. First, for many workers, human ailments or hazardous environmental conditions constitute the only legitimate focus for a program. Thus, concern with tuberculosis or water pollution is a program, but disease casefinding or food handler training is not. Such workers frequently classify casefinding, food handler training, and similar concerns as a "subprogram," "component," "project," or "technique."

To simplify terminology and logic, any area or scope of concern may be considered a program for the purpose of evaluation of performance. Thus, disease casefinding, food handler training, and professional education can be evaluated, although their immediate objectives do not have direct impact on a human ailment or environmental hazard.

A second common ambiguity results when the work "program" is further specified by adding a content area, such as "school health program." To some workers, a school health program means correction of defects; to others, measurement of height and weight or immunization; and to yet others, school health may connote certain areas of instruction.

Both sources of ambiguity may be removed by stating the objectives of the program and listing the activities performed and resources used.

If this is done, the result is a statement that the program consists of resources a, b, c, used to perform activities d, e, f, which, in turn, are designed to attain objectives g and h. This definition, therefore, permits widely varying scopes of work to be defined properly as programs.

Objective. A situation or condition of people or of the environment which responsible program personnel consider desirable to attain. To permit subsequent evaluation, the statement of an objective must specify (a) what—the nature of the situation or condition to be attained, (b) extent—the quantity or amount of the situation or condition to be attained, (c) who—the particular group of people or portion of the environment in which attainment is desired, (d) where—the geographic area of the program, and (e) when—the time at or by which the desired situation or condition is intended to exist.

Within the framework of our definition are three kinds of objectives, each meeting the basic definition.

1. Ultimate objective. A condition which is desired in and of itself according to the value system of those responsible for the program. Reductions in morbidity and mortality are examples of conditions that are typically regarded as inherently desirable.

2. Program objective. A statement of that particular situation or condition which is intended to result from the sum of program efforts. It may or may not be considered inherently desirable, that is, an ultimate objective.

3. Sub-objective. A subordinate or sub-objective is an objective which must be attained before the program objective may be obtained. A sub-objective is seldom inherently desirable.

Most programs have several sub-objectives. All sub-objectives are related in time to each other and to the program objective; that is, the program planner believes they must be accomplished in a particular order. Frequently, two or more sub-objectives must be attained simultaneously. In some programs sub-objective 1 must be accomplished before sub-objectives 2, 3, and 4 may be accomplished, and 2, 3, and 4 may have to be accomplished simultaneously in order that sub-objective 5 may be obtained, and so on. Other writers have used such terms as "intermediate objectives" or "activity goals" to describe sub-objectives.

There is a commonly used distinction between long-range and short-range objectives. The phrases are not recommended because they can be ambiguous, as the following examples illustrate.

In some circumstances long range refers to a program objective and short range to a sub-objective. Thus the long-range (program) objective might be a 90 percent reduction in the prevalence of tuberculosis after 5 years and one short-range (sub-) objective might be that all people with tuberculosis know how to follow a prescribed chemotherapeutic regimen.

In other instances long range and short range refer to amounts of the program objective that can be expected at any given stage. The long-range objective might be a 90 percent reduction in the prevalence of tuberculosis after 5 years and the short-range objective might be its reduction by 20 percent after 1 year.

The meanings of the concepts are different in these two examples. In the first, the short term objective is actually a sub-objective which might be wholly attained and still not imply any attainment of the program objective. In the second, the short-range objective represents partial attainment of the program objective. The distinctions used in this paper make it possible to describe plans and outcomes without differentiating between long-range and short-range objectives.

Activity. Work performed by program personnel and equipment in the service of an objective. Activity as we use it does not imply any fixed amount or scope of work; it may be applied with equal validity to such diverse efforts as writing a letter or providing comprehensive health care. An activity can usually be subdivided into more specific activities. Providing comprehensive health care, for example, could be subdivided into providing curative health care and providing preventive health care; these, in turn, are capable of further sub-division and specification.

Probably the greatest cause of confusion and difficulty in both planning and evaluating health programs is lack of a clear and consistent distinction between an activity and an objective. James[5a] has made the distinction in terms of an analogy to a bird—the activity is flapping wings, the objective is being at some desired place. Activities consume program time and resources whereas objectives do not.

The distinction between objectives and activities may be further clarified by an analogy between the logic of an experiment and the logic of a program plan. In an experiment, the investigator asks whether a cause-effect relationship can be demonstrated. He performs some procedure on a group of subjects (cause) and predicts that a specific result will or will not occur (effect). The experimental procedure is linked to the expected outcome by an hypothesis. The hypothesis can be stated in an "if . . . then" form; that is, if treatment A is provided, then effect B will result. Program planning parallels the logic of an experiment. After identification and analysis of needs or problems, a program objective is established and decisions are made about the activities to be undertaken. A program objective is parallel to the experimenter's expected result or effect, and the program activities are parallel to the experimental procedure or cause. The planner hypothesizes that a given method or set of activities will lead to the attainment of the objective; if a certain activity is performed, then the desired objective will be achieved. The hypothesis can be tested only by evaluation.

Resource. Personnel, funds, materials, and facilities available to support the performance of activity. Resources, like activities, may be described with varying levels of specificity.

Program assumption. An hypothesis concerning the nature of relationships among the various aspects of a program. Every program plan includes three major kinds of assumptions.

1. The assumption that use of resources as planned will result in the performance of planned activity.

2. The assumption that performing planned activity will result in the attainment of the desired objectives. Similar assumptions link subdivisions of program resources to the sub-set of activities they support and, in turn, to the program sub-objective they are intended to establish.

3. The assumption that each sub-objective must necessarily be attained before the program objective can be attained and that attainment of all sub-objectives will result in attainment of the program objective.

A Program Overview

It is helpful at this point to describe the logical planning of a program if such limiting factors as financial and technical constraints could be ignored. Assume that a program objective as we have defined it has been established; that is, a statement has been formulated that the program is intended to attain a given situation or condition in a particular group of people or portion of the environment, in a given geographical area, by a particular time, and to a particular extent. Ideally, the planners, having specified the objective of a program, would then specify the conditions that would have to occur before the objective could be attained. Each of these necessary conditions is a sub-objective.

The planner then identifies alternative activities which might be effective in attaining the objectives. He considers the anticipated costs and effectiveness of each alternative. Finally, the planner selects the best alternatives in terms of his assessments of program appropriateness. adequacy, effectiveness, and efficiency. Current approaches to select- ing objectives and activities include planning-programing-budgeting, cost-benefit analysis, systems analysis, and operations research.

The final phase of planning is assignment of resources to support the activity selected.

It has already been indicated that the total program plan contains many assumptions about the relationships among resources, activities, and objectives. In a very real sense, evaluation of effectiveness is the determination of the extent to which these assumptions are true; eval- uation assesses (a) whether the expenditure of resources did lead to the performance of planned activity, (b) whether each activity did attain its intended outcome or sub-objective, (c) whether each sub- objective was necessary to attain the next higher sub-objective, and (d) whether attainment of all sub-objectives was sufficient to accomplish the program objective.

Application of the Model

To conduct an evaluation of program effectiveness using the model proposed involves a series of actions. The process is divided arbitrarily into three steps.

Step 1. Describing the Program

The program description consists of naming the program to be eval- uated and specifying the program objective or objectives, sub-objec- tives, activities, and resources. If these things have already been done in the planning phase, this step in evaluation is relatively simple and may require only copying them from the program plan. However, it is rare in current health practice to find written program plans with ob- jectives spelled out in sufficient detail and precision to permit evalua- tion of effectiveness.

Specification of objectives. Specification of the program objective or objectives and sub-objectives may prove especially troublesome if these concepts are new to health workers. Drawing up a sequence of objectives may improve understanding.

The time sequence of objectives may be placed on a horizontal line, with an ultimate objective at the extreme right. At left is the initial condition or sub-objective that, in the opinion of program planners, must exist if the ultimate objective is to be attained. Other planners might formulate a still earlier sub-objective. The initial sub-objective is arbitrarily chosen to represent the first new condition that the planner believes must be attained before the succeeding conditions can occur. Everything to the left of the initial sub-objective is taken as a given, that is, it is assumed to take place without program intervention.

Between the initial sub-objective and the ultimate objective are the intervening sub-objectives or necessary conditions. Many sub-objectives are possible if each is stated specifically, or all sub-objectives can be grouped under two or three general headings (fig. 1). There are disadvantages, however, in specifying either a very small or very large number of sub-objectives.

The first task in describing a program to be evaluated is to state its objective. The program objective may or may not be an ultimate objective from a health professional's point of view. A program may encompass an entire line, or any portion of such a line. Nevertheless, the program objective is an arbitrary point on a line that is expected to culminate in an ultimate health objective. Thus one program might include only the portion of the line that includes the first three intervening sub-objectives (fig. 1).

An evaluation of program effectiveness must include measurement of the condition that is specified in the program objective. In addition, it should include measurement of as many sub-objectives as available time and resources permit. In general, we recommend that several sub-objectives be measured in order to locate the source of trouble if a program is less effective than desired. Measurement of a large number of sub-objectives can consume great quantities of time and possibly of other resources. Should an administrator wish to evaluate the effectiveness of several programs and have limited resources for evaluation, he may prefer to measure attainment of program objectives only for all programs, returning to measure sub-objectives for those programs manifesting lowest effectiveness.

FIGURE 1. TIME SEQUENCE OF OBJECTIVES

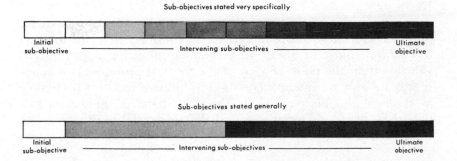

Sub-objectives stated very specifically

Initial sub-objective ———————— Intervening sub-objectives ———————— Ultimate objective

Sub-objectives stated generally

Initial sub-objective ———————— Intervening sub-objectives ———————— Ultimate objective

No dictum can yet be given as to the optimal number of sub-objectives since an infinite number of previous conditions (sub-objectives) are necessary for a given condition (objective) to occur. Suppose sanitarians are attempting to increase restaurant operators' knowledge of defects in their operations. One necessary condition (sub-objective) for acquisition of information is that the operator understand the sanitarian's vocabulary. But a necessary condition for the operator to understand is that he pay some attention to what is being said, and a necessary condition for his paying attention is that he be physically exposed to the message (he be physically present and capable of hearing, seeing, and thinking). The ability to perceive and think, in turn, is contingent upon the functioning of nervous tissue which, in turn, is contingent upon more basic biochemical balances. Biochemical function is contingent upon atomic motion which is dependent on subatomic motion and so on.

Although this is reduction to absurdity, it is clear that a somewhat arbitrary division will be needed to determine the number of sub-objectives to be measured. The cutoff point would seem to be the point where the apparent disadvantages of expending further resources on measurements would about equal the apparent disadvantages of assuming that doubtful conditions will in fact be realized. Specifying too many sub-objectives may make the evaluation too costly and detailed; specifying too few may yield insufficient information about weak aspects of the program. Most administrators assume that restaurant operators are not deaf, blind, and mentally defective, but many will be unwilling to assume that operators will automatically pay attention to what the sanitarian says. In that instance, the adequate functioning of sense organs would be accepted as a given rather than as a sub-objective and would be to the left of the initial sub-objective, but the operator's attentiveness would be a sub-objective.

The nature of ultimate objectives, program objectives, and sub-objectives is illustrated by combining examples from Hutchison[3] and Knutson.[6]

In a discussion of programs of early casefinding, Hutchison cites a program with an ultimate objective. He considers that alteration of the natural course of disease in a favorable direction is intrinsically valuable from the point of view of the medical profession—although it may be only an intermediate or sub-objective for such professions as theology and philosophy. On the other hand, a number of sub-objectives (which he terms intermediate) are crucial to program effectiveness but are not in and of themselves intrinsically valuable, such as (a) that people come for screening, (b) that cases of illness are detected, and (c) that persons with the disease follow prescribed treatment. Sub-objectives a, b, and c are desired not because of their inherent value but because the ultimate objective cannot be attained unless each of them is attained.

Knutson refers to a hypothetical health education program, whose objective is some desired behavior of people to whom the program is directed. He lists a number of sub-objectives for his program which he, like Hutchison, terms intermediate objectives: (a) the people must be exposed to the material, (b) they must give the material their attention, and (c) they must understand the words and concepts. If the objective (behavior of target audience) referred to by Knutson were that people come for screening, that objective would be identical with initial sub-objective specified by Hutchison. The sub-objectives specified by Knutson, then, occupy a portion of the program line to the left of Hutchison's initial objective (fig. 2).

FIGURE 2. RELATIONSHIP OF KNUTSON AND HUTCHISON
PROGRAM LINES

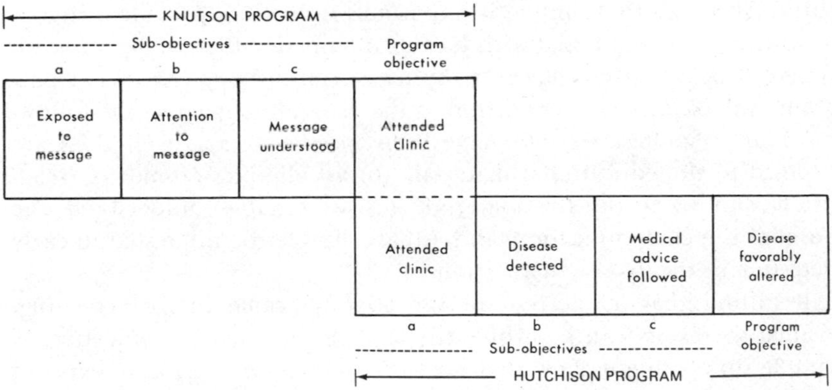

The program objective for Knutson's health education program is the initial sub-objective of Hutchison's broader disease control program. Knutson's sub-objectives are taken as givens in the Hutchison example.

The importance of correctly stating the program objective may be illustrated by another example. Assume that the health education program within a larger disease control program is to be evaluated. The true objective is that all members of a particular group residing in a given area come to a clinic for a particular screening test on a specified date. Figure 2 shows that the adjacent objectives, in elaborated form, are that all members of the group understand the words and concepts of the educational material and that all positive cases of disease in the group are detected.

If either adjacent objective were mistakenly stated as the program objective, the results of subsequent evaluation would be misleading. In the first instance, the program would be judged as more effective than it actually was, since many people may indeed have understood the words and concepts, but nevertheless failed to attend the clinic—failed, that is, to take the desired action. In the second instance the program would be judged as less effective than it actually was, since failures of diagnosis would incorrectly be attributed to the health education program. Therefore, it is essential to state as the objective of the program the precise outcome that is desired and expected to result from the activities to be evaluated.

To illustrate further the usefulness of measuring attainment of sub-objectives, consider a program similar to the health education program discussed previously. The true objective was that stated in the previous example, and 50 percent of the specified group attended the clinic. Although that finding is important, it does not provide a clue as to why the program failed with half its intended audience. Such knowledge can be acquired, however, by measuring attainment of the program's sub-objectives. In addition to the program objective, the following four sub-objectives may have been specified: (a) all eligibles are exposed to the educational material, (b) all eligibles attend to (read, listen, and so forth) the material, (c) all eligibles understand the point of the communication, and (d) all eligibles be interested in early detection of the disease in question.

Recalling that 50 percent of the eligibles came in for screening, evaluative results can be arbitrarily assigned to each sub-objective. A sample survey might show that for each 100 eligibles: 95 were exposed to the material; of those, 90 paid attention to it; of those, 65 adequately understood the point of the communication; and of those, 35 were interested in detecting disease early. Finally, all 35 satisfying all four sub-objectives came in for screening. Thus, the first two sub-objectives were attained with a total loss of 10 percent of the eligibles. Some attention might be given to reducing this loss. However, more important is the additional loss of 55 percent (25 and 30 percent respectively) that occurred in attaining the third and fourth sub-objectives. Thus, of all 90 people attending to the program material, more than 60 percent

(55 of 90) failed to understand the message and to become interested in early detection. Clearly, activities to accomplish these two sub-objectives need to be strengthened.

It may be noted that 50 percent came in for screening, but only 35 percent were interested in early detection. This suggests that personal interest is important but not absolutely necessary to obtain participation. Perhaps further study would show that some people came in because of the influence of relatives or friends. The planners might wish to build on such a finding in subsequent programs.

The preceding discussion and examples have implied an objective that is identical for each person in the program population. However, for some programs, the objective for each member of the target group may be different as those in mental health and home care programs.

In these, it would be more appropriate to state a separate objective (and sub-objectives) for each person to be served. In such programs the attending physician may establish a unique objective for each patient; for example, by the end of some time period, Mr. A will return to work, Mr. B will bathe and dress himself. The program objective can then be summarized as all, or some proportion of, program clientele will attain their unique objectives within specified periods.

Thus far, the discussion of objectives has focused on only one kind of content objective associated with programs. However, two other kinds of objectives need to be recognized.

Each health worker in a program will have personal objectives, such as advancement in rank or title, a higher salary, respect of his peers, popularity, and so forth. These may or may not be consistent with program objectives.

In addition to these personal objectives, every agency or organization has what may be called survival programs—a set of activities undertaken to insure the stability and continued existence of the agency. Certain public relations and public service activities are examples of survival programs.

Concern with personal satisfaction and organizational survival will act as constraints in planning programs, in the setting of priorities, and in the selection of objectives and activities. In this sense, they do not interfere with evaluation of program performance although knowledge of constraints may be useful in interpreting evaluation results. If desired, however, our model could be applied to the evaluation of employee morale or organization survival "programs."

The attention given to program objectives is deemed necessary because rarely have objectives been stated clearly when evaluation is desired and because it is difficult but extremely important to distinguish betweeen objectives, sub-objectives, and activities.

Some reasons for lack of predetermined objectives have been described by Selznick.[7]

> Once an organization becomes a "going concern," with many forces working to keep it alive, the people who run it can readily escape the task of defining its purposes. This evasion stems partly from the hard intellectual labor involved, a labor that often seems but to increase the burden of already onerous daily operations. In part, there is the wish to avoid conflicts with those in and out of the organization who would be threatened by a sharp definition of purpose, with its attendant claims and responsibilities.

The threat engendered by making program objectives explicit becomes intensified when one seriously proposes measuring attainment.[8-10] We do not see any ready way to eliminate all threatening aspects of evaluating program effectiveness, but we do believe that the threat can often be overcome if the benefits can be perceived as outweighing the costs.

Specification of activities. When the program objectives and sub-objectives have been stated, the next task in step 1 is to specify all program activities, linking each to the objective or sub-objective it is intended to accomplish. There are two reasons to do this. First, making activities explicit can serve as a check on the adequacy and completeness of stated objectives. If a planned or continuing activity cannot be linked to any stated objective or sub-objective, either a necessary objective or sub-objective has been omitted, or the activity is unnecessary. Conversely, if a stated objective or sub-objective has no activity linked to it, either an essential activity is not being planned or performed or the stated objective or sub-objective is not necessary to the program.

The second reason for including activities in the program description is to determine the extent to which they were performed as intended. For this purpose, activity must be carefully specified—what is to be done, by whom it is to be done, and when and where it is to be done.

If an objective or sub-objective is not attained, either an activity was not performed as planned or the assumption linking the activity and the objective or sub-objective was not valid. Of course, if the activity was not performed or not performed properly, the linking assumption must remain untested.

Specification of program resources. The final task in step 1, specification of program resources, makes it possible to determine if resources were used as planned. If planned activities were not performed, knowledge of whether resources were used will allow determination of the validity of assumptions linking resources and activities made in the planning process.

In summary then, the first step in evaluating program effectiveness requires a clear statement of the program objectives, the specification of a reasonable number of sub-objectives, specification of program activities, and a description of program resources.

Step 2. Measurement

A complete treatment of steps 2 and 3 is not possible in this paper. The interested reader is referred to standard texts which cover the material in detail.[11-14] In addition, consultation from experts such as statisticians and behavioral scientists will often be helpful in completing steps 2 and 3.

Step 1 outlined a method for describing programs to permit evaluation of program effectiveness. Step 2 requires identification of the kinds of evidence needed to determine that an objective or sub-objective has or has not been achieved.

In general, valid and reliable measures of program accomplishment are needed. Briefly, validity of a measure is the extent that an obtained score measures the characteristic that it is intended to measure. The terms "sensitivity" and "specificity" applied to diagnostic tests are components of validity. Reliability of evidence is the consistency or repeatability of a score.

We are concerned with validity and reliability because test scores do not always measure consistently what they are intended to measure. Suppose a series of measures are obtained on a group of persons or restaurants or on samples of water. A range of scores will be obtained. Differences in scores may reflect true differences in the characteristic being measured, but different scores may reflect other factors. If the measure is of people, responses may not only reflect the item being measured but also such transitory factors as mood or fatigue. In measures of the physical environment, factors such as variations in the administration of a test and the care with which instruments are read will also affect scores.

Another possible source of variation in scores exists in measurements of complex concepts such as health status, morbidity, or cleanliness. Such concepts are composed of many specific sub-concepts. For example, good health might include almost an infinite number of measurements of the functions of various organ systems. It is unlikely that any one test will measure all functions. A test of two or three functions applied to a group of people might show that some are healthier than others without giving recognition to the fact that had tests been made of other functions, results might have been different.

Because test scores are determined not only by true differences in what is being measured but also by other causes, it is never completely safe to accept a test score at face value. When possible, evidence should be obtained that the test is valid (it measures what it is intended to measure) and that it is reliable (successive administrations of the test or administration by different persons yield similar scores).

· In selecting a measure of accomplishment, the evaluator may know of valid and reliable measures or he may search the literature for relevant measures that others have used. If he fails to locate an acceptable measure, he may have to develop a unique measure which satisfies the basic criteria of measuring instruments. However, if his resources do not permit the development of a measure for certain objectives, he may be forced to omit some measures from the evaluation, thus reducing the resultant amount of information bearing on the success of a program.

When to measure. The program objectives and sub-objectives state the time period in which the measures are to be applied. Although one tends to think of evaluation as being conducted over a relatively short period, evaluation will be most valuable if it is conceived as a more nearly continuous process. Since attainment of sub-objectives occurs in a time sequence, attainment of each should be measured soon after attainment is expected.

How to measure. In deciding how to make the needed measurements, two problems are particularly important: how to avoid bias and the problem of sampling.

The possibility of bias is great if one evaluates his own work. This possibility is especially great if observational rather than physical measures are used, such as reporting the cleanliness of an object or the satisfaction of a patient. Bias can be reduced by using physical measures when possible, or if observation or judgment is necessary, by having more than one person judge.

Sampling procedures are often used in evaluating a program since it is rarely feasible to measure the attainment of objectives in every person in the target group or at every location. In such cases, a probability sample which accurately represents the total population must be selected.

The size of the sample required depends on such technical considerations as variance in the distribution of the quality being measured, the amount of change expected as a result of program activity, and the level of certainty desired when inferring that what is true of the sample is also true of the population from which it was drawn.

Collecting the data. Data on the attainment of objectives and subobjectives as well as on the performance of activities and use of resources must be collected at times indicated in the program description.

Step 3. Determining Effectiveness

In evaluating effectiveness the question is not merely were the program objectives accomplished but to what extent can achievement of the objective be attributed to the activities of the program?

Analysis of program effectiveness can be simplified by using a set of ratios involving the three program variables: resources, activities, and objectives.

Simplest is the ratio of actual resources to planned use of resources, $\frac{AR}{PR}$.

Slightly more complicated is the ratio of actual program activities performed to planned activities, $\frac{AA}{PA}$.

The ratio that indicates attainment of objectives is still more complex. We denote this ratio as $\frac{AO}{PO}$. AO is the net attainment of the objective attributable to program activity and PO is the attainment desired less the status that would have existed in the absence of the program. It might be imagined that the proper comparison would be between actual status of the objective when evaluation is performed and the status of the objective that had been planned. However, such a comparison is not valid since it does not take account of effects on the program of activities and events outside it. Evaluation should assess the extent to which achievement of the objective can be attributed to activities performed in the program.

Therefore, it is necessary to find a way of comparing the net accomplishment attributable to the program with the accomplishment intended for the program. One way of doing this is to determine the status of the objective at the time of evaluation and then to subtract from it an estimate of what the status would have been had the program not been undertaken. For example, if a program operator finds that 90 percent of a group of clients are immune to a disease following the conduct of a program, he cannot properly take credit for all 90 percent, but only for those who would not be immune had his program not been undertaken.

What is true for the actual status of the objective, the numerator, is also true for planned attainment, the denominator. One must subtract from planned attainment that portion of the desired status that would have occurred in the absence of the program. For example, suppose it was desired that 90 percent of a population be immune to a disease. Evaluaton shows that 80 percent actually became immune but that half, 40 percent, became immune through activity outside the program (visits to physicians and so forth). Program effectiveness would then be $\frac{80-40}{90-40} = \frac{40}{50} = 80$ percent.

Another example based on actual data will show how the ratio may be computed. In a food service sanitation program consisting of inspections, a rating system was used as the measure both of the problem and the objective. The objective was that the average sanitation rating of food establishments in the county will be at least as high as 90 by July 1, 1966. On July 1, 1966, the average rating was 85.7.

Additional data showed that the average rating in an uninspected section of the county was 81 on July 1, 1966. If we use the rating of 81 as an estimate of what the countywide rating would have been without the program, the program effectiveness ratio becomes $\frac{85.7-81}{90-81} = \frac{4.7}{9} = 52.2$ percent.

How is it possible to estimate the status of the objective in the absence of the program? The most certain way is to use a control or comparison group similar to the one exposed to the program. The control group procedure maximizes confidence in judging the results that may be properly attributed to the program.

Control groups are not always feasible in evaluations of health programs, but they could be employed more often than they currently are. For example, when a new program cannot be initiated throughout a jurisdiction, it may be possible to begin it in several places selected at random and to use the remaining areas as controls. Or alternate procedures to accomplish objectives might be applied systematically in different parts of the jurisdiction, as is done in clinical field trials to test whether one procedure is superior to another.

However, if a strict control group is not feasible, a control group can be approximated by comparing community status before and after the program with information about nearby communities not exposed to the program. While this is not an ideal procedure, it may provide guidance as to the impact of the program.

A major danger in using natural groups as comparisons or controls is that an available group, within or outside the community, may not be similar to the study group in crucial respects. The laboratory practice for minimizing this danger is to assign subjects randomly to treatment and control procedures. Sometimes this practice can be used in evaluating health programs, but often it will be impossible because treatment must be given to or withheld from whole groups.

Baseline measures are helpful when random assignments to experimental (program) and control groups cannot be made. If baseline measures show that the program and comparison groups were similar at the beginning of the program, one may be more confident that the status of the comparison group at evaluation represents what would probably have occurred in the program group without the program. If the groups differ at the beginning, one should be much less confident.

Where no comparison group can be devised, it may still be possible to obtain information on the probable impact of program activity on the objective. One can, for example, formulate alternative explanations for the outcome of the program and see whether available facts support the alternative explanations. Suppose, for example, one wishes to determine whether a decline in the incidence of tuberculosis in a community can properly be attributed to an ongoing tuberculosis control program but the community in question cannot be compared with another.

The operator might examine other possible explanations for the falling incidence. He might consider improved nutrition and improved housing as two possible alternative explanations and investigate whether nutrition and housing indeed improved over the period being considered. If neither improved substantially, he could with greater confidence attribute the reduced incidence of tuberculosis to his program. If one or both alternative hypotheses were borne out by evidence, he could not attribute the outcome to his program. At that point he could, however, use the analysis of cross-tabulations to study the interrelationships among the alternative explanations and thus throw more light on the relative contribution of each explanation to the program objectives that were attained.[14]

The conclusion that program activities caused program outcomes requires a judgment that can never be made with absolute certainty. After using control groups or testing alternative hypotheses, however, one can make a more confident judgment than would be legitimate without the use of such procedures.

Use of Findings

Most evaluations of programs will reveal imperfect success in attaining objectives and sub-objectives. Evaluation does more, however, than demonstrate degree of attainment. It also pin-points where problems exist. Our model for evaluation of programs assumes that programs have been planned to expend resources to enable activities to be performed and that the activities are intended to cause the attainment of sub-objectives and the program objective.

A program may be less effective than planned for several reasons.

1. Resources were not used as planned.

2. The assumptions linking resources to activities were invalid.

3. Activities were not performed as planned.

4. The assumptions linking activities to sub-objectives or objectives were invalid.

5. The assumptions linking sub-objectives to the program objective were invalid.

Locating program difficulties requires measuring each of three program variables: resources, activities, and objectives and sub-objectives. If evaluation can pinpoint the problems, subsequent program planning should proceed more effectively than it could in the absence of evaluation. Thus, in the hands of the thoughtful administrator, evaluation of program effectiveness can improve planning of programs and thereby increase program effectiveness.

REFERENCES

1. Paul, B. D. Social Science in Public Health. Am. J. Publ. Hlth. 46: 1390-1396, 1956.
2. MacMahon, B.; Pugh, T.; and Hutchison, G. B. Principles in the Evaluation of Community Mental Health Programs. Am. J. Publ. Hlth. 51: 963-979, 1961.
3. Hutchison, G. B. Evaluation of Preventive Services. J. Chronic Dis. 11: 497-508, 1960.
4. Freeman, R. B. Public Health Nursing Practice. Philadelphia: W. B. Saunders, 1963, p. 289.
5. James, G. Administration of Community Health Services. Chicago: International City Managers Association, 1961, ch. 6, pp. 114-134; (a) p. 118.
6. Knutson, A. Pre-testing: A Positive Approach to Evaluation. Public Hlth. Rep. 67: 699-703, 1952.
7. Selznick, P. Leadership in Administration. New York: Row, Peterson, 1957.
8. Bergen, B. J. Professional Communities and the Evaluation of Demonstration Projects in Community Mental Health. Am. J. Publ. Hlth. 55: 1057-1066, 1965.

9. Stanley, D. T. Excellence in Public Service—How Do You Really Know. Public Admin. Rev. 24: 170-174, 1964.

10. Herzog, E. Some Guidelines for Evaluative Research, Children's Bureau Publication, No. 378, U. S. Department of Health, Education, and Welfare, 1959.

11. Selltiz, C., Jahoda, M., Deutsch, M., and Cook, S. Research Methods in Social Relations. New York: Henry Holt, 1960.

12. Cronbach, L. J. Essentials of Psychological Testing. 2nd ed. New York: Harper & Row, 1960.

13. Kerlinger, F. N. Foundations of Behavioral Research. New York: Holt, Rinehart & Winston, 1966.

14. Hyman, H. Survey Design and Analysis. Glencoe: Free Press, 1955.

This investigation was supported by Public Health Service research grant no. CH00044 from the Division of Community Health Services.

Section III

Evaluation Techniques and Indexes

The PERT System: An Appraisal of Program Evaluation Review Technique

DANIEL D. ROMAN

PROGRAM Evaluation Review Technique, better known as P.E.R.T.,[1] represents a significant step forward in the development of managerial science. The system, developed jointly by the Navy Special-Projects Office and Booz-Allen-Hamilton, in conjunction with the Fleet Ballistic Missile Program, has had its major impetus and success in association with the Polaris missile.

PERT is essentially a planning and control concept designed to: focus managerial attention on key program developmental parts; point up potential problem areas which could disrupt program goals; evaluate progress toward the attainment of program objectives; give management a prompt mechanical reporting device; and, finally, aid and facilitate decision-making. In the accomplishment of these stated objectives, PERT uses TIME as a common denominator to reflect three categories of factors which influence success—time, resource applications, and required performance specifications.[2] The explanation of the PERT program, as set forth in this paper, represents a considerable over-simplification of the system. The basic purpose is to examine PERT as a development in management science. The mechanical composition is therefore not covered in detail.[3]

The Mechanics of PERT

Essentially, PERT is an attempt at quantification of program planning and control. An important characteristic of PERT, as distinguished from existing systems, is the attempt to systemize and mechanize the planning and control process. The *innovation of the system* would seem to lie in the addition of mathematical embellishments, the use of computers and variations of known scheduling methods, such as Gantt Charts, "goes-into," and minus day scheduling. The system goes beyond the traditional Gantt Chart scheduling, but still uses the principle of this technique. In the PERT variation, the Gantt-type bars that indicated various phases of activities measured against a time scale have been eliminated.

The Network

The fundamental tool used in the PERT approach is the network or flow plan. The composition of the network is a series of related events and activities. Events (required sequential accomplishment points) are most frequently represented by circle or square symbols. Activities are the time consuming element of the program and are used to connect the various events. They are shown in the flow plan as arrows. A simplified model of the flow plan is illustrated in Figure 1.

FLOW PLAN

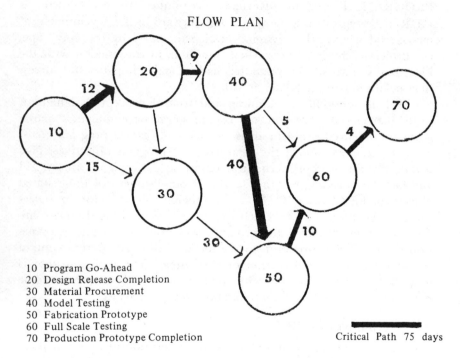

10 Program Go-Ahead
20 Design Release Completion
30 Material Procurement
40 Model Testing
50 Fabrication Prototype
60 Full Scale Testing
70 Production Prototype Completion

Critical Path 75 days

FIGURE 1.

The number of events shown on any flow plan should reflect significant program accomplishments (such as administrative, intellectual or hardware) and should be in some approximation to the complexity of that program. It should also be noted that some events may depend only on one single prior event, while in other situations there may be an interrelationship of several events leading to the accomplishment of an ultimate objective.

Estimating Elapsed-Time Between Events

To determine the elapsed-time between events, the activity time, responsible engineers evaluate the situation and submit their estimates using three possible completion assumptions: optimistic completion time, most likely completion time and pessimistic completion time. Optimistic completion time is predicated on minimal difficulties. The most likely completion time represents the most accurate forecast based on normal developments. Pessimistic time is estimated on maximum potential difficulties.

Based on the three time estimates, a simple formula[4] can be derived which will give the activity time to be used in the system flow plan. The application of the formula gives a time with a 50% chance of realization.

ACTIVITY TIME

O = Optimistic Completion Time
M = Most Likely Completion Time
P = Pessimistic Completion Time

Assuming $O = 6$ weeks, $M = 8$ weeks and $P = 16$ weeks, the activity time can be computed, using the formula:

$$\frac{O + 4M + P}{6} = \text{Activity Time} \qquad \frac{6 + 32 + 16}{6} = 9 \text{ weeks}$$

The formula is based on the probability distribution of the time involved in performing the activity.[5] Once the network has been established and all activity times computed, the information on activities and events can be translated into dates based on a program start time.

The Critical Path

The critical path of the program is established by the longest possible time span along the system flow plan. To determine the critical path, data and events are organized in sequence. The starting point for plotting the critical path is the final event in the total network. From the final event, related events are placed sequentially, working backward, until the present is reached. Where the network is simple the critical path can be computed and determined manually. In more complex situations a procedure for sequencing events can be programmed on an electronic computer.[6]

In Figure 1, the heavy line indicates the critical path in the network. If the proposed final completion date is to be bettered, indicated by event 70, reappraisal and curtailment of activity time must take place along the critical path.

Inasmuch as the critical path takes the longest time and is the determinant for the project completion, other events may conceivably be completed before the time they are actually needed. The time differential between the scheduled completion of the non-critical events and the time that they are actually required is called the Slack Time. Where excessive Slack Time exists in the program, a re-evaluation should take place. It should be determined which resources, and in what amount, could be transferred to other activities. This, in turn, could shorten the Critical Path or better balance the allocation of resources assigned to the project.

Program Review and Reporting

Once the schedule has been established, frequent review by program participants is required to assess actual progress against planned accomplishment. Inputs are then assembled and programmed into the computer, which prints out the status report of time interval estimates versus actual reported progress.

Reporting can be done bi-weekly, for example, on all items shown in the network or flow plan. The currency and frequency of the reporting promptly alerts management to the events which are deviating from the basic program plan. Where corrective action is not possible and the scheduled date of an objective event has been changed, it will become necessary to recompute the entire program to determine the current anticipated completion dates of all events.[7]

PERT as a Management Tool

There are many dramatic implications of PERT relative to management. Initially and perhaps most important, it focuses management's attention on the importance of planning and control and the coordination of these functions by means of tangible and systematic inputs, audits and reports.

Too often planning and/or control are performed on a segmented basis with inconclusive results and little direction toward a well-defined objective. PERT eliminates uncoordinated segmentation and brings an integrated methodology into program planning. PERT indicates every event critical for program performance and shows the related activity time before the next sequential event (s) can take place. Most control systems also indicate time span and sequence but lack the specificity of PERT in drawing direct links between the events, the time and the responsibility for functional performance.

While individually none of the ideas employed by PERT represents startling innovation, the total approach takes a major step forward in managerial technique. An appraisal of the system would seem to indicate some significant advantages over existing approaches; these are discussed in the next section.

Participation

The program is planned in detail by the participants. Planning inputs in the PERT system flow upward to be assembled and evaluated as a composite working document. Frequently, in the traditional planning approach basic premises may flow downward and lead to unrealistic assumptions and commitments when program boundaries are predetermined before detailed participation is requested. (When the program performers are given limitations such as commencement and completion dates, performance specifications to be met, budget restrictions, and the like, participation may be only partial, even illusory.)

In the PERT system, no master plan formulated by management, the project office or a central planning staff is forwarded to the working levels as a compulsory program plan. The people who will ultimately have to meet the program objectives are active contributors from the outset. This can promote teamwork, facilitate communication, encourage a proprietary interest and foster orderly, intelligent planning. After the program ground rules have been established, the people who have participated in the planning are the same people who do the work and report and forecast accomplishment in relation to the original plan.

Perspective, Programming and Interrelationship of Events

PERT departs from normal programming where only key milepost developments are depicted. The PERT network shows the interrelationship between all vital program functions. In short, it attempts to give total program perspective.

The events that are shown on the network or flow plan are broken into meaningful, related segments. The activity time between events may vary from zero to several days or months. As an example, if the activity time is indicated on the network as zero, it alerts the participants to the fact that instantaneous action must take place between certain events before additional sequential development or activity can occur. The flow plan fixes each group's participation time and responsibility and draws attention to each event or chain-event dependency.

Morale and Performance Review

The PERT concept applied to planning and control literally demands the active participation of high level functional personnel. In general practice the detail planning and subsequent control work is usually delegated to secondary staff people. Since the "doers" and the "planners" are different it has often happened that the direction of the plan and the actual direction of the program were only loosely related. By divorcing or estranging planning and performance, the performers felt only a mild sense of obligation to adhere to program boundaries.

PERT has changed this insofar as planning and performance cannot be disassociated. The event and activity time injected in the flow plan represent firm commitments by the person(s) responsible for performing the work. The importance of fulfilling the commitment seems to be a reflection of professional pride and competence. Therefore, an intelligent appraisal and evaluation of the situation is encouraged before events and activities are injected into the entire program. It would be reasonable to assume that if the program segments are well conceived the total program plan should be proportionately better. A good plan well conceived and forcefully executed can be a strong factor in building up organization esprit de corps.

Another consideration is the awareness by technical and scientific personnel that management now has a yardstick of performance evaluation and a means of frequent review. The proximity of planning and performance in one jurisdiction, accountable to an interested management, can stimulate accomplishment and bolster morale.

PERT Schedules Intellectual Activity

A constant source of irritation in program planning is the scheduling of intellectual activities. Scientific and administrative personnel have traditionally been loath to accept time limitations on creative work. As a consequence, scheduling has normally dealt more successfully with tangible accomplishments than with creativity. PERT attempts to show all significant program accomplishment points, including the scheduling of research, administrative activities and decision making. From present indications, it appears that PERT is achieving the scheduling of these points with more than minimal success. The acceptance of this type of scheduling can perhaps be attributed to psychological forces associated with the participative activities, the explanation of total program goals shown in series on interrelated events and increased morale.

PERT and Computers

One of the more important aspects of the PERT system is that its design permits use of the computer. The information is quantified and assembled and programmed into the computer where it can be quickly translated and accurately reported to management for rapid decision making. The quantification and programming of the information into the computers in this new application represents one of the foremost innovations of PERT.

Some of the PERT Problem Areas

In the past several years many new ideas, techniques and tools have been introduced on the business scene. Preliminary successes and elaborate publicity on some of these concepts have led management, in many instances, to embrace them with almost an appalling fanaticism. Quite often acceptance has been on the basis of insufficient study regarding adaptability to the unique problems of a particular business situation. Results have many times been disappointing and costly. Potentially good managerial tools have fallen into disrepute and have become the victims of fadism because of promiscuous application.

While the PERT system holds great promise and obviously can be useful in certain applications, words of caution against uncritical application are appropriate. Many problems pertaining to PERT still have to be solved. Some of the more critical problem areas are the human element, lack of correlation between progress and expenditure and some questions on scheduling practices.

The Human Element

After the total plan has been established, events identified and activity time estimated, the program can be reasonably quantified. However, the basic premises, such as the critical events and the estimated completion times continue to be based on personal evaluation—the human element.

Each contribution to the total program must be carefully analyzed. Incompetent evaluation, general optimism or pessimism can permeate the individual estimates and lead to skewing of the total program. It frequently happens, for example, that representatives of finance and manufacturing are conservative, whereas representatives of engineering and sales may lean toward fairly consistent optimism. Personal variations also exist within functions. Based on functional and personal variations, it would appear that some calibration of individual inputs is necessary to obtain a moderately accurate program forecast.

Another area where the human element cannot be ignored is the review periods when progress is interpreted in relation to schedule. Again, taking into consideration the varying dispositions of the contributing individuals, difficulties can be encountered as a consequence of poor status evaluation. For instance, many times a solution, although elusive, appears imminent and the fact that the problem has not been solved is discounted when giving information to the reviewer. Subsequent scheduled completion dates may not be satisfied because the imminent solution still has not been uncovered. The result may be a slippage of the entire schedule without any prior warning or opportunity to take corrective action. Of course, the converse can be true. While it is not common, completion of a program phase before its schedule time without adequate notification can lead to an uneconomical utilization of resources.

Training of personnel and constant performance evaluation can encourage more accurate forecasting, but it can never completely eliminate the human element. Cursory examination of PERT can obscure the fact that the critical premises are based on personal estimates. As long as this is so, no amount of scientific quantification or methodology can eradicate a foundation built on human error.

Lack of Correlation Between Progress and Expenditure

At least three basic ingredients are in every developmental program: Time, Function and Cost. If these three ingredients are not meaningfully interpreted, it is impossible to determine properly the true program status. A fundamental weakness of the PERT system as it now exists is the failure to correlate progress and expenditures.[8]

If schedule is the sole criteria for status determination, misleading assumptions may develop regarding the progress of the program. Schedules in many instances can be maintained at an accomplishment ratio disproportionate to ultimate function and cost considerations. Without cost inputs it could be possible to maintain schedules, at least initially, by large allocations of expensive resources. Later in the program, when remaining funds were inadequate or exhausted, the cost discrepancy would become apparent and the total status and net accomplishment would have to be reappraised. To date, PERT has not satisfactorily solved this very important problem.

Scheduling Practices

Where program review indicates a slippage of a critical event, re-scheduling takes place and new inputs are fed into the computer. Proportional changes are then made in the remainder of the program.

Again the human element in the problem cannot be ignored. The computer cannot think; it can only interpret information at a programmed rate. A computer cannot possibly accurately determine the net effect of the slippage of one critical event on all subsequent events. A critical development may slip schedule-wise, and in many instances proportional slippage does not take place in subsequent events. Related events and activities must be studied and analyzed in relation to new developments. Some events may be affected in direct proportion, other events may slide downstream disproportionately, while in still other instances events may not be adversely affected at all.

Another disturbing element in the PERT process is the method of determining the schedule pattern. The activity time computed by the formula $\dfrac{O + 4M + P}{6}$ represents an estimated average time. Average time assumptions may be adequate under certain conditions. But when they are predicated on an estimate of optimistic, most-likely and pessimistic times they can be skewed in one direction or the other by very high optimism or pessimism.

Quite often on the non-critical paths of the flow plan there is Slack Time. However, there is no Slack Time in the critical path and therefore, there does not appear to be sufficient schedule flexibility in the critical path to allow for unforeseen contingencies. Unless contingency time is initially calculated in the estimated activity times of events along the critical path, serious scheduling difficulties can be encountered.

Finally, it is not clear whether the final event shown on the network represents the committed contractual completion date. Professional schedulers normally build flexibility into the schedule and also provide contingency time between the final scheduled event and the actual requirement time.

Reporting to Management

Under PERT, reporting to management is on a highly systematic basis. The reports are printed out by the E.D.P. equipment on all events programmed into the computer. Most intelligent management is based on the exception principle. Busy managers do not have the time to examine endless information that does not require action and decision. Again, the human element must be injected into PERT. Reports must be condensed and recast for management to point up trouble spots with comprehensive analysis and evaluation of the difficulties. Mechanical reporting to date is neither discriminating nor elucidating enough.

Conclusions

The PERT system has primarily been used in association with program control on military contracts. The Government and defense contractors have been seeking means to correlate program planning and control into some meaningful system which will relate Time, Function and Cost. PERT has thus far not solved the Cost correlation problem, but has had signal success in relating accomplishment to Time and Function. The enthusiastic reception of PERT by the military services in defense contracting is evident in current requirements for PERT or PEP type planning and control systems as a prerequisite for the granting of new military business. If no other justification for the adoption of the system existed, this would exert sufficient pressure for the general adoption of the concept.

As currently conceived, the system is far from perfect. It has not been extensively tried in broad areas of operations planning and control. With some modifications and innovations, it might prove to be a very effective tool. As yet, the system is couched only in general terms as an experimental device in a relatively narrow application. Many of the firms using the system are exploring variations and adapting embellishments peculiar to their specific problems.

Uninhibited acceptance could lead to ultimate disillusionment. For example, small concerns with limited resources may find the system too complex and costly for adaptation. The outstanding criterion of success of the system has been with the Polaris missile. The installation cost of the system and its administration should be projected against potential benefits to be derived.

One of the greatest attributes of the concept is the acceptance of the idea and the participation by scientific, technical and administrative personnel. At this stage it may be too early to go overboard on that account since the idea is unique and has been highly publicized in defense contracting. It is even possible that the initial control groups may have responded to the stimulus of attention, à la the control group in the Hawthorne experiments.

Despite the existing weaknesses in the present system, it is a commendable step. PERT forcefully drives home to management the importance of planning and control. It takes an integrated methodological approach in solving an interrelated problem by encouraging participation and giving perspective; and finally it does attempt to simplify and quantify managerial decision making by elaborating and modifying several of the known managerial tools.

NOTES AND REFERENCES

1. The Air Force has also adapted a similar system under the designation, Program Evaluation Procedure (P.E.P.).
2. Fazar, W. Advanced Management Systems for Advanced Weapon Systems. (Presentation Abstract) Washington: U.S. Navy Special Projects Office, 1961.
3. Detailed information on the mechanics of the PERT system is available through the Special Projects Office of the Department of the Navy, Washington 25, D.C.
4. Barrett, B. B. Basic Principles of PERT/P.E.P. An address before the Controls and Planning Association, Los Angeles, March 22, 1961. For additional calculations in computing activity time, see Malcolm, D. G., Roseboom, J. H., Clark, C. E., and Fazar, W. Application of a Technique for Research and Development Program Evaluation. Operat. Res. 7:651-652, 1959.
5. Estimating the time distribution is more fully discussed in PERT Summary Report Phase 1. Washington: Special Projects Office, Bureau of Naval Weapons, Department of the Navy, 1958, p. 6.
6. Malcolm, et al., op. cit., p. 653.
7. PERT Summary Report Phase 1. Washington: Special Projects Office, Bureau of Naval Weapons, Department of the Navy, 1958, p. 13.
8. Research teams are now working on this problem.

15

Operations Research in Public Health

STIG ANDERSEN

THE spectacular progress of public health in certain parts of the world during the last century, and notably in the last half century, was a result of a cumulative interaction between a large number of factors, many of them associated with economic progress and the development of science. The prospering society could afford to buy more and more public health services, and improved public health in turn accelerated economic progress. At the same time, the technical means of the public health services were created and developed more or less in step with the increasing capacity of a prosperous society to apply them.

The situation in the less industrial countries by mid-twentieth century corresponds in some respects to the situation a hundred years earlier in Europe and the United States. Their economies cannot afford to buy adequate public health service, and the state of their national health hampers progress. The decisive difference, however, is that a large part of the inventions and experience in techniques gained elsewhere are available now to all nations to apply in logical systems as and when possible.

This relative preponderance of technical knowledge over economic capacity is the social fact which necessitates a new type of research. The research which is needed most at this time is not inventive. These societies are not in pressing need of new techniques and new inventions. Their demand is for systems composed of currently available techniques which give the optimal utilization of scarce economic resources. Research that satisfies this demand can be called operations research, at some risk of criticism from other employers of the term.

After a start in the military field in the 1940's, the techniques of operations research have been developed mainly in the field of industrial management. There is little likelihood that operations research in public health can reach a stage, for many years to come, where it can utilize directly many of the mathematical programing techniques which have been developed for military and industrial purposes. However, the basic concept of research into total systems which, in principle, can be translated into mathematical models can and should be adapted to the needs of public health services research. The name operations research implies research into some or all aspects of conducting or operating a system, a business, or a service, while treating the system as a living organism in its proper environment; thus it distinguishes itself from laboratory research.

Following are the major phases in operations research, adapted from Churchman and associates[1] and Houlden: [2]

1. Formulating the problem, including definition of the objectives.
2. Collection of data relevant to the problem.
3. Analysis of data to produce a hypothesis and a mathematical model to represent the system under study.
4. Deriving solutions from the model.
5. Choosing the optimal solution and forecasting results.
6. Testing the optimal combination of interventions, with controls built into the system to keep continuous check on the hypotheses.
7. Recommending implementation of the solution, including the control system.

The concept of an operations research team is an important aspect of the process. No one single person possesses all the necessary skills and experience to conduct worthwhile operations research. Usually a team in industry comprises scientists in the fields of mathematics, statistics, economics, and engineering, in addition to experts in the special field under study. Some teams also include a professional logician or a specialist in the science of scientific methods.

Applications to Public Health

The need for applying operations research to public health has been recognized by a few public health administrators in the United States and in the United Kingdom, for example, Committee on Enquiry[3] and Bailey,[4,5] particularly with respect to hospital planning.

Undoubtedly many public health administrators use methods implicitly akin to operations research. But I hope to demonstrate that explicit adoption of the operations research approach would benefit public health services of developing economies. It may be seen that operations research may be applied not only to the solution of detailed problems within the services but, more importantly, to larger systems within them and to the entire system of the public health service in the nation.

A modest attempt to apply operations research to one system within India's Public Health Service is being made by India's National Tuberculosis Institute in developing the national tuberculosis program. The institute is only at the beginning of its efforts, and only a few aspects have been described in published papers. Andersen and Piot[6] summarize the operations research approach of the NTI. Raj Narain[7] summarizes the extent of the problem; Waaler and associates[8] attempt a first formulation of an epidemetric model, and Banerji and Andersen[9] and Andersen[10] deal with certain sociological and economic aspects. A provisional "optimal combination of interventions" is suggested by Piot.[11]

The present paper attempts to foresee some of the types of problems which an operations research team in public health would face. These are divided into the seven major phases of operations research listed above, with the Indian experience as background.

Formulation of the Problem

The first and perhaps one of the most formidable challenges to the operations research team is the precise and explicit formulation of the problem. What is the system under study? Does it comprise the entire health field in the nation? Or can the team at least confine itself to that part which is under direct public control? How does the team define the boundaries of its field towards other public undertakings, the expenditure for which can be considered alternative to expenditure for public health? Can it evaluate public health output without comparisons with results of alternative investments? It is not unlikely that it may be found necessary to confine the first stages of a system analysis to one or a few local areas, and perhaps even, to begin with, to a given total budget, so as to reduce the total number of variables.

Even if, by this and other means, the system under study is brought down to manageable proportions, the team is left with an equally arduous task: the definition of objectives. At first glance it may appear puzzling that this should be part of the researcher's function. It is usually, and rightly, considered outside the province of the scientist, as a scientist, to decide or interfere with the objectives of a service, which are determined by the executive and ultimately by the people and its elected assemblies. However, in modern complex societies the popular will and even the executive's objectives are not necessarily transparent, and they are usually difficult to translate into scientific terms.

Conceivably the administrative and political heads of a public health service could be assumed to want "the maximum utilization of the given resources towards the promotion of health among the people," but the operations research team would require far more specific objectives than that. A major obligation of the team in the first stages of its work is to guide the executive toward very specific definitions of objectives. (If the team never achieved anything else, this would in fact be an extra-ordinarily valuable contribution.)

The team must stimulate the executive to define the objectives by presenting the logical alternatives. For example, taking a starting point in the above statement of objective, What is meant by "given resources"? Cannot the resources planned to be expended on health services be increased or reduced if the expenditure can be shown to be more or less profitable than assumed? What is meant by "promotion of health"? One might particularly wish to emphasize one of two entirely different aspects: (1) the state of health itself in a certain distribution in the population, which again might be viewed according to (a) absence of illness and (b) presence of positive health, or (2) the existence in reasonable proximity to the thus distributed population of a confidence-inspiring health service. Again, "among the people" must be far more sharply defined; assuming that equality is a guiding principle, are qualifications to the general equality principle to be considered permissible, for example, emphasis on highly productive groups or on children versus old people? Among the most difficult problems are those of the dynamics of the objectives: Should target dates be set? Or should the formulations be more dynamic and relate to the development over a period? If so, which period? And should they be related to the concomitant economic, demographic, and other social development?

Already at this stage the team will have to start considering the terms of the solutions, particularly on the output side. When the team—and the executive—have agreed on a set of general objectives, these have to be specified, perhaps in the form of indices, some of which probably can only be formulated in the course of data collecting.

Collection of Data

The collection of data is inextricably related to the formulation of objectives and the formulation of the hypothesis. Data collection, no doubt, is bound to be extensive, but it must also be strictly economical and strictly relevant to the objectives and the hypothesis. Data collection in present-day public health services research is perhaps relatively overdeveloped. A wealth of material, no end of official reports, and a considerable amount of scientific data become available every year, but this material is rarely, if ever, related to clearly formulated objectives and hypotheses, and it is therefore of far too little value for decision making. For this very reason, the operations research team will have to supplement existing data considerably. But it should only collect data that are strictly necessary for its other functions, and it should not be hesitant about making informed guesses when it finds that data collection on a particular subject is out of proportion in cost to the importance the data will have in the total system. Naturally, the team will rely extensively on sampling techniques. This is particularly true for a large part of the output functions, where a good deal of the information is to be collected among the general population.

On the input side, cost of services, training of personnel, handling medical stores, administrative and technical operations, the number of observations will often be too small for sampling. The major part of the data to be collected under this phase will be on the system as it now works and the results that are now obtained. But under many circumstances it will probably be necessary to supplement these data with a limited amount of data of a more experimental type. Such public health "experiments" have for example been found useful by India's National Tuberculosis Institute, which is conducting a series of comparisons of organizational approaches to tuberculosis control in a number of primary health unit blocks in southern India. The detailed protocols for these so-called operational investigations are available.[12]

For its data collection functions the research team will have to employ special investigators. Depending on the fields in which data are particularly lacking, medical officers, various kinds of paramedical technicians, accountants, social investigators, and demographic investigators may be needed. Most of these specialists must be given special courses in interviewing techniques.

One phenomenon must be mentioned in this context: the effect of observation on that which is observed. This is a difficult factor to deal with in all scientific inquiry, but it is particularly disturbing in operations research where experimental conditions cannot, in fact shall not, be established.

This observer effect must be kept constantly in view, both in the data collection and the test runs (where all devices must be employed to minimize its influence) and in the analysis, where the effect which nevertheless remains must be accounted for.

Analysis and Hypothesis Formulation

The formulation of the hypothesis or the construction of the model to represent the system under study may be considered the pivotal procedure of operations research in the fields where it is now relatively highly developed. By far the largest part of existing literature on operations research deals with the mathematical and statistical aspects of this phase of operations research. However, Eddison and associates[13] have reviewed operations research in industrial management in largely nonmathematical terms.

There is also no doubt that the pioneers in operations research in public health must strive, within a few years, to reach the stage where at least simple models depicting a public health service can be constructed. Such models will probably be input-output models of the type which are particularly employed in econometric research. However, for a system as complex as an entire national health service, with inputs that can only with the greatest difficulty be translated into common terms, and particularly with outputs of which the units vary from, say, average nutritional status of a population to satisfaction of the average health service consumer, it is unlikely that comprehensive and useful models, mathematically formulated, will result from the first few years of the research team's efforts. This does not by any means defeat the purpose of adopting operations research techniques in public health.

First, for some time, invaluable contributions can be made by the other phases of the research: the careful formulation of the problem and the objectives, the purposeful, economical collection of data, the precisely formulated and carefully evaluated test runs.

Second, while it may not be possible initially to formulate the model or the hypotheses mathematically, the operations research team can think mathematically, that is, logically, in making the formulation under this phase. Its members will think in terms of hypotheses, assumptions, parameters, and prognoses precisely expressed and systematized. By committing themselves they will expose themselves to the test of verification.

The model is a simplified explicit description of the existing services, the elements and factors of which it consists, and the relationships between them. It summarizes the input of resources: money, material, personnel training; preventive, curative, and educational services; and administrative, decision-making, and evaluating machinery; it outlines the geographic and functional distribution of such resources. It summarizes output partly with regard to operational achievement, public participation in services, and numbers of relevant health personnel actions (again geographically and functionally distributed) and partly in relation to fulfillment of declared objectives, including disease control, health promotion, demographic change, consumer satisfaction, and economic effects.

The construction of such a model, even if vastly simplified, is in itself complex. However, the research team cannot be satisfied before it has at least broadly outlined the relationships of the interactions of the public health system with the partly supplementary, partly competitive relationships between investments in public health and alternative investments.

The operations research team will, certainly in the first phases of its work, severely limit the scope of the model. As mentioned under definition of objectives, the team would perhaps also start with the assumption that present allocation of resources to the total public health service is an unchangeable parameter. Furthermore, it would restrict the measurement of objectives fulfillment in the model to a few simple indices. Finally, but not least, the team would attempt to construct the whole system on the basis of a manageable number of key variables. One of the several functions of the team is the selection of what is to be considered, at least provisionally, the key variables of the system. In such a complex system as a health service, no model or hypothesis can ever be expected to comprise all the innumerable interdependent variables of which the system consists. Among them, the team must choose the key variables, that is, the variables which if changed bring about the largest effect in the total system.

Though observation plays a considerable role when this choice is made, there can be no doubt that insight and more or less intuitive understanding of the system will be of decisive importance. This is the situation where all team members, with wisdom and patience, even humility, must sort out what is true insight from what is mere prejudice.

It is in the formulation of these hypotheses that teamwork is put to its acid test. There can be no strict delimitations of the functions of each team member. The logistics and methodology may well be largely contributed by the mathematician and the statistician, and the material knowledge by the public health administrator, the epidemiologist, the economist, and the sociologist, but unless they all gradually get a considerable grasp of each others' subjects they will be unable to make their full contribution.

Examples of factors which would be part of the model are:

Input: The total health budget, its geographic and functional breakdown, inflow and outflow of personnel, quantity and quality of training, inflow, storage, and consumption of durable and nondurable goods, and distribution of all types of health services and institutions.

Output: Operational achievements seen from the side of the services, including participation and attendance, vaccinations performed, number of childbirths assisted, wells constructed, drugs distributed. Otherwise the output part of the model can probably afford to be rather sketchy and give four or five indices, for example, demographic: crude or age-specific death rates and birth rates; epidemiologic: prevalence of two or three major diseases; and educational: at least one index of health educational status.

Derivation of Solutions From the Model

The manipulation of the model consists of a long continuous series of theoretical input changes in the model and calculation of the probable output changes. For example, input changes range from replacement of female health visitors with males and simplification of procedure for indenting supplies to major shift of emphasis from curative to preventive services and radical reforms in the organizational machinery or in the training of health personnel. The solutions theoretically carried out—on paper and in digital computers—will have the form of combinations of interventions in the existing system. The number of possible combinations of interventions, naturally, is virtually infinite.

However, several factors will restrict the number of combinations deemed worthy of study. First, the team's choice of key variables in the system (which may, admittedly, be revised in the course of the process of deriving solutions) will limit the number of even theoretically possible solutions. Second, the economist will constantly keep the team in check as to what is economically feasible; the public health administrator will have a similar function on administrative subjects; the epidemiologist will restrain enthusiasm, for example, concerning the possibilities of eradication of specific diseases; the sociologist will no doubt often have to remind the team of what is socially, psychologically, and politically acceptable; and the statistician and the mathematician will, among other tasks, certainly see that the imagination of the team does not transgress reasonable limits of calculability.

Finally, and most importantly, the common sense of all team members will restrict the field of theoretical study to sufficiently few combinations to make it possible to derive solutions before the administrators become too impatient about the results.

When this is said, however, one should not forget that it is exactly in the play of the creative imagination of the team, together with its scientific restraint, that hope lies for considerable improvement of the system under study. Within reasonable limits of realism and practicability, the team should play a free game with the multiple factors and relationships involved, combining and recombining until theoretically optimal combinations are approached. This "game" will consist of an iterative process of changing the value of a small number of variables while keeping the remaining variables constant. In this process, the team will pursue a number of intervention combinations, appearing virtually equally good, until it ends up with perhaps 5 or 10 combinations of which the output results seem to be of comparable magnitude.

Choice of Solution and Prognosis

Thus arriving at a limited number of intervention combinations, the team faces the choice of one of these solutions for testing. Under some circumstances the team may find it desirable and possible to test more than one solution.

Before making this choice the team consults the executive. The various intervention combinations are likely to differ from each other, particularly in two major respects: (a) the degree of departure from the existing system will vary, and (b) the solutions will differ in the degree to which they are calculated to fulfill each of the three, four, or five major objectives.

The team is now in a position to present the executive with a set of specified proposals for interventions, with details of changes needed in the system and consequences of these changes.

Once the choice of one or several combinations of interventions is made, the team works out the details of implementation of input changes and details of the prognosis of results, operationally as well as in terms of fulfillment of objectives.

These details should in the first instance be worked out only for the test run; they should specify the exact timetable of implementation. One would hazard to guess that much of the intervention would emphasize changes in training and would comprise a series of manuals detailing the functions of all personnel engaged in the public health services in the area.

Crucial to the solution is the prognosis. This prognosis will partly forecast the change in operational achievements and partly, the change in results (mostly in indices) with respect to the declared objectives. The task is, at least in principle, relatively simple as far as operational achievements are concerned: for example, specified changes in attendance at outpatient departments, a certain change in turnover of such and such drugs in the medical stores depot, a given number of new closed and chlorinated wells in so many villages distributed according to a given plan over the area.

But more difficult by far, both principally and practically, is the team's task of forecasting the results with respect to the general objectives, as it cannot afford to omit any of the major aspects of health and disease. For example, while incidence of smallpox may not necessarily figure in the model describing the existing situation, the forecast cannot exclude an opinion on the prospect of smallpox outbreaks.

One of the obstacles for the output forecast is the relatively slow development of health status, health consciousness, health action, or health habits. Even rather radical changes in several aspects are not observable in less than 5 or 10 years. The team will therefore probably have to select a range of indices with varying reliability and varying sensitivity so that changes in at least some of them are observable after a rather short time, say 2 years. If these indices are then, as one would expect, relatively unreliable, one must await their gradual confirmation by more reliable, but less sensitive, indices.

The form of the prognosis will largely be statistical and conditional, with results expressed, for example, as 19 in 20 chances of a value being within certain limits provided the operational achievement attains a given value and within certain other limits if the operational achievement attains such other value.

The Test Run

The test run is not a central part of operations research in industrial management, but it probably should play a key role in the application of operations research to public health services. Unlike industrial researchers, the team will be confronted with a large number of factors which will not be within their ambit of control, although the demand for health services is probably as foreseeable as the demand for, say, nylon stockings.

The most important characteristic of the test run is that, while limited geographically, it is true to life in every possible aspect. Of course, the observer effect will play a role; it is also inevitable that the personnel executing the test will know that they participate in a special program and that this will influence their behavior. These factors must be rigorously controlled, and in the evaluation of the test run they must, as far as possible, be taken into consideration.

Obviously, the test run is in no way spectacular, no showpiece. The test operators are, with as little fuss as possible, given new instructions to follow. In many cases these may not be strikingly different from existing ones, though probably often more explicit. The test run will also normally be within, or not significantly exceed, previous budgets, since the operations research team will always keep strictly within the limits of what is nationally applicable. Indeed, it is conceivable that the team will have arrived at a lower budget, put to better use than the previous one.

The test run area should be of manageable size, but it should be sufficiently large to provide observations for proper statistical inference.

The major difference between the test run and the final national implementation is that the former has a more intensive control system. Even the final implementation will have, of course, a carefully planned control system, but to derive full benefit from the test run the team will require a particularly good apparatus through which information on all aspects of the operations and their results are fed back. This feedback will continuously be analyzed and compared with the prognosis. Whenever key variables attain values outside the predetermined limits of variation, these new values must be fed into the model and the hypotheses, and the model solved anew. The question will soon arise as to what extent to allow changes in the test run programs, if they are wide of the mark. In principle, the test run should be allowed to run itself out without modification and new test runs in new areas applied if need be, but the team may have to compromise.

Although the operators and operations should themselves report on their performance, the test run will need additional staff to conduct sample investigations of the results (mainly interviews of population) and even local statistical assistance to cope with the data acquired.

Recommending Implementation

The last link in the chain of operations research is application of the solution to the whole system and establishment of evaluation machinery with an apparatus for new decision making when the key variables change beyond predetermined limits. In industry (and in the military field), such implementation follows more or less automatically after the final solution has been derived and tested, though even here the stockholders may insist on having their last say. In a public service, there may well be other obstacles to a rational solution.

This rationality may be questioned by the executive or by the public. Even when the rationality is recognized, the solution may be considered politically unacceptable to special groups or certain political parties, including the party in power. However, in principle, such factors should already have been taken into consideration by the research team. This is one of several justifications for the inclusion of a sociologist. Failure to have the scheme accepted can rightly be blamed on a team that did not appreciate the political climate in which it worked. For example, it is of little use if the team concludes that the whole health service, including general practitioners, should be nationalized, if the feelings and power of the medical profession or the public are such that this part of their solution is not feasible.

The recommendation for national implementation would probably in many cases, notwithstanding a successful test run, be in the form of recommendation for gradual extension, with a large pilot area to begin with, where the realism of the test-run-modified solution is put to a final test.

Minor Uses of Operations Research

Operations research is holistic. However, whole systems usually consist of many smaller ones. A national public health service is itself only a sector of a whole socioeconomic system, and the public health service in its turn comprises numerous large and small sectors and units, within many of which one can well visualize good use being made of operations research. Work on subsystems has, it would seem, far lower priority than the efforts described in the preceding paragraphs, but a team working in a country on a major effort might find it worthwhile to gain experience from small systems.

One example of a subsystem which would no doubt be fertile ground for operations research in many countries is the medical stores system. Considerable loss in operational efficiency is sustained in some countries because the medical stores take months, even years, to expedite indents, and this often occurs at the same time that the stores have to dispose of, and occasionally even destroy, items which have become obsolete.

The team might also try to solve subordinate problems within the main system before or as part of the whole solution. Examples are optimal size of area and population to be covered by midwife, smallpox vaccinator, or basic health unit; ideal vehicle for local health workers; administrative management solutions leaving maximum time for technical personnel to use their skills; architectural design of hospitals and health centers; queueing in outpatient departments and hospital waiting lists; integration of specialized services developed on an emergency basis outside the general health services.

The Operations Research Team

Operations research can be a more or less continuous process, or it can be a valuable one-time effort. Once a team has gone through the procedure described above, the service will presumably have been considerably improved. For a small national health service, such a procedure, or perhaps gradually a more simplified one, could be repeated at economical intervals. For a large country, for example the three or four largest in Asia, operations research could be perpetual. The team here would be employed, perhaps equally, in overall systems research and in work on subsystems.

With such a variation in the requirements, it is difficult to suggest general rules for the size and composition of the operations research team. However, some features would be more or less common to all such teams. The minimum composition is probably a public health administrator, an epidemiologist, a mathematician, a statistician, and a social scientist. Larger teams should probably also comprise a sanitary engineer and an educationist, and the general social scientist should be replaced by an economist and a sociologist. To these must be added, because the team must have its own data collection apparatus and test-run evaluation system, a number of investigators of various categories, perhaps 10, 20, or more, and perhaps as many junior statisticians and statistical clerks.

Finally, if the team cannot rely on outside assistance in computer programing, it must have its own programer, with full-time use of statistical processing machinery and part-time use of a digital computer.

Many skeptics will say, "This is just common sense, with a superstructure of fine new words." Operations research is very little but common sense. This is perhaps even more true when it is admitted that in the first stages of applying operations research in public health services, mathematical models may be of limited relevance. The essence of operations research is that logical thought, combined with careful observation and methodological analysis, should form the basis for decision making. Adoption of such a principle may not appear revolutionary, but in an irrational world the public health service that carries it out to its full logical consequence, abiding by its sometimes exacting commands, would be likely to find itself vastly improved. The methodological study of alternative courses of action can, of course, be given many names; probably most operations researchers would be proud to have their science known as the science of common sense.

Other skeptics assert that operations research can never replace experience. Human experience is a more or less unconscious collection of data and analysis of data by an individual or a group of individuals. But experience is often unreliable, is often narrow and biased. Scientific methods can remove the bias and insure that data are properly systematized to give a true picture of the past and a more reliable forecast of the future, including the probable outcome of intended executive action. They can also give a measure of the so-called imponderables by calculating probabilities of occurrences.

REFERENCES

1. Churchman, C. W., Ackoff, R. L., and Arnoff, H. L. Introduction to Operations Research. New York: Wiley, 1957.
2. Houlden, B. T. (Ed.) Some Techniques of Operational Research. London: Hazell Watson & Viney Ltd., 1962.
3. Committee of Enquiry (Guillebaud Committee) into the Cost of the National Health Service: Report. London: Her Majesty's Stationery Office, 1956.
4. Bailey, N. T. J. Operational Research in Hospital Planning and Design. Operat. Res. Quart. 8: 149, 1957.
5. Bailey, N. T. J. Operational Research. In Welford, A. T., Argyle, M., Glass, D. V., and Morris, J. N. (Eds.) Society, Problems and Methods of Study. London: Routledge & Kegan Paul Ltd., 1962.
6. Andersen, S., and Piot, M. The Operations Research Approach. In Souvenir of the 18th All-India Tuberculosis and Chest Diseases Workers' Conference, Bangalore. 1962.
7. Narain, Raj. Size and Extent of the Tuberculosis Problem in Urban and Rural India. Indian J. Tuberc. 9: 147-150, 1962.
8. Waaler, H. T., Geser, A., and Andersen, S. The Use of Mathematical Models in the Study of the Epidemiology of Tuberculosis. Am. J. Publ. Hlth. 42: 1002-1013, 1962.
9. Banerji, D., and Andersen, S. Bull. WHO. In press.
10. Andersen, S. Some Aspects of the Economics of Tuberculosis in India. Indian J. Tuberc. 9: 176-180, 1962.
11. Piot, M. Outline of a District Tuberculosis Programme. Indian J. Tuberc. 9: 151-156, 1962.
12. National Tuberculosis Institute. Protocols for Operational Investigations. Bangalore, India, 1961. (Mimeo.)
13. Eddison, R. T., Pennycuick, K., and Rivett, B. H. P. Operational Research in Management. London: English Universities Press, Ltd., 1962.

16

On Indices for the Appraisal of Health Department Activities

ANTONIO CIOCCO

AMONG the forces contributing to the ecologic pattern of disease in a community, one cannot overlook the efforts of the organized health agencies. Through the application of knowledge of the natural history of various diseases these agencies have sought to raise the health level of the community by influencing, in one way or another, the incidence, prevalence, and severity of disease.

It is the purpose of this paper to describe major historical aspects of the development of statistical indices for the appraisal of such organized community health activities and to discuss certain principles to be considered in the formulation of adequate indices of accomplishment.

Some 30 years ago, Wade Hampton Frost[1] noted that ". . . the health officer occupies the position of an agent to whom the public entrusts certain of its resources in public money and cooperation, to be so invested that they may yield the best returns in health; and in discharging the responsibilities of this position he is expected to follow the same general principles of procedure as would a fiscal agent under like circumstances." His thesis was that the demonstration of accomplishment should be supportd by a simple and unquestioned theory about the activity under study in conjunction with adequate statistical data, ". . . for while the facts expressed in a statistical record constitute only a part of the evidence required, they constitute the part which can be most conveniently and forcibly presented and are essential to any quantitative statement of results achieved.

"If we really desire to submit our judgement of what is being accomplished to this final test of statistical evaluation we must set about collecting statistics which will serve the purpose."

It may seem remarkable that Frost wrote in this vein as late as 1925. His statement implied, first, that not all statistics on health and disease in the community were appropriate to measure the results achieved by health departments and, second, that the logical bases for a quantitative evaluation of these results were often lacking. As we shall see, both implications find considerable justification even today.

Evaluation by Mortality and Natality Statistics

The formal gathering of statistics originated several centuries ago to provide government with data on the conditions of the governed. The collection of data on population, births, deaths, and other demographic characteristics was initiated primarily to furnish the state with information on which to base policy decisions. Graunt's interest in vital statistics (1662), of which he is considered the founder, resulted in part from his preoccupation with what now is called urban planning or redevelopment.[2] The Memoires des Intendants, summarized in the classic work of Moheau (1778), were the seventeenth and eighteenth century equivalent of Reports of the President's Council of Economic Advisers. The statistics on deaths were used simply to describe existing conditions and hardly ever to evaluate governmental efforts in the field of health. Perhaps this was so because no one expected that governmental effort could do much about improving health conditions. Where, instead, governmental effort was considered to be deciding, as in the maintenance of an adequate food supply, pertinent statistics were employed to measure the results. Thus, Graunt pointed with pride to the data which showed that in London only a few persons died of starvation.

The statistical index which first served to measure the health condition of the community and which was already in use in Graunt's time was the mortality rate or its equivalent. (With Halley's contribution (1693), mortality was also measured in terms of survivorship and average life expectancy.) However, until the middle of the nineteenth century, students of vital statistics emphasized the regularity of the age distribution of deaths year after year and, save for epidemic years, the relative constancy of mortality from year to year in any one locality. Süssmilch,[3] in the late eighteenth century, attributed such regularity to a "Divine Order," while Quetelet,[4] 100 years later, attributed the same regularity to "natural law." So far as can be determined, mortality did occur at a fairly constant rate during this period. This constancy in rate, incidentally, encouraged the use of life tables and the extension of mathematical actuarial theory. It is of interest to speculate whether the growth of insurance companies in the eighteenth century would have been as marked if the annual rate of mortality had not been constant.

Interest in the variation in mortality and survivorship rates existed, but mainly to identify etiological factors. In the works of Graunt,[5] of Süssmilch,[6] and of Quetelet,[7] differences in mortality were examined in terms of sex, urbanism, climate, topography, and other physical and social environmental conditions to discover causes of variation, not to measure the effectiveness of community health work or to determine policy in this field.

Data were collected simply to describe the health problems, since there were no organized community health activities, and especially since ideas on what to do about the problems were lacking. Quetelet's *La physique sociale* (1835), the best example of midnineteenth century quantitative study of community health problems, makes it clear that the major preoccupation was with mortality. The impression is obtained that survival was the primary goal of the community. In a chapter devoted to statistical measurement of the prosperity of a population, Quetelet suggested use of the index: number of births divided by number of deaths in a specified unit of time. He pointed out that when this index is above unity, health conditions of the population are favorable; when it is less than unity, conditions are unfavorable. Some 70 years later Raymond Pearl was to reintroduce this index, which he called the Vital Index of Population.

This index provides a limited interpretation of the health conditions of a community since the numerical value of the index for a community with high mortality and high natality could be the same as that for a community with low mortality and low natality.

Public Health Movement

The Public Health Movement and the bacteriologic discoveries which began almost simultaneously in the middle of the nineteenth century brought ". . . to the mind of the average man the conception that life and death are not merely dispensations of divine providence but lie within the control of the human mind and the human will. . . ."[8] This was a marked change in social attitude and it was reflected in a changed approach toward the collection of statistics related to health problems. The new approach was characterized by:

Attention to Cause of Death With Particular Reference to Infectious Diseases. Interest in the publication of data on deaths by cause led to the study of classifications of causes of death by the first International Statistical Congress (1853), and eventually in 1900 to the adoption of the International List of Causes of Death which, with revisions, is in use today.

Comparisons of Mortality Rates Between Localities for Purposes of

Stimulating Community Action to Improve Environmental Conditions. Spurred by the conviction, so ably presented by Chadwick (1842) and others, that the removal of filth and the correction of insanitary conditions would reduce epidemics and mortality from the epidemic diseases, the higher mortality for one community in comparison to that of another was regarded as an indication that the former required additional sanitary action. No longer were comparisons among communities made solely to reveal possible reasons for differences, but they were made in order to emphasize the amount of work to be done by the community with the higher mortality. Pettenkofer's[9] (1873) remarks in comparing Munich's mortality with that of London illustrate this point. "If it was possible in London, in historical time, to reduce the death rate from 42 to 22 per thousand, we are well justified in hoping that in Munich too, we may be able to come down with our death rate, from 33 to 22. All we have to do is find out what factors and measures have contributed in London to this propitious result and to apply them intelligently to our conditions in Munich."

Consideration of the Amount of Sickness. Systems of compulsory reporting of selected communicable diseases were initiated in many communities to provide the health authorities with data on the number of cases of disease and their distribution in the population. In addition, increasing interest was expressed in the sickness and disability which accompany disease. Pettenkofer[10] estimated the reduction in number of days of sickness and in costs that would result from a reduction in number of deaths. (He assumed 34 cases of sickness for every death, 20 days of disability for every case of sickness, and a total of one florin per day of disability in loss of wages and expenditure for medical and hospital care.) John Shaw Billings, while still a military medical officer in 1878, suggested to the Surgeon General of the U.S. Army that the population census of 1880 include information on sickness because: "As is pointed out by the Royal Sanitary Commission of England, however complete the registration of deaths may be it cannot give a fair estimate of the sickness which is not fatal, it cannot indicate where or how these are to be prevented, it cannot tell the cost which it is worth incurring for their diminution." Actually, this suggestion that the 1880 census include information on sickness was followed, and for the first time in this country statistics on sickness and disability became part of the measurements of health problems.

In brief, it would appear that in conjunction with increasing knowledge about specific diseases, with greater assurance that certain diseases could be prevented and with wider acceptance of the view that health was not simply the absence of death, data were collected on specific causes of death and on sickness and were utilized as indices of required activity for the solution of health problems. These historical associations and all that they entail must be borne in mind in order to understand the factors which have brought about the development of the indices of health department activities in current use.

Statistical Appraisal of Health Department Activities

In this country, the growth of governmental health activities, which to a large extent resulted from the Public Health Movement, manifested itself in terms of increase in both numbers of health departments and types of activities. Chapin[11] described well the evolution in types of activities: "The sanitarians of the nineteenth century, up to about 1870, were, except for maritime quarantine, occupied chiefly with the problems of municipal cleanliness. . . . The attempt to control contagion became the chief function of the health department for the next fifty years. . . . During the last twenty years or so [Chapin was writing in 1921], a new phase of public health work has been evident. Attention is being directed more and more, not only to persons, *but to individual persons.* Education has become one of the most important factors, and it is the education of the individual which is aimed at. Cure also must be personal and individual. The great health movements, like the movement against tuberculosis and that against venereal diseases, the hookworm campaign in the South, the prevention of infant mortality and the medical supervision of school children, all seek out the individual, teach right ways of living and offer treatment." Today we can add to this list such movements as those aimed at the control of cancer, heart disease, and mental disorders.

At the same time, ideas regarding the collection and utilization of statistics to appraise health department activities began to be formulated in a more definitive manner. Shattuck[12] in 1850 had recommended sanitation surveys along the lines of his report on Massachusetts. Both in this country and in the United Kingdom, community surveys were actually carried out. They attempted to measure the health problems of the community and indirectly appraised the activities of the government. The most far-reaching of these surveys in this country, from the standpoint of the development of statistical indices, was that undertaken by the American Public Health Association's Committee on Municipal Health Department Practice (now Committee on Administrative Practice) in cooperation with the U.S.

Public Health Service and the Metropolitan Life Insurance Company.[13] This survey, which obtained data on the health activities of 83 cities, was the origin of the establishment of the Association's Evaluation Schedule "for use in the study and appraisal of community health programs." Until a few years ago, the use of this schedule included the calculation of indices for purposes of comparing one community with another. In the 1947 schedule,[14] for example, formulas for calculating over 130 ratios or indices were provided, and suggestions were made for comparing 32 of these ratios with either ideal or the best of observed indices. It is revealing to note the kinds of indices which are suggested: percentage of hospital beds in approved hospitals; population per practicing physician and per practicing dentist; percentage of population in communities over 2,500 served with approved water and with approved sewerage systems; percentage of rural school children served with approved water supplies and with approved means of excreta disposal; percentage of food handlers reached by group instruction program; percentage of restaurants and lunch counters with satisfactory facilities; percentage of bottled milk pasteurized; percentage of children under 2 years given immunization for diphtheria, smallpox, whooping cough; newly reported cases per tuberculosis death; tuberculosis deaths per 100,000 population; percentage of tuberculosis cases reported by death certificates; percentage of contacts of newly reported tuberculosis cases examined; percentage of syphilis cases reported in primary, secondary, and early latent stages; contacts reported per 100 cases in primary, secondary, and early latent stages; percentage of reported syphilis contacts examined; peurperal deaths per 1,000 total births; percentage of antepartum cases under medical supervision before the sixth month; percentage of women delivered at home under postpartum nursing supervision; percentage of births in hospital; deaths under 1 year of age per 1,000 live births; deaths from diarrhea and enteritis under 1 year per 1,000 live births; percentage of infants under nursing supervision before 1 month; percentage of entering school children examined with parent present; percentage of elementary school children with dental work completed; deaths from motor accidents per 100,000 population; deaths from home accidents per 100,000 population; cents per capita spent by the health department.

In more recent revisions of this guide (1955),[15] suggestions are made to collect data that may be used to calculate the above types of indices but less emphasis is given to the calculation of indices. In line with newer public health practices, community agencies are asked questions such as: How many children were served last year in well-child conferences, under age 1, 1 to 2 .. 5 to 6? However, they are not told to calculate ratios or averages. Greater interest in certain chronic diseases, such as cancer, heart disease, diabetes, mental hygiene, industrial hygiene, health education, social services, and rehabilitation, is demonstrated by expansion of sections devoted to these activities; but suggestions for the appraisal of activities are usually in the form of questions such as: "What detection center and cancer clinic facilities are available in the community?" "Does the educational program reach: (a) physicians, (b) nurses, (c) dentists, (d) general public?"

The changes in public health activities described previously by Chapin[16] brought about introduction of indices which serve *to measure the operations of the health departments rather than the bearing of these operations on the health of the community or the survivorship of its people.* Some of these indices are easy to interpret in terms of the effectiveness of health department activities to reduce disability or prolong life. In these terms, the percentage of children under 2 years of age given immunization for diphtheria has meaning. There is evidence of the effectiveness of such immunization to prevent diphtheria (provided that the organism remains unchanged) and consequently, if all of the children have been immunized at a young age, we can anticipate that the prevention of sickness and death from diphtheria has been accomplished. It is less easy to interpret, in terms of reduction of sickness or death, an index such as the proportion of food handlers who have received group instruction, or an index based on the number of persons who receive educational material. Greenberg and Mattison[17] (1955) point out that the latter index may be used as a measure of a step in the evaluation of the effectiveness of health educational literature in eventually reducing morbidity and mortality. This view would assume that the succeeding steps actually will achieve the final objective of the health department activity. The burden of proof for such an assumption is on the users of the index.

Apparently, the formulation of statistical indices currently suggested or employed to appraise health department activities are based both on the degree of knowledge of the factors which affect health and on tenets which underlie current public health practices. It is interesting to note also:

(1) Mortality rates still occupy a central place among appraisal indices as shown by the number of these rates mentioned. In part, this may be due to the noticeable lack of data on sickness and disability which only very recently is being remedied. In part, it may be due to a

continued preoccupation with survival on the part of the community. In this respect, it may be that the general public lags behind the public health worker who has set as his objective to achieve something more than absence of disease. On the other hand, the public health worker has shown only limited interest in the collection of data on sickness and disability, let alone on other signs of variation in health status.

(2) Indices for the appraisal of health department activities aimed at such chronic conditions as cancer, heart disease, and mental disorders tend *to measure activities directed at health professions and facilities rather than at the disease status of the community*. For example, questions are asked regarding the existence of special provisions for the continuous care of children with rheumatic fever and the agencies responsible for those provisions, but not regarding the number of children with rheumatic fever in the community, the number under continuous care, the number not under care and the reasons for this, or regarding the disability experience of both groups. When mortality or morbidity statistics are available on some of these chronic disease conditions, they are employed mainly for comparisons among communities in order to explore possible etiological factors rather than to appraise the relative effectiveness of the activities of the communities. This approach is similar in many respects to the situation observed a century ago. Again, it could be an indication of a feeling of helplessness regarding any measure of prevention or control.

(3) A new feature of the current utilization of appraisal indices is that of comparing observations in the community with standards established by experts. Some of these standards represent objectives more or less theoretically possible, as would be the case of setting the standard of infectious diseases rates at zero; others represent generalization of experiences which are considered to indicate adequacy, as in setting the standards of relative number of general hospital beds equal to that found in the 12 states with the highest relative number; others represent the rationalizations of the hopes and convictions of students of the subject. The tendency to follow this approach reveals perhaps that public health workers still retain faith in someone's ability to achieve complete understanding of the means of meeting community health problems. It seems unnecessary to point out that such an approach could be dangerous. It could lead to blind reliance on authority, or worse yet, to a smug satisfaction with conditions which satisfy current opinions.

Interpretation of Statistical Indices of
Health Department Activities

As should be clear now, many statistical indices have been introduced to appraise health department activities. The multiplication of these indices corresponds to the increase in number and scope of health department activities. The construction of an index is mechanically a simple procedure. But the interpretation to be given to variations in the numerical value of an index is ordinarily a complex analytical operation, involving an understanding of the elements of the index, the phenomenon it actually measures, the factors which influence variations in the phenomenon, and the relationships between the phenomenon and the health status of the community. Even when dealing with an index such as the infant mortality rate, long recognized as being a sensitive measure of well-defined objectives of health agencies, the interpretation of differences among communities is not so simple. For example, in Pennsylvania 62 of the 67 counties do not have a local health department or carry out organized local health activities. The median infant mortality rate of these counties in 1956 was 22.7. In the neighboring state of Ohio there are 13 counties with full-time health departments, in New York there are 16 counties with full-time health departments. The medians of the infant mortality rates in these counties with health departments in 1956 were 24.6 for Ohio and 22.9 for New York. In other words there are a number of counties in Pennsylvania which have no organized local community health activities yet which have a better record in terms of infant mortality than do counties with health department activities. Similar observations can be made regarding other indices and other comparisons. The point is that *comparisons among communities or within communities require a logical analytic approach*. In the case of the comparisons just cited, it may well be that communities with well-trained physicians and a population characterized by a high level of education and understanding of health problems will have a low infant mortality even though health agencies do not exist. The appraisal of health department activities must take into consideration the specific role of the health agency as well as the general effects of progress in public health concepts. These concepts are acquired by the community as part of its social evolution, in which the health department participates.

In seeking for quantitative indicators of the effectiveness of the operations of health agencies, the same logical approach is required as for the measurement of the effects of any procedure on the behavior and reactions of groups of mice or men. This was emphasized some time ago by Edgar Sydenstricker,[18] who in 1926 outlined certain principles which should guide the measurement of public health work. According to his views: (1) "Specific activities, rather than the program as a whole, should be measured first." (2) "The objectives and methods of a public health effort should be clearly defined." (3) "Principles of experimentation should be applied." (4) "The use of 'experimental' and 'control' groups or areas should be followed."

These principles, which parallel those set forth relative to physiologic experimentation by Claude Bernard in 1865, were further amplified and illustrated in the Pittsburgh Conference on Methods in Public Health Research in 1950.[19] It is unnecessary to discuss them in great detail but certain of their consequences deserve elaboration since they are pertinent to the topic of this paper. They are those referable to (1) formulation and selection of numerical indices, (2) comparisons of effectiveness of health activities among and within communities.

Formulation and Selection of Appraisal Indices. Any reaction or behavior manifestation of the population group or of the health department which can be counted or measured may be used as the basis for an index. This may be expressed in the form of a ratio—proportion of school beginners immunized—or an average—mean duration of life. It means that the numbers of indices which can be formulated are many, and the issue is to select among the many possible indices those that satisfy best the logical requirements of all measurements and, specifically, of measurements of the effectiveness of health department activities. Logical requirements of measurements in field studies were stated at the 1950 Pittsburgh Conference of the Public Health Study Section: "The measurements used should be: 1. Objective; 2. Repeatable by different observers and at different times; 3. Efficient in terms of clear and mutually exclusive divisions, undistorted scale, and broad range of values to be recorded; 4. As simple, generally available, easily performed, and inexpensive as possible; 5. Accurate in sensitivity and specificity; 6. Tested in pilot study."

In line with these requirements, a first consideration pertinent to the selection of an appraisal index is that the elements of the index, the counts or measurements of the things or activities under scrutiny, are objective, reliable, accurate, and easily obtainable. All things being equal, the most appropriate data would be those derived from some routine operation which is independent of the specific health department activity. To the extent that birth and death certification, disease

reporting and registration, governmental· census, school and other institutional records, etc. are reliable and accurate, they provide data
that are easily obtained and objective, i.e., persons involved in the
activity cannot interject bias in the observation. For certain specific
activities, however, such as "classes for expectant mothers," it is difficult to obtain routine independent data that could conceivably relate
to an appraisal of this activity which seeks to engender a wholesome
attitude about pregnancy and childbirth. To obtain direct or indirect
measurements for the evaluation of such activities requires that either
a mechanism for independent objective appraisal be established as part
of the activity or that independent objective appraisals be carried out
from time to time. In either case, a research project must be undertaken with appraisal as its purpose.

A second consideration pertinent to the formulation of indices is
availability of knowledge about the properties of the ratio or average
employed, and of the factors which are related to variations in its numerical value. Mortality, morbidity, case fatality rates, ratios of health
facilities and personnel to population, and so on measure with greater
or less precision many aspects of the interaction between man and his
total environment. To use these rates or ratios as indicators of the
effectiveness of health department activities assumes that their characteristics and the factors related to their variation are understood and,
furthermore, that the health department activity is also a factor in
that variation. As an illustration, the ratio of hospital beds per 1,000
persons is correlated with the ratio of physicians per 1,000 persons; both
are highly correlated with the degree of wealth and with "cultural"
facilities, such as centers of learning, available in the community. Any
attempt at appraising some specific health department activity, even
one devoted to the adminstration of Hill-Burton funds, through the use
of the ratio of hospital beds per 1,000 persons must take into consideration the dependency of both number of hospital beds and health department activity on the wealth and high level of education in
the community. Similarly, the validity of using an index based on per
capita expenditure for the health department as a measure of acceptance
of the health department by the community depends on the means by
which the budget of the community is decided upon, and the extent to
which the health department's activities are a factor in the decisions
reached. Knowledge regarding the infant mortality rate and the factors
related to its variation has served to give this rate the standing of a
general index of health department activity. High mortality among
infants is due in large part to infectious diseases and is indicative of the

incidence and prevalence of these and other diseases with a common origin in ignorance, poverty, lack of sanitation, and of good hygienic practices. Use of the infant mortality rate as an index which appraises health department activities aimed at improvement of sanitation, raising of hygienic standards, and prevention and control of infectious diseases is amply justified in principle. However, as has been mentioned, community actions in addition to health department activities play a role in the variation in the numerical value of this index.

A third and most important consideration in formulating appraisal indices is that of establishing the nexus between an index and the objective of the activity it is supposed to measure. This nexus can be correctly perceived only when the objective of the health department activity is stated precisely and unequivocally. Confusion is often created when a variety of objectives are included under a term that could be understood to mean a single activity, e.g., well-child conference, mental hygiene, or cancer control. For example, cancer control programs in this country may have a number of different specific objectives, from the maintenance of a tumor registry to the operation of diagnostic services. An index of appraisal for the former should be based on the completeness and accuracy of the registry, for the latter it should be based on the accuracy, stage, and timing of diagnosis, on the load it carries for the community, or, if its function includes follow-up, the outcome of the diagnoses. For the registry an index based on cancer morbidity, incidence or prevalence would make little sense; it might be appropriate under certain conditions for services.

Comparisons Among Communities and Within Communities. It has been mentioned that with the development of the public health movement, comparisons among communities were employed to indicate what could be accomplished. For this purpose such comparisons may be worth while, particularly if differences among communities serve to stimulate the public health authorities to probe more deeply into the specific health department activities which may have resulted in the observed differences. But it is precisely at this point that difficulties are encountered, for an appraisal of *specific* health department activities requires the disentanglement of the action of the health department from pertinent conditions in the community. Even when dealing with such a well-established measure as diphtheria immunization, comparisons cannot be easily interpreted. Differences among communities in diphtheria mortality obviously will reflect differences in the operation of the health agency. However, the factors which relate to the differences in activity may be of many kinds: personnel, facilities, cooperation of the medical society, public acceptance, and level of diphtheria experience in preceding years. Unless in some way the factors that affect differences are taken into consideration, such comparisons have meaning only to reveal that one community has more problems than another. Comparisons become even more difficult to interpret, for example, when dealing with the number of defects found at school health examinations for the prevention of which there are no specific health department activities. For such indices, it is not immediately obvious what factors to take into account to achieve meaningful comparisons.

On the surface, long-term comparisons in the same community would seem to offer easier interpretation. Observations are made at one initial point of time, a public health measure is introduced, and changes in the health condition are observed. Again, suppose we take as illustration a well-established procedure such as diphtheria immunization. The case or mortality rate at a certain point in time is measured, the immunization program is introduced, and the changes in the rate are observed. In this instance the community serves as its own standard of comparison. This is valid *if no other changes in the community occur which may produce the same effects.* For a specific procedure such as diphtheria immunization, this would not be expected, yet even for such an activity the results in one community might or might not be related to direct action by the staff of the health department. As an example of the former, the well-known antiyaws campaign in Haiti might be cited because it achieved practically universal compulsory treatment. In other instances, the results could be due to the indirect effects of the educational efforts of the health department which have led to action on the part of parents, of medical practitioners, etc.

When dealing with less specific health department activities, particularly those that concern some aspect of social behavior, it becomes more difficult to determine whether or not changes in health conditions are a product of the health department's activity. In such circumstances, a comparison group, a standard, or "control" is definitely needed.

Establishing criteria for the selection of comparison groups which will provide a basis of meaningful interpretation is a particularly difficult problem. One such criterion is obviously that the "experimental" and "control" groups should be selected without bias. However, it is necessary to secure the cooperation of the group which is going to submit to the experiment. This attitude of cooperation, however, can itself prejudice the experiment. Furthermore, it is difficult to find two groups that are alike in all but the activity under study. If this activity is to be publicized and is stated to be something "good," how can one expect the "control" group not to want it also? Except for the Newburgh-Kingston study of fluoridation and reduction of dental caries, there have been few situations in which this problem has been successfully met. Several approaches to this problem might be attempted. I shall describe two which we outlined for specific situations.

In the first of these, it was felt that for political reasons once its use was announced no community could be deprived of a prophylaxis procedure even though it was still very much in the experimental stage. This is a view which public officials as well as medical practitioners hold when a new drug or procedure catches the public's fancy. To avoid political repercussions and still achieve some means of evaluating the procedure, the following steps were suggested: (1) measurement of the status of the population of the total area containing the several communities with respect to the disease condition under study; and (2) introduction of the prophylaxis procedure gradually, a few communities at a time, the selection of the communities to follow a plan whereby certain communities would serve as "controls" for a given period of time.

In the second, efforts were being made to improve simultaneously the general economic condition and the health program of certain areas of a country. In developing possible designs for the evaluation of the program the following considerations seemed important:

(1) Improvement in the economic and educational level is anticipated throughout the whole country. Therefore, we must expect that the effects of this improvement in terms of increased demand for health services and increased realization of health problems will be country-wide.

(2) The study area will be most affected by these anticipated economic and social improvements and consequently will be expected to reveal a higher increase in demand for health services and in realization of health problems than other areas of the country. However, within this area there will also undoubtedly be variations in the degree of economic and social improvement.

(3) When the details of the program are publicized, other areas within the country will seek to adopt one or more aspects of the program.

In view of these considerations, it seemed rather hopeless to set up fixed "control areas." That is, there was no point in asking the question: Has the utilization and quality of services improved more in the study area than in area X (where area X is comparable to the study area except for the program)? Instead, the question was rephrased as follows: Has the utilization and quality of services improved at a greater rate than expected, relative to economic changes, in those parts of the study area and in other areas where the program has been put into effect than in the areas of the country in which the program has not been put in operation?

To answer this question means that we must (a) obtain indices both of economic and social development and of improvement in health services for all the communities of the country for the period in which comparisons are desired; (b) measure the relationship between improvement in economic and social conditions and improvement of health services in all of the country where the essential parts of the program have been put in operation and where they have not; (c) make comparisons of changes in health services primarily between those areas in which similar changes in economic and social conditions have taken place.

Summary

This review of the development of health department appraisal indices and outline of some of the logical criteria required for the correct interpretation of variations in these indices reveal a number of points that are important for establishing quantitative measures of the effects of community health activities.

The existence of information on mortality led to the utilization of mortality statistics, first, as a measure of the health status of the community; later, as a tool in the search for etiological factors and as a means of arousing the community to action; and, finally, as an index of achievement of community health work.

Increase in knowledge about etiological factors of certain causes of death, demonstrations of the preventability of certain disease conditions, and a growing community realization that health is not simply absence of death were accompanied by the initiation of routine procedures to collect data on specific causes of death, sicknesses, immunity status, etc., and to utilize these data for the construction of indices to measure health needs of the community as well as the achievements of its health agency.

Meanwhile, spurred on by a broadening definition of health, community health agencies have moved toward activities which are less directly or immediately concerned with death or infectious diseases.

As a result, available mortality and morbidity statistics have become less useful and less appropriate for the construction of indices to measure achievement, and are being replaced by data on the amount of health department operations and on the extent of health facilities and personnel in the community. In formulating appraisal indices of activities derived from the broader concepts of public health, the focus of interest has shifted from a consideration of the health status of the community to that of volume and kinds of health services and facilities provided. Consequently, variations in these indices are difficult to interpret in terms of the adequacy with which health needs of the community are being satisfied.

It is also difficult to assess, from these and other appraisal indices, the actual contribution which the activities of a health agency has made in meeting certain health and disease problems of the community. Each health agency is an integral part of the community, and changes in philosophy and activities of an agency are reflected in, and reflect, changes in philosophy and activities of its community. By the direct examination of changes in the numerical value of the indices, it is not always possible to identify which changes in health status (or whatever else is measured by the indices) are due specifically to health department activities and which are due to general community evolution. On this point, a question may well be raised as to the importance of differentiating precisely between the activities of the health department and those of its community. In answer, it is to be noted that such differentiation is important, not only for theoretic reasons but also for reasons of practical policy. When faced with the problem of recommending expenditures to improve the health of communities it would be well to know if expenditures for the expansion of health department activities are effective without corresponding efforts to accelerate social evolution.

To overcome these difficulties, to formulate appraisal indices which can be correctly interpreted, requires the application of sound investigative methods. Some of the logical criteria to be considered in constructing indices and in comparing communities both in time and space have been examined and their application illustrated. The illustrations make it clear that a community agency sincerely interested in measuring the effects of its activities on the health of the people *must be willing to establish a research program for this purpose.*

An essential step in the planning of such research is to recognize the principle that the focus of appraisal is not the volume of facilities and services but the measurement of the health needs and status.

Fulfillment of this principle requires that at least two conditions be satisfied: (1) statements of the immediate objectives of specific health department activities and (2) systematic collection of data on the health problems of the community. Some health department activities are aimed directly and specifically at the elimination of certain causes of death, others at prevention of certain diseases, others at reduction of certain disabilities, others at promotion of certain health practices, and others are intended simply to observe accepted norms of administration. Explicit statements regarding the immediate aims of a number of specific activities are frequently lacking, and sometimes the impression is gained that all these aims are gradations of a single aim such as prolongation of life or promotion of health. To determine how well specific activities meet their stated objectives and how well these objectives meet the health problems of the community requires data on mortality, sickness, disability, health practices, and attitudes. The means for the collection of these data exist in all communities, but the organization and, for want of a better term, interest is often missing. A true appraisal of community health activities, measurements of achievements and goals, is obtained only when specific aims of these activities are contrasted with corresponding data on the health needs and problems of the community.

REFERENCES

1. Frost, W. H. Rendering Account in Public Health. Am. J. Publ. Hlth. 41: No. 8, part II, 1951.
2. Graunt, J. Natural and Political Observations Made Upon the Bills of Mortality. Edited with an introduction by Wilcox, W. F. Baltimore: Johns Hopkins Press, 1939.
3. Süssmilch, J. P. Die gottliche Ordnung in der Verandergung des menschlichen Geschlects, aus der Geburt, dem Tode und der fortpflanzung Desselben. Berlin: Buchladen der Realschule, 1761-1762.
4. Quetelet, L. A. J. La Physique Sociale. Brussels: C. Muquardt, 1869.
5. Graunt, op. cit.
6. Süssmilch, op. cit.
7. Quetelet, op. cit.
8. Winslow, C.-E., A. The Evolution and Significance of the Modern Public Health Campaign. New Haven: Yale Univ. Press, 1933, p. 2.
9. Pettenkofer, M. Von. The Value of Health to a City, Two Lectures Delivered in 1873. Bull. Hist. Med. 10: 473-503, 593-613, 1941.
10. Ibid.
11. Chapin, C. V. History of State and Municipal Control of Disease. In A Half Century of Public Health. New York: Am. Publ. Hlth. Ass., 1921, pp. 133-160.
12. Shattuck, L. Report of the Sanitary Commission of Massachusetts, 1850 (Reprinted less appendix). Cambridge: Harvard Univ. Press, 1948.

13. American Public Health Association, Report of the Committee on Municipal Health Department Practice. Public Health Bulletin No. 136. Washington: Government Printing Office, 1923.

14. American Public Health Association, Committee on Administrative Practice. Evaluation Schedule, 1947.

15. American Public Health Association, Committee on Administrative Practice. Guide to a Community Health Study, 1955.

16. Chapin, op. cit.

17. Greenberg, B. G., and Mattison, B. F. The Whys and Wherefores of Program Evaluation. Canad. J. Publ. Hlth. 46: 293-299, 1955.

18. Sydenstricker, E. The Measurement of Results of Public Health Work. Annual Report of the Milbank Memorial Fund, 1926, pp. 1-35.

19. Conference on Methods in Public Health Research. Am. J. Publ. Hlth. 41: No. 8, part II, 1951.

17

Approaches to the Quality of Hospital Care

MINDEL C. SHEPS

INCREASING attention is being paid to the problems of improving and of appraising the quality of health services in general[1-8] and of hospital care in particular. The general problems of measurement and evaluation in all these areas are similar.[9-16] Basically, they involve finding valid and reliable measurements of quality and interpreting these measurements when made.

Purposes of Hospital Evaluations

Evaluations of hospital quality may have different purposes. The methods and standards selected must be related to the particular purposes for which they are being applied. The most familiar purpose is regulatory. Such an appraisal is designed to match an institution against specified standards that determine its acceptability for the purposes of the regulatory or accrediting agency. It is intended to correct abuses and raise the general level to an acceptable minimum. Various national bodies, now united in the Joint Commission for the Accreditation of Hospitals, have evolved minimum acceptable levels of facilities, equipment, administrative and professional organization, and professional qualifications. They have also made use of some numerical indexes of organization and performance. All of these have been set forth in the commission's Standards for Hospital Accreditation.

The requirements of licensing boards, health insurance funds, and other organizations serve a similar purpose. Regulatory appraisals set minimum or desirable levels by excluding institutions that fail to qualify. At the same time, this provides protection for patients and students who go to acceptable institutions.[17-20] As yardsticks, these standards have one division that divides hospitals into two classes only—good enough or not good enough.

Improvement of Quality

The second purpose of appraisals is a closely related one—that of serving as a stimulus for the improvement of quality. Licensing and accrediting assessments serve this purpose as well as that of regulation. Hospitals also make self-appraisals for this purpose. The standards used may be minimum or optimum levels, similar to those used for regulatory purposes, or may provide for comparisons among physicians in the same institution. One of the chief instruments for such appraisals has been the medical audit.[21-25]

The basis of the audit is a review of hospital records according to such criteria as qualitative judgments of the care given and examination of diagnostic errors,[26-29] as well as such numerical indexes as mortality rates, rates for the incidence of specific complications, removal of normal tissues at operations,[30-32] consultations, cesarean rates, and the rates for certain tests by diagnostic category. The term "professional service accounting" has been suggested for the compilation of these rates and "medical audit" for their evaluation.

Program Evaluation

The third, and more recently recognized, purpose for quality appraisal, is to study the effects of specific programs or procedures on the quality of care. Generally we may refer to this purpose as program evaluation. Certain procedures, such as clinical-pathological conferences, are believed to improve the quality of hospitals. Large-scale complex programs, such as regionalization, are under trial. It is essential that their effectiveness be examined. We need to know in detail the effect of such procedures on the care received by patients. Program evaluation is the attempt to study this effect, by seeing whether a difference or an improvement in quality is associated with a certain procedure or program.

In other situations the purpose of a program evaluation may be to see whether a certain institution is giving "good" care. Such an appraisal is basically an evaluation in which the judge compares what he finds with what in his mind seems desirable and possible.

For regulatory purposes, it is desirable to establish criteria which actually do differentiate between acceptable and unacceptable institutions. They must be discriminating at the level where the regulating agency feels the line must be drawn. To help in improving the quality of hospital care, the criteria used must discover the most important problems and reflect progress in meeting them. Criteria used for these purposes may be useful in program evaluation, but more refined measuring tools are also needed. A scale which only says "good enough" or "not good enough" is inadequate. What is needed is a scale that measures values along a continuum extending from one extreme to the other. The measurements used must be sensitive to those aspects of hospital quality that may be affected by the program.

Reference has been made to some of the standard methods in use. It has recently been stated that the statistics used in judging hospitals are usually meaningless, often illogical and frequently unscientific."[33] For example, postoperative mortality ratios are based on deaths within 10 days divided by the total number of operations performed. Thus, deaths after 10 days are omitted, and on the other hand procedures of varying risks, such as dental extractions and neurosurgery, are indiscriminately lumped together.

Moreover, there is a question regarding the validity of the standards by which some of the indexes are evaluated.[33-36] A top limit of 3 to 4 percent is set for cesarean sections, but current clinical practice and results justify consideration of a higher level. Many of the standards were derived empirically, and their validity was not adequately established. Progress in clinical practice, in any case, calls for frequent revision and revalidation of the standards. The standards to be used, therefore, should be at levels which move according to changing medical knowledge.

The American College of Surgeons and the Professional Activity Study Group in Michigan are cooperating on a new approach to the audit as a measuring device and on the development of new indexes.[36] A number of new indexes of hospital or medical care have recently been described.[37-39] Studies currently in progress in the Rochester Regional Hospital Council, the North Carolina General Practice Study, and the Boston Evaluation Study may produce other indexes.

Other methodological developments of interest have been the application of the time study technique to hospital nursing[40] and a statistical analysis of the items included in hospital licensing regulations.[41]

Problems of Measurement

Hospital care is multidimensional. It is a service provided by a coordinated group of professional, technical, and other workers under the direction of a physician. The quality of the care received by patients is affected by the adequacy of the hospital facilities and their maintenance, by the administrative and professional organization of the hospital, by the competence of the personnel, and by the interpersonal relations among the staff as well as between the staff and the patients.

Any consideration of evaluation, therefore, must recognize the large number of factors involved in patient care. It has been frequently suggested that an appraisal form for hospital quality be developed. Some have extended this concept to include deriving a final score or number to represent the quality of a given hospital. Such a composite index would obscure important differences. Moreover, it would be impossible to choose the items to be included and the relative weights for them on a basis that was generally applicable. On the other hand, a number of measurements can be made and each of these allowed to stand by itself, thus producing a profile of the hospital.[42] We do not try to represent the health status of an individual by a single figure such as 90 percent of the optimum, but rather, we say something like:

"This patient's health, in general, is excellent, except for mild obesity and a hemoglobin of 10 grams."

Similarly, would it not be meaningful and helpful for the final report of a study to state not that "the quality is good" but rather something of this sort:

"Differences found in the following indexes were highly significant . . . No differences were observed in . . . The quality of physicians' services was significantly higher . . . The differences in social service were not significant . . ."

An exhaustive discussion of all the aspects of hospital care that could be included in such a profile will not be attempted. Instead it is proposed to deal with some of the methodological problems involved.

The main techniques used in appraisals of hospital quality can be divided into:

- The examination of prerequisites or desiderata for adequate care.
- Indexes of elements of performance.
- Indexes of the effects of care.
- Qualitative clinical evaluations.

By Set Standards of Care

According to the first approach, it is assumed that it is possible to select prerequisites for adequate care and that improvement of these factors leads to improved care. These prerequisites are minimum or optimum levels of facilities, equipment, professional training, and organization. As examples we may mention:

- The provision and appropriate maintenance of adequate physical facilities.

• The existence of special facilities, such as blood bank, bone bank, special laboratory and diagnostic facilities, premature nursery, and artificial kidney.

• An effective organizational structure, both administrative and professional.

• Standards and functioning of service departments such as records, laboratories, and libraries.

• Numbers of personnel by size of hospital—interns, residents, nurses, social workers, physical therapists, nutritionists, technicians.

• The availability of specialized personnel for consultation and of facilities for consultation with others, as in certain regional programs.

• Arrangements for ward rounds, refresher courses, continuing education.

• Minimum qualifications of personnel.

• The existence and functioning of internal controls, such as tissue committee, obstetrical committee, and medical audit.

The use of this approach implies the hypothesis that, given certain facilities and standards, the desirable quality of care is achieved. This hypothesis should be recognized and tested explicitly so that valid criteria can be used in a more informed fashion and to better purpose.

Consideration of the norms used for these desiderata raises such questions as, should they be national averages, regional averages, minimum adequate levels or optimum levels, or, should the search for standards be abandoned and the findings on various hospitals simply compared with each other? The answer depends partly on the purpose of the appraisal. In program evaluation, for example, it may be preferable to use flexible indexes applicable to different types of hospitals and to different periods, rather than to adopt any fixed standard of desirability.

Similar considerations led Stouman and Falk,[10] in their proposals for international health indexes, to abandon the search for standards. If one has valid measurements for a characteristic, then intelligent, directed application of these measurements in some situations will provide useful information as to their variability and their significance without a norm.

The argument will perhaps be made clearer by an example. When we use an index such as weight of children, we need a knowledge of norms to assist in diagnosis of a particular child. However, if we want to test the effect of a certain vitamin on weight, we need to compare the gains made by children receiving the vitamin and those not receiving it. Knowledge of the norms is here irrelevant.

By Elements of Performance

The second approach to quality uses indexes intended to reflect one or more elements of performance. Indexes may be defined as "one or a set of measures . . . used to measure indirectly the incidence of a characteristic that is not directly measurable."[43] Patient care is such a characteristic. Its quality cannot be measured quantitatively, except by the arbitrary allotment of a certain number of points to a qualitative judgment. It is difficult to define; it is complex and intangible. It is therefore natural and logical that much of the effort to evaluate this quality has been focused on the development of indexes, for example:

• Utilization rates for specific procedures by category, such as admission chest X-rays as an index of preventive services, or rectal examination in specified groups of patients.

• Utilization rates of certain laboratory and other diagnostic procedures, by category.

• Indexes which would reflect the promptness and discrimination with which new procedures or drugs are used in the hospital.

• Referral rates and patterns.

• Autopsy rates.

• Cesarean rates.

• Pathological reports on surgical specimens.

• Correlations between preoperative and postoperative diagnoses and between ante-mortem and post-mortem diagnoses.

• Accuracy of diagnostic procedures.

• Average length of hospital stay by diagnosis. It may be hypothesized that in a well-organized service where the staff members work with purpose and integration, hospital stay will be shorter, on the average, for certain types of cases.

• Listing specific diagnostic and therapeutic procedures expected for each type of case and matching records against them.

Good indexes are objective, reliable, and valid. By the reliability or precision of a measurement, we mean the degree of agreement among repeated measurements of the same things. Numerical indexes, such as rates or ratios, would appear to be relatively precise—anyone counting the number of autopsies done out of all hospital deaths should get the same rate provided that a hospital death is defined without ambiguity. Reliability is more difficult to achieve in indexes that require measurement rather than counting, as has been shown when different physicians measure the same enlarged livers,[44] or the same reactions to tuberculin tests.[45] Agreement on interpretation of X-ray films, even when repeated by the same physician, is far from perfect.[46] Quality indexes that depend on such assessments or on diagnosis, however made, must be tested for precision. It is an error to assume that because they are numerical they are precise.

The use of these performance indexes depends on an assumption that they are valid for an assessment of hospital quality. Presumably this involves the hypotheses (a) that each index does measure an element of patient care, and (b) that one or a number of these indexes are highly correlated with the intangibles of care. These hypotheses can and should be examined in the light of clinical information and by statistical analysis.

Again, the desirability and validity of the yardstick for these indexes must be examined. We can all agree that the higher the proportion of correct diagnoses, the better the quality of medicine. But what proportion ought we to expect in 1955 in different hospitals?

Other standards are even less definite. There can be too many laboratory tests as well as too few; too few cesareans as well as too many. Discriminating standards would be based on studies of the relation between good patient care and the resultant number of procedures by category of case. The development of appropriate yardsticks thus involves studies to estimate desirable levels for the various indexes and the expected variation. These levels should be adaptable for different types of hospitals and capable of reflecting progress in clinical medicine.

By the Effects of Care

A third approach to appraising hospital quality is the use of indexes intended to measure the effects of quality of care on patient health. The outcome of specific therapy is influenced by many factors in addition to that of treatment, factors such as age, sex, nutrition, stage of the disease, and the emotional state of the patient. The use of these indexes may therefore be highly misleading. It necessitates a careful evaluation of concomitant factors and an attempt to control them.

Some instances of such indexes are in fairly common use. They include:

• Specific mortality ratios such as postoperative, puerperal, and neonatal.

• Survival rates of premature infants in a specified weight range.

• The incidence of preventable complications such as postoperative infections.

These indexes would seem to be relatively precise if their basis is carefully defined. A postoperative mortality rate depends only on the careful definition of postoperative deaths and of the types of surgery counted. However, the validity of this rate as an index of the quality of surgery would still need to be established. The definitions used are highly relevant to this validity. But even then questions remain:

Does the death rate within 10 days after major chest surgery really reflect the quality of care?

What about the effect of such patient characteristics as diagnosis, complicating illnesses, age, sex, and nutritional status?

Objective indexes of the kinds discussed therefore require careful definition and evaluation. They hold considerable promise for the appraisal of hospital quality, but they are not yet the ideal measuring tools. At best, they are indirect and partial indicators of the basically intangible characteristic with which we are concerned. In a given organizational setting, with access to given standards of consultation and services, doing a certain number of laboratory examinations, one can have numerous shades in the range of quality of care, depending on the skill, the judgment, the experience and the character of the persons involved and on their relationships with patients. This end product is what one really is trying to evaluate in any assessment of patient care. It is for this reason that some workers have tackled the problem of evaluating quality directly through the fourth approach, namely a clinical evaluation.

By Clinical Evaluations

Makover[47] included a clinical evaluation in his study of medical groups associated with the Health Insurance Plan of New York. The continuing HIP evaluation program has adapted some of his techniques as well as adding new ones. According to a preliminary unpublished report by M. A. Morehead, delivered at the 1954 New England regional meeting of the American Public Health Association, records from six clinical fields are selected and scores assigned on the completeness of records, diagnostic management, treatment, and reporting. Although performance is measured against prepared standards, the final score depends on the judgment of the consultant making the evaluation.

More recently, another type of combined appraisal was made by Goldmann and Graham.[48] To an analysis of the availability of service and utilization of service, they added qualitative ratings of the efficiency of service organization and of a random sample of patient records.

Clinical evaluations are in the end subjective and thus less precise than some of the indexes previously discussed. However, they may be more valid since they are a direct approach to the characteristic we want to evaluate, the quality of patient care. Quality, though intangible, is not an abstraction. Nor is judgment of quality capricious or a purely personal whim. While agreement could not be expected to be complete, there are, in numerous situations, widely accepted concepts of what is meant by good care.

The reliability of qualitative judgments can be tested, and they can be subjected to statistical analysis.[49-51] To make relatively precise estimates of quality, it is necessary to have the findings of several independent judges. This permits an assessment of the degree of agreement among judges;[52-53] it allows for an objective test of the reliability of the evaluations and diminishes the effect of individual bias. Although more difficult than assessing the precision of interpretations of objective tests, it is the same in principle.

At times, agreement on judgmental evaluation is better than agreement on definitions and criteria. Reynolds[44] describes such a case. A group of clinicians attempting to outline criteria for ambulation of patients with infectious hepatitis could not reach agreement after a lengthy discussion of weighting procedures. But analysis of "paired comparisons" by which each man gave his preferences between the criteria in all possible combinations of two, resulted in good agreement on the ranks to be assigned them. Thus, it may be that several clinicians would agree more readily on the relative ranks of a number of hospitals than they would on the weights to be given various objective indexes in computing a quality score.

Judgmental assessments are resorted to in other fields. In some food industry situations the taste of a product must be evaluated. Objective tests give some information, but to answer the important question, "how does a particular process affect the taste," one must in the end resort to tasting the food. If it is necessary to study the effect of different ingredients and preparation procedures on the palatability of ice cream, the only way out is to ask a number of judges which product tastes better to them.

From such tests, valid results may be obtained notwithstanding the problems related to nonagreement among a group of judges and the lack of consistency on the part of an individual judge. The validity is also dependent on such controls as randomization of the tests and the judge's ignorance of which particular product he is testing.

Accordingly, it would appear that appropriate experimental and statistical procedures would enable more meaningful results to be obtained from qualitative evaluation of hospital care. In general, qualitative judgments are expressed through either ranking or scoring.

In ranking, a number of units are placed by each judge in order of his preference and the various ranks analyzed for consistency.

In scoring, a scale of quality is established, and each judge assigns the score that he considers appropriate.

These techniques may be combined in various ways. Thus, individual scores can be given on quality in different clinical fields, and the findings combined into one overall score. The subjects may then be ranked according to the scores obtained.

As already emphasized, the use of these techniques depends on replication, that is, on securing at least two separate evaluations of the same set of units. This is not the same as asking a committee to make a combined appraisal. Only through separate evaluations is it possible to assess the consistency of the individual judgments and to arrive at a relatively unbiased estimate. The value assigned results from combining the different judgments, and is more reliable and objective than the opinion of a single individual. A committee of experts would emerge with one final appraisal, but this would not allow the internal checking suggested. It is even possible with such a panel that one or two members could influence the others so that the final assessment would not be truly a consensus.

If qualitative appraisals of hospital care are made, the particular aspect of care to be studied might be medical, surgical, obstetrical, nursing, social work, or a combination of these and others. Well-qualified, experienced practitioners in the field under study should make the evaluation. Although most clinicians, medical and other, would probably prefer to base their opinions on actual observations of patient care, a properly selected random sample of clinical records may provide adequate information. If various clinical fields were reviewed, replication would be desirable in each field. The evaluations in the major clinical fields could then be crosschecked to test the consistency among them.

It is obvious that such qualitative judgments would have meaning only as comparisons among different hospitals or subdivisions of hospitals. The rank or score would have no absolute value but merely a relative value within the groups appraised. Direct comparisons are unavoidable when we operate without a scale or yardstick. However, this only makes explicit the fact that comparison lies at the basis of all measurement. Measurement has been defined as "the assignment of numerals to things so as to represent facts and conventions about them . . . under a consistent set of rules."[54]

The operations to which any measurements can be subjected depend on the rules that can be made and on the validity and reliability of the values obtained. However, with any measurements we make comparisons. If we measure height, we compare the height of the subject with the markings on an arbitrary scale. These markings have meaning only in terms of established norms, of earlier results on the same subject, or of readings obtained from another subject. When we don't have a ruler, we can stand two subjects next to each other and make the comparison directly. Similarly, any index of quality may be measured against a yardstick, or the values obtained on several hospitals may be directly compared.

The Basis of Comparison

Any of the four approaches to quality, therefore, involve comparisons, either indirectly through the use of standards or directly. In program evaluations the basis of comparison is vital. If a specific procedure has an effect on quality, it must be revealed in differences. To find such differences, the hospital under study must be compared with something, either with other hospitals or with itself before inception of the program. When differences exist, it is of paramount importance to isolate differences related to the program itself from differences owing to such other factors as changes in time, economic differences, cultural differences, and so on. The selection of a basis of comparison or control is crucial in this attempt.

The basis of comparison and the indexes to be used, in fact the plan for evaluation of a new procedure or program, should go hand in hand with planning the program itself. Ideally, before the new procedure is instituted, several similar hospitals would be chosen. By random selection, half would become experimental units for the new program, and half, controls.[55] A careful study of patient care would be made in all the hospitals before instituting the new program and again at a suitable time after the program was in effect. Medical and social progress occurring during this period might produce changes in both experimental and control units. But the changes might be different, and it is these changes that would be compared.

Such an experiment would be relatively simple if it tested only one procedure at a time. Thus one could, for example, estimate the effect of providing small hospitals with special courses for laboratory technicians by comparing changes in the accuracy of their results in certain procedures. More complex programs should also be amenable to this type of experiment.

However, there are cases where this does not apply. The effects of an existing program are to be evaluated, or a hospital plans to embark on a new program, and a study is to be made of quality before and after. The institutions then are self-selected and thereby are different from other hospitals. The before-and-after case does not make the problem simpler. A comparison within the one hospital at two different periods necessitates control of secular changes related to the passage of time or changes owing to extraneous factors that may have come into play.

This situation has parallels in population studies, in public health research, and in clinical research. Analytical studies of what exists, rather than of a planned experiment, call for a more critical evaluation of the findings, and the conclusions must be more tentative. This is even truer when the analyses are retrospective, being made after the fact.[56-59] However, in some cases it may be possible to select suitable controls for comparison[60] and to test their suitability by an examination of variables that might affect the result. The careful selection and critical analysis of the controls[61] are basic to the validity of the findings.

An important step in program evaluation, therefore, is the search for suitable controls and for methods of eliminating some of the many variables that affect the quality of care. This is especially difficult because hospitals are highly complex institutions, and patient care is an intangible quality, influenced by many variables.

It is therefore possible that no comparable units could be found for nonexperimental situations. In the event of failure to establish acceptable controls, or even as a complement to comparisons made with controls, there is another avenue of approach that might prove fruitful. One might formulate a hypothesis such as:

"Characteristic x is usually found only in teaching hospitals. A random sample of nonteaching hospitals in comparable communities will show low values for x, but an examination of hospitals in our group will reveal significantly higher values."

Characteristic x might be laboratory services of a certain type, or rehabilitation services, or one of the quantitative indexes considered. Such an approach, of course, adopts the rest of the country as controls. As in other situations, purely descriptive studies may be used as a basis for planning future experiments.

Many references have already been made to testing the validity of various indexes. This could be done in various ways. One would be through a statistically controlled clinical analysis of each index. Another would be through seeking correlations among various measurements[37,62] including qualitative appraisals. Thus, correlations might be sought among two or more measurements which are believed to measure practically the same thing. It might be found that a relatively simple, inexpensive objective test showed a high correlation with the results of the qualitative judgments, or, more likely, that a combination of such tests did so. Once the validity and applicability of such indicators were established, there would be many instances where they could be used instead of more difficult, expensive, and cumbersome techniques.

Conclusions

Most of the work done to date in the appraisal of hospital quality has been related to the purposes of correcting abuses, setting minimum standards, and stimulating improvements in quality. The field of program evaluation is just beginning to be explored.

Techniques used in quality evaluations vary with the purposes of the particular study. The quality of care can be evaluated through a multidimensional approach which results in a profile of the hospital. The main basis of the appraisal can be the use of one or a combination of: examinations for prerequisites for good care, indexes intended to measure elements of performance, indexes intended to measure the effect of care by results obtained, and qualitative clinical judgments.

Any indexes and standards used in such appraisals would be clearly defined, based on comparable data, and examined for their reliability and validity. Qualitative clinical appraisals should also be tested in a similar fashion and statistical controls and analysis applied to them as well.

Correlations among different indexes and judgments used should be attempted.

Appraisals which are intended to examine the effects of specific procedures or programs should be planned before the inception of the program.

The selection of an appropriate basis of comparison is crucial to program evaluation.

The development of practical and valid methods of measurement will involve the expenditure of considerable money and time. However, in view of efforts and money now being spent on programs to raise quality, it would seem essential to direct some of those resources toward the development of appropriate methods with which to judge their effects. Collaboration of clinicians, administrators, and statisticians is necessary for such a development.

A critical analysis of the particular methods used should be an explicit objective of a quality evaluation.

REFERENCES

1. Reed, L. S., and Clark, D. A. Appraising Public Medical Services. Am. J. Publ. Hlth. 31: 421-430, 1941.
2. Goldmann, F. The Adequacy of Medical Care. Yale J. Biol. & Med. 19: 681-688, 1947.
3. The Quality of Medical Care in a National Health Program. A statement of the Subcommittee on Medical Care, American Public Health Association. Am. J. Publ. Hlth. 39: 898-924, 1949.
4. American Public Health Association, Subcommittee on Medical Care. The Quality of Medical Care: Concepts, Standards, Methods of Evaluation and Improvement. New York: The Association, 1954 (Processed).
5. Weinerman, E. R. Appraisal of Medical Care Programs. Am. J. Publ. Hlth. 40: 1129-1134, 1950.
6. Improving the Quality of Medical Care. Dublin, T. D.: The Training of Personnel; Clark, D. A.: Group Medical Practice; Kaiser, A. D.: Regionalization of Hospitals; Daily, E. F.: Sound Principles of Administration. Am. J. Publ. Hlth. 39: 314-339, 1949.
7. Lee, R. I., and Jones, L. W. The Fundamentals of Good Medical Care. Chicago: Univ. of Chicago Press, 1933.
8. Evaluation and Health Practice. Editorial. Am. J. Publ. Hlth. 40: 868-869, 1950.
9. Youmans, J. B. Experience with a Postgraduate Course for Practitioners: Evaluation of Results. J. A. Am. M. Coll. 10: 154-173, 1935.
10. Stouman, K., and Falk, I. S. Health Indices. A Study of Objective Indices of Health in Relation to Environment and Sanitation. Quart. Bull. Health Organ., League of Nations, 5: 901-1081, 1936.
11. Methods in Public Health Research. Proceedings of a conference held under the auspices of the Public Health Study Section, National Institutes of Health, in conjunction with the Graduate School of Public Health, University of Pittsburgh. Am. J. Publ. Hlth. 41: 1-117, 1951, pt. 2.
12. Evaluation Studies Which Have Contributed to School Health Services and Education. Am. J. Publ. Hlth. (Year Book 1951-52) 42: 125-129, 1952, pt. 2.
13. Yankauer, A. Designs for Evaluation Needed in the School Health Field. Am. J. Publ. Hlth. 42: 655-660, 1952.
14. American Public Health Association, Medical Care and Statistics Sections, Joint Committee on Medical Care Statistics: Medical Care Statistics. New York: The Association, 1953 (Processed).
15. Sheps, M. C., and Sheps, C. G. Assessing the Effectiveness of Programs in Operation. Study Group Reports, Committee IV on Research, National Conference on Care of the Long-Term Patient. Baltimore: Commission on Chronic Illness, 1954, pp. 93-104 (processed).
16. Cowles, J. T. Current Trends in Examination Procedures. J.A.M.A. 155: 1383-1387, 1954.

17. Commission on Hospital Care: Hospital Care in the United States. New York: Commonwealth Fund, 1947.
18. Gonzalez, J. Medical Staff Organization Vital to Accreditation. Hospitals, 27: 104-106, 1953.
19. Crosby, E. L. The Goal of Accredition. Mod. Hosp. 78: 74, 1952.
20. Gundersen, G. Benefits of Hospital Accreditation to the Medical Profession. J.A.M.A. 154: 917-918, 1954.
21. Ponton, T. R. The Medical Staff in the Hospital. Revised by MacEachern, M. T., Chicago: Physicians Record Co., 1953.
22. Hill, F. T. The Staff Audit and the Consultation Ratio. J. Maine M.A. 42: 58-60, 1951.
23. Mortrud, L. C. The Control of Professional Practice through the Medical Audit. Hospitals, 27: 91-93, 1953.
24. Krause, C. D. The Merits of a Medical Audit. Mod. Hosp. 81: 85-86, 1953.
25. Perdew, W. C. Are Your Patients Properly Cared For? A Medical Audit, or Analysis, Helps the Staff Answer This Question. Mod. Hosp. 71: 84-88, 1948.
26. Cabot, R. C. Diagnostic Pitfalls Identified During a Study of Three Thousand Autopsies. J.A.M.A. 59: 2295-2298, 1912.
27. Swartout, H. O. Ante-mortem and Post-mortem Diagnoses. New England J. Med. 211: 539-542, 1934.
28. Pohlen, K., and Emerson, H. Errors in Clinical Statements of Causes of Death. Am. J. Publ. Hlth. 42: 251-260, 1942; 33: 505-516, 1943.
29. Redlich, F. C., Dunsmore, R. H., and Brody, E. B. Delays and Errors in the Diagnosis of Brain Tumor. New England J. Med. 239: 945-950, 1948.
30. Miller, N. F. Hysterectomy: Therapeutic Necessity or Surgical Racket. Am. J. Obst. & Gynec. 51: 804-810, 1946.
31. Doyle, J. C. Unnecessary Ovariectomies: Study Based on Removal of 704 Normal Ovaries from 546 Patients. J.A.M.A. 148: 1105-1111, 1952.
32. Doyle, J. C. Unnecessary Hysterectomies: Study Based on 6,248 Operations in 35 Hospitals During 1948. J.A.M.A. 151: 360-366, 1953.
33. Myers, R. S. Professional Activity Study. Hospital Statistics Don't Tell the Truth. Mod. Hosp. 83: 53-54, 1954.
34. Letourneau, C. U. The Legal and Moral Aspects of Unnecessary Surgery. Hospitals, 27: 82-86, 1953.
35. Robson, S. M. Why Pick on the Surgeons? Mod. Hosp. 82: 57-58, 1954.
36. Professional Activity Study. Slee, V. N. Statistics Influence Medical Practice; Mooi, H. R. Doctors Do Take Records Seriously; Hoffman, R. G. We Must Ask the Right Questions to Get the Right Answers; Erickson, W. Small Hospitals Benefit by the New Approach; Van der Kolk, B. Did They Have Pneumonia— Or Didn't They; Farr, V. Record Librarian Lists Advantages; Eisele, C. W. Opinions are No Basis for Objective Analysis. Mod. Hosp. 83: 53-64, 1954.
37. Ciocco, A., Hunt, G. H., and Altman, I. Statistics on Clinical Services to New Patients in Medical Groups. Pub. Hlth. Rep. 65: 99-115, 1950.
38. Furstenberg, F. F., Tayback, M., Goldberg, H., and Davis, J. W. Prescribing an Index to the Quality of Medical Care: A Study of the Baltimore City Medical Care Program. Am. J. Publ. Hlth. 43: 1299-1309, 1953.
39. Lembcke, P. A. Measuring the Quality of Medical Care Through Vital Statistics Based on Hospital Service Areas. I. Comparative Study of Appendectomy Rates. Am. J. Publ. Hlth. 42: 276-286, 1952.

40. Wright, M. J. Improvement of Patient Care. A Study at Harper Hospital. New York: G. P. Putnam's Sons, 1954.
41. O'Malley, M., and Kossack, C. F. A Statistical Study of Factors Influencing the Quality of Patient Care in Hospitals. Am. J. Publ. Hlth. 40: 1428-1443, 1950.
42. Kossack, C. F. To Measure the Quality of a Hospital. Mod. Hosp. 81: 77-79, 1953.
43. Hagood, M. J., and Price, D. O. Statistics for Sociologists. Rev. ed. New York: Henry Holt and Co., 1952, pp. 138-143.
44. Reynolds, W. E. Some Problems of Clinical Measurement in the Study of Chronic Diseases, in Research in Public Health. Papers presented at the 1951 Annual Conference of the Milbank Memorial Fund. New York: Milbank Memorial Fund, 1952, pp. 76-88.
45. Meyer, S. N., Hougen, A., and Edwards, P. Experimental Error in the Determination of Tuberculin Sensitivity. Pub. Hlth. Rep. 66: 561-569, 1951.
46. Birkelo, C. C., Chamberlain, W. E., Phelps, P. S., Schools, P. E., Zacks, D., and Yerushalmy, J. Tuberculosis Case Finding. A Comparison of the Effectiveness of Various Roentgenographic and Photofluorographic Methods. J.A.M.A. 133: 359-366, 1947.
47. Makover, H. B. The Quality of Medical Care: Methodology of Survey of the Medical Groups Associated with the Health Insurance Plan of New York. Am. J. Publ. Hlth. 41: 824-832, 1951.
48. Goldmann, F., and Graham, E. A. The Quality of Medical Care Provided at the Labor Health Institute. St. Louis: Labor Health Institute, 1954.
49. Savage, I. R. Bibliography of Nonparametric Statistics and Related Topics. J. Am. Stat. A. 48: 844-906, 1953.
50. Bradley, R. A. Some Statistical Methods in Taste Testing and Quality Evaluation. Biometrics, 9: 22-38, 1953.
51. Mason, D. D., and Koch, E. J. Some Problems in the Design and Statistical Analysis of Taste Tests. Biometrics, 9: 39-46, 1953.
52. Moroney, M. J. Facts from Figures. Baltimore: Penguin Books, 1951, ch. 18.
53. Bradley, R. A. Some Notes on the Theory and Application of Rank Order Statistics. Blacksburg: Virginia Agricultural Experiment Station of the Virginia Polytechnic Institute, undated (Processed).
54. Stevens, S. S. On the Theory of Scales of Measurement. Science, 103: 677-680, 1946.
55. Greenberg, B. G., Harris, M. E., MacKinnon, C. F., and Chipman, S. S. A Method for Evaluating the Effectiveness of Health Education Literature. Am. J. Publ. Hlth. 43: 1147-1155, 1953.
56. Hill, B. A. Observation and Experiment. New England J. Med. 248: 995-1001, 1953.
57. Dorn, H. F. Philosophy of Inferences from Retrospective Studies. Am. J. Publ. Hlth. 43: 677-683, 1953.
58. Cochran, W. G. Matching in Analytical Studies. Am. J. Publ. Hlth. 43: 684-691, 1953.
59. Greenberg, B. G. The Use of Analysis of Covariance and Balancing in Analytical Surveys. Am. J. Publ. Hlth. 43: 692-699, 1953.
60. Wright, J. J., Sheps, C. G., and Gifford, A. E. Reports of the North Carolina Syphilis Studies. IV. Some Problems in the Evaluation of Venereal Disease Education. J. Ven. Dis. Inform. 31: 125-133, 1950.

61. Densen, P. M., Padget, P., Webster, B., Nicol, C. S., and Rich, C. Studies in Cardiovascular Syphilis. II: Methodologic Problems in the Evaluation of Therapy. Am. J. Syph., Gonor. and Ven. Dis. 36: 64-76, 1952.
62. Platt, P. S. The Validity of the Appraisal Form as a Measure of Administrative Health Practice. New York: Am. Publ. Hlth. Assoc., 1928.

Dr. Sheps presented this material at a joint session of the Medical Care Section of the American Public Health Association and the American Association of Hospital Consultants at the annual meeting of the American Public Health Association in Buffalo, October, 1954.

18

Measuring Social Restoration Performance of Public Psychiatric Hospitals

CHARLES E. RICE, DAVID G. BERGER,
LEE G. SEWALL, and PAUL V. LEMKAU

CURRENT interest in assessing the performance of psychiatric hospitals is linked with the widespread conviction that, in expending their energies in day-to-day operations, social organizations may fail to attain the efficiency expected of them. A corollary belief is that systematic observation of such organizations may lead to recommendations for improving their performance.

At first sight it may appear necessary to use radically different methods of evaluating organizations with such diverse purposes as education, national defense, health and welfare, and industrial production. However, with the development of formal systems of operations research, logistics analysis, and management science, certain common dimensions of analysis have been found useful in assessing different types of social organization. One such dimension is organizational goals.

To use a goal orientation in appraising social organizations, it is necessary to determine the pattern of goals during a given period of operation, to define each goal, and to select the best available measures of organizational results to reflect effectiveness in the attainment of each goal.

Medical Audit Plan

The Medical Audit Plan for Psychiatric Hospitals, a research program designed to develop a method for appraising the effectiveness of public psychiatric hospitals, is being readied for application in a series of hospitals. The staff of the plan has been working to derive a set of goals that will represent the objectives of public psychiatric hospitals in our culture. Results of a nationwide survey indicate that, in the opinion of both the professional and lay public, social restoration and care of patients, protection of patients and public, education and training, research, and effective administration are prominent purposes in these institutions. This paper deals with social restoration, an important dimension in evaluating hospital performance.

To measure the social restoration performance of public psychiatric hospitals, it was necessary first to define social restoration in terms of hospital-patient events and then to develop a workable system for recording and measuring these events so that the procedure could be tested in a series of hospitals. If the system proved practicable, a rudimentary program for estimating social restoration performance would be formalized.

If the formal program proves to be applicable in public psychiatric hospitals, it could be the "foot in the doorway" to hospital evaluation, making it possible to catalog differences in treatment programs, staff programs, staff patterns, patient populations, structural features, and so on, in a series of public psychiatric hospitals, and to learn which hospital characteristics occur most frequently in combination with "satisfactory" social restoration results. A system of empirically based standards for the operation of such institutions could then be described in terms of social restoration. Other goals could be treated similarly.

Definition of Social Restoration

The principal purpose of the psychiatric hospital is often defined as the successful return of patients to the community. What, however, is a "successful return"? Is return to the community successful if the patient leaves the hospital by escape or unauthorized absence, if his posthospital behavior is severely disorganized, if he is subsequently readmitted or admitted to another institution, if he spends 10 years in the hospital before being discharged, or if he dies within a week after discharge? The definition we seek must establish the limits of hospital responsibility in the events and behavior which occur during and after the patient's release from the hospital. It must also conform to the basic principles of psychiatric hospital operation, so that the events and behavior observed have meaning and application in a large number of hospital settings.

The medical audit plan defines the social restoration goal of public psychiatric hospitals as maximal success in authorizing the release of patients who will not only remain in the community but also will make a favorable community adjustment.

The three levels of social restoration may be expressed as follows:
• To what extent is the hospital authorizing the return of patients

to the community for the purpose of establishing extrahospital residence? With some minor reservations, this is akin to a "discharge rate" and may be designated level 1, the first and most rudimentary level of social restoration.

• To what extent do patients whose release from the hospital is authorized remain in the community? Quantification of this level would represent a "readmission rate." Adjustments must be made, however, for patients dying in the community after release from the hospital, as well as for patients subsequently admitted to other institutions. Level 2 of social restoration represents the capacity of the hospital to discharge patients who will remain alive in the community.

• To what extent is the hospital authorizing release to the community of patients who prove capable of a satisfactory extrahospital adaptation? The nature of the patient's adjustment to the community is the subject of level 3. No familiar statistic is applied to this level, which reflects the limited effort of public psychiatric hospitals in the followup of patients.

Before formulating a program for measuring the three levels of social restoration, two ancillary concepts are needed, the patient cohort and the description of the time intervals comprising the total study period.

Patient Cohorts

The study of hospital effectiveness in terms of social restoration focuses on patients departing from the hospital. Whether the hospital administrator is interested in the success of his hospital in releasing a selected class of patients, such as schizophrenics, married females, or alcoholics, or in the movement of all patients from the hospital to the community, the essence of the problem is identification of the reservoir of patients available for release. Cohorts of patients, made up of groups with distinctive traits or characteristics, such as those in a particular diagnostic rubric or within a prescribed age range, are a useful concept for this purpose.[1]

In this project, two cohorts are used for measuring the social restoration performance of psychiatric hospitals: an admission cohort, assembled by assigning to it all patients admitted during a given time interval; and a resident cohort, made up of all patients in the hospital the day the research program is installed. By classifying patients in the resident cohort according to length of hospital stay, a series of second-order resident cohorts will be formed. In this way, a 1-year resident cohort as well as 2-year and longer cohorts will be identified in each hospital.

Interest in the admission and resident cohorts in each hospital centers on various forms of patient movement, both within and from the hospital, as well as on the type of adjustment in the community demonstrated by patients discharged from both cohorts.

Since the rate of discharge for newly admitted patients is generally greater than for patients who have been in residence for a protracted period of time, an estimate of hospital success in the restoration of all types of patients is important. To use only recently admitted patients for estimating hospital success provides only a partial picture. The research program is designed to discover features in the hospital system which vary with social restoration performance. If the estimate of social restoration is based on a limited portion of the hospital population, such as a resident or an admission cohort, it would be necessary to decide what portion of hospital resources were expended in serving the specified cohort. Accurate apportionment of this expenditure in retrospect would be an extremely delicate task. The use of two cohorts provides a global picture of hospital social restoration capacity as well as one which should prove more rigorous and economical in operation.

Time Schedules

The study of a hospital's social restoration functioning may be divided into three time phases: collection, observation, and follow-up.

• The collection phase, necessary only for the admission cohort, is the period during which this cohort is assembled. It occupies the first 183 days, or 6 months, of project work in the cooperating hospitals. The admission cohort includes all patients entering the hospital during this interval except patients dying within 48 hours of admission.

• During the observation phase, each patient in both the admission and resident cohorts will be followed for a maximum of 274 days, or 9 months, to determine what happens to him (death in the hospital, transfer, discharge, and so on). For all resident cohort patients, the observation phase begins on the day the study is installed in the hospital; for admission cohort patients, on the day of admission during the collection phase.

The first day of a patient's hospitalization is symbolized by $P(A)1$ (A refers to admission). Each day of his hospital stay is similarly symbolized; for example, his 100th day of hospitalization is represented by $P(A)100$.

For all resident patients, $P(A)1$ is the first day of the study; it is as though all of these patients were admitted on the first day of project work in the hospital. For both resident and admission patients the observation phase extends, potentially, from $P(A)1$ to $P(A)274$. The observation phase is terminated whenever a change, such as death, occurs in any patient's status. Nine months, or 274 days, is merely the upper limit or time boundary for this phase.

• In the follow-up phase, for both the admission and resident cohorts, each patient placed on convalescent leave or given an authorized discharge by $P(A)274$ will be followed in the community for a period up to 9 months after release.

If we let $P(R)1$ (R stands for release) represent a patient's first day in the community, then the follow-up phase for him can extend to $P(R)274$ if he continues to adjust at some level throughout the 9 months. The followup phase closes for patients who are reinstitutionalized, or die, before $P(R)274$. It would be interesting to observe reinstitutionalized patients throughout the follow-up period, but this study is planned so that observation is discontinued when a significant change in a patient's status occurs.

The three time phases described are fundamentally "time samples" of on-going hospital-patient events. The time intervals are admittedly arbitrary, but limits must be imposed to measure hospital performance. The scheme outlined requires 2 years to carry the three phases to their prescribed time boundaries.

Measuring Social Restoration

Social restoration may be measured at three levels: by the number of patients who return to the community, by the length of their stay in the community, and by the posthospital adjustment of those remaining in the community.

Level 1

In level 1 of social restoration, the problem is to determine how many members of a given cohort are returned to the community during the observation phase of the study. To discover what happens to patients during this phase, patients in the two cohorts were subdivided into seven classes, as follows:

(1) d, died in the hospital by $P(A)274$.

(2) t, transferred from the hospital by $P(A)274$.

(3) r_{AMA}, released "against medical advice" by $P(A)274$.

(4) r_{elope}, released via elopement (escape or unauthorized absence) from the hospital by $P(A)274$.

(5) r_{MHB}, released with "maximum hospital benefit" by $P(A)274$.

(6) r_v, placed on trial visit, sometimes termed "convalescent leave" or "parole," but not including "day care" or "night care," by $P(A)274$.

(7) h, patients who had none of the above experiences but who remained in the hospital throughout the observation phase, although they may have been granted short leaves of absence, such as weekend passes.

Classes 1-6 include cohort patients discharged or released from the hospital, using the terms "discharge" and "release" in a broad sense. Classes 5 and 6 differ from classes 1-4 in that patients released with maximum hospital benefit and patients placed on trial visit are released because the hospital has decided they are "ready" to return to the community, at least on a trial basis. These hospital-approved releases are designated as R. Therefore R represents the number of cohort patients discharged with maximum hospital benefit or placed on trial visit before $P(A)274$.

Classes 1-4 include patients withdrawn from a cohort by means other than a hospital-approved release. W represents the number of these patients in a cohort.

To summarize, if N represents the total number of patients in a cohort, then $N = R + W + h$. A patient can be classified only according to the first event in his hospital experience after he enters the study. For example, a patient discharged with maximum hospital benefit is classified as r_{MHB} (or R) even if he is readmitted to the hospital a few days following his discharge.

These patient movement categories were developed for the medical audit plan research program and represent the minimum number of categories needed to appraise the social restoration performance of State hospitals. They do not conform to the category structure of any State hospital system but resemble most closely the classification instituted by the mental hospital statisticians participating in the work of the Model Reporting Area for Mental Hospital Statistics.[2] While the categories have been reduced to a minimum, there will be settings where certain categories have no utility. This will be especially true for patients released against medical advice, since a number of States do not use the designation r_{AMA} for patients who leave the hospital on their own insistence. As with any classification procedure, the essential requirement is that category definitions be followed faithfully by each cooperating hospital.

Discharge rate. The extent to which a hospital gives its patients an opportunity to return to the community can be measured by two basic indices, a discharge rate and a length-of-stay measure. A discharge rate constitutes our primary level 1 index.

The term "hospital-approved release rate" is a more realistic and meaningful measurement of hospital functioning at level 1 of social restoration than the term "discharge rate" because it is based on cohort patients whose release is approved by the hospital. It also avoids "inflation" of the usual discharge rate, which happens when "patients discharged from the hospital" include discharges via death, transfer, and elopement.

Another advantage of the "hospital-approved release" concept is its inclusion of patients placed on trial visit. Although these patients remain on the hospital books and are technically not discharged, they represent "releases to the community," and should be included in any measure of the social restoration effectiveness of a hospital. In many respects, the major difference between the status of patients discharged as having received maximum hospital benefit and patients placed on trial visit is administrative definition. By and large, both classes of patients are released into the community because the hospital believes they are "ready" to attempt to adjust to community living.

The discharge rate is usually computed by dividing the number of patients available for release during a given period of time by the total number of patients in the cohort:

$$\frac{\text{Discharges}}{\text{Discharges} + \text{nondischarges}} \qquad [1]$$

(or total number of patients in the cohort)

If the concept of "hospital-approved release" is used, this ratio must be refined, so that it would read

$$\frac{\text{Authorized discharges}}{\text{Authorized discharges} + \text{nonauthorized discharges} + \text{nondischarges}}$$

(or total number of patients in the cohort) $\qquad [2]$

If the symbols R, W, and h are substituted in ratio 2, it would read

$$\frac{R}{R + W + h} \text{ or } \frac{R}{N} \qquad [3]$$

Ratio 3 contains yet another pitfall. Patients who die, transfer, or elope from the hospital (W's) are removed from the cohort and are not available for authorized discharge throughout the entire observation phase of the study. Inclusion of these patients in the denominator of the index results in a misleadingly low index of hospital performance. A correction factor is needed to modify the denominator so that it will more accurately represent the number of cohort members with an equivalent "availability" or exposure time for authorized discharge. When the exact date of departure of W patients is unknown or difficult to obtain, it is customary to assume that they are leaving the cohort uniformly throughout the observation period. This is tantamount to saying that W patients are spending, on the average, one-half of the observation phase in the hospital or that there are, in another sense, only one-half as many patients in the W category as there are in fact. The usual corrected denominator is on the order of

$$N - \tfrac{1}{2}W \qquad [4]$$

However, since the exact date of withdrawal of W patients will be recorded for each patient in the study cohorts, assumption of a uniform rate of departure is not necessary. The sum of the days spent in the hospital by each patient withdrawn from the study divided by the number of such patients will produce an average period of exposure to hospital-approved release for patients leaving the hospital by means other than authorized discharge. Dividing the average exposure period by 274, the number of days in the observation phase, will give the average proportion of the observation phase which the W patients spent in the hospital before withdrawal from the cohort. Subtracting this proportion from unity will give the average proportion of the observation phase during which the W's were not exposed to the risk of a hospital-approved release. Symbolically, this correction would be expressed as

$$C = 1 - \frac{\dfrac{\text{Sum } Li}{W}}{274} \qquad [5]$$

The only unfamiliar term is Li, which represents the number of days a withdrawn patient spends in the hospital before release. Multiplying C by W will yield the number of patients who were not available for release due to their withdrawal from the cohort. If the correction is integrated into index 3, the refined discharge rate, symbolized by $1a$, becomes

$$1a = \frac{R}{N - (C \times W)} \qquad [6]$$

The denominator represents the number of cohort members who were in the hospital for an approximately equal time during the observation phase, and the index yields that proportion of these patients given hospital-approved releases.[3] This proportion may be multiplied by 100 if a percentage is desired.

Table 1 shows hypothetical data on movement of patients and the computation of level 1 indices for each of two hospitals. Over a given length of time hospital A released 35 percent of the cohort patients who had spent equal periods of time in the hospital, while hospital B released 49 percent, or nearly half, of the cohort patients with equal exposures to hospital-approved release. The level 1 index would be computed for both admission and resident cohorts; thus, a hospital would be characterized by several indices.

TABLE 1. CALCULATION OF PRIMARY LEVEL 1
INDEX BASED ON HYPOTHETICAL DATA

	Hospital A	Hospital B
(1) N (total number in cohort).	360	250
(2) r_{MHB} ("maximum hospital benefit" discharges).	22	26
(3) r_v (trial visits).	94	88
(4) $R=(2)+(3)$.	116	114
(5) d (deaths).	18	14
(6) r_{AMA} ("against medical advice" discharges).	16	10
(7) t (transfers).	14	10
(8) r_{elope} (elopements).	7	5
(9) $W=(5)+(6)+(7)+(8)$.	55	39
(10) $h=(1)-(4)-(9)$.	189	97
(11) Average number of days in hospital for W's.	120	155
(12) $C=1-\dfrac{(11)}{274}$	0.56	0.43
(13) $1a=\dfrac{R}{N-(C)W}=\dfrac{(4)}{(1)-(12)\times(9)}$	.35	.49

Length of hospitalization. The primary level 1 index was developed in terms of the number of patients released into the community by a hospital during a given period of time and is essentially a refined release rate. A somewhat different way of considering social restoration at level 1 is to ask, "How long are patients kept in the hospital?" The answer to this question involves a length-of-stay measure.

The secondary level 1 measure is merely the average length of stay of R and h cohort patients during the observation phase of the study. In the secondary level 1 approach, measurement is restricted to R and h patients. Inclusion of patients withdrawn from the cohort for reasons other than hospital-approved release would give a lower, and often less meaningful, result. For example, if a given cohort lost many of its members by death during the observation phase, a low mean length of stay would result.

If we let $1b$ represent the secondary level 1 measure, then

$$1b = \frac{\text{Sum } Li(R,h)}{R + h} \qquad [7]$$

The mean length of stay is computed for the admission cohort of a hospital and also for each resident cohort. For the resident cohort, the measure does not include the time spent in the hospital prior to the start of the study. This is a legitimate limitation because operation of the hospital system during the observation phase is the subject of the study. Any inferences about the relationship between hospital programs and hospital results will perforce be limited to the period which coincides with the observation phase. However, for purposes other than this research program, it might be more useful to calculate the average length of total hospital stay for the entire body of resident patients.

Collection of data for level 1 poses no particular problem other than stratifying the resident cohort by length of hospital stay and recording certain basic demographic information on these patients before the day the study is officially launched. From this point on, during the observation phase, it will be necessary to record the exact dates of admission and release for all patients in both admission and resident cohorts and to obtain the same demographic data on the admission cohort as on the resident cohort.

Level 2

The extent to which a hospital gives its patients a chance to return to the community is only part of the social restoration story. Patients released from the hospital have not necessarily been "socially restored"; they have only been given the opportunity to achieve this status. Follow-up activities, to learn what happens to patients released into the community, are essential for evaluating the "true effect" of hospitalization. Therefore, all cohort patients given a hospital-approved release (r_{MHB} or r_v) within the observation phase of the study will be followed in the community up to 9 months, or 274 days, after their release.

These R patients may be subdivided into smaller groups according to what happens to them following their release into the community. For example, they may die; they may return to institutionalized status, to the same or a different psychiatric inpatient facility or to a prison, a nursing home, or a home for the aged; or they may remain in the community throughout the follow-up phase of the study. This breakdown is valid for both the trial visit and maximum hospital benefit patients of both admission and resident cohorts.

The R group of a cohort will be broken down as follows:

(1) Rd, number of R patients who die in the community by $P(R)274$.

(2) Ri, number of R patients reinstitutionalized by $P(R)274$.

(3) Rs, number of R patients remaining in the community throughout the follow-up phase of the study.

As in the observation phase of the study, a patient is classified only once, according to his first hospital experience.

Readmission rate. The primary level 2 index is based on the question. "To what extent do patients whose release from the hospital is approved remain alive in the community?" This suggests use of a readmission rate analogous to the release rate developed for level 1, based on Ri, the number of R individuals of a cohort reinstitutionalized during the follow-up phase.

The primary level 2 index is

$$2a = \frac{Ri}{R - (C \times Rd)} \qquad [8]$$

where C in the denominator is a correction term. This correction is analogous to that used in the level 1 index and is necessary because some individuals will die in the community and thus will be withdrawn from the R group. The treatment of the Rd cases is similar to the treatment of the W's in level 1. The level 2 correction term is computed by dividing the average length of community stay, prior to death of the Rd individuals, by 274, the maximum potential duration of the follow-up phase, and then subtracting this result from unity.

The denominator of the primary level 2 index represents the number of R individuals in a cohort who had "equal exposure to the risk of reinstitutionalization." This index is computed for the admission cohort of a hospital and for each resident cohort. Subsequent admissions of cohort members to other institutions, as well as readmissions to the study hospitals, are recorded.

The computation of the level 2 index, symbolized by 2a, may be illustrated by an example based on hypothetical data from two hypothetical hospitals (table 2).

TABLE 2. CALCULATION OF PRIMARY LEVEL 2
INDEX BASED ON HYPOTHETICAL DATA

	Hospital A	Hospital B
(1) R (number of hospital-approved releases).	116	114
(2) Rd (number of released patients dying in the community during followup phase).	8	14
(3) Ri (number of released patients who were reinstitutionalized during followup phase).	28	40
(4) Rs (number of released patients who remained in the community throughout the followup phase).	80	60
(5) Average number of days in community for Rd patients.	37	55
(6) $C = 1 - \dfrac{(5)}{274}$	0.86	0.80
(7) $2a = \dfrac{Ri}{R-(C \times Rd)} = \dfrac{(3)}{(1)-(6) \times (2)}$	.26	.39

For hospital A, 26 percent of the released patients who had "equal exposure to the risk of reinstitutionalization" had to return to an institution during the follow-up period. The figure for hospital B is 39 percent. Unlike the level 1 index, a low level 2 value represents "better hospital performance."

Although hospital B was giving more of its admission cohort patients a chance to return to the community than was hospital A, relatively fewer of hospital A's patients had to be reinstitutionalized during the follow-up phase. Therefore, it would be misleading to conclude, on the basis of the level 1 index, that hospital B was doing a better job than hospital A in "socially restoring" its patients.

Length of community stay. As in the secondary level 1 measure, the question "How long do those cohort patients who are released from the hospital remain in the community?" leads to a measurement of length of stay in the community.

This measure is simply the average number of days spent in the community by reinstitutionalized and authorized release members of a cohort during the follow-up phase of the study. The cohort members who died in the community are omitted from this computation because their inclusion would lower the value produced. This value might merely reflect the fact that a hospital has released a large number of elderly patients who died soon after their release and thus had no chance to remain in the community for the entire follow-up period or to be readmitted to the hospital. The secondary level 2 measure is computed for both the admission and resident cohorts of a hospital, as follows:

If $2b$ symbolizes the secondary level 2 measure, then

$$2b = \frac{\text{Sum } Lc(Ri,Rs)}{Ri + Rs} \tag{9}$$

where the numerator represents the number of days spent in the community by the reinstitutionalized and authorized release cohort members $(Lc = \text{days in community})$ during the follow-up phase of the study, and the denominator represents the number of members of these cohorts.

Records of readmissions of previously released members of the patient cohorts are obtained from the daily roster of admissions in each cooperating hospital. The procedure for recording admissions to other institutions as well as deaths in the community is described under level 3.

Level 3

Measurement of the social restoration performance of hospitals in terms of the number of patients given an opportunity to resume community living and of the number of these patients who remain in the community provide valuable clues to hospital effectiveness. These measures, however, leave a number of important questions unanswered. For example, "Is hospital performance successful if discharged patients remain in the community because they or their families balk at returning them to the hospital or because the patients or their families find readmission procedures too complex?"

The most direct measure of hospital success and the measure which furnishes a qualitative estimate of the social restoration effectiveness of the hospital is the posthospital adjustment of patients in the community. To know how well patients adjust after they leave the hospital, however, is not enough. Information on their prehospital experience is needed as a baseline for evaluating their posthospital adjustment. With reliable information on both prehospital and posthospital adjustment, inferences can be drawn about the impact of the hospital experience on patients. In this way, patients serve as their own controls, and the role of the hospital in contributing to changes in the community adjustment of patient cohorts is evaluated.

At this point in the program, a number of decisions had to be made. Since it is more difficult and expensive to collect information on the community adjustment of patients than to record their movement in a hospital setting, the project staff adopted two basic tenets: (a) that community residents familiar with the patient and his adjustment, rather than the patient himself, serve as sources of information; and (b) that the information sought have to do with broad "areas of social living" rather than with symptom portraits or mental status examinations. Patients most often enter a public psychiatric facility because of public or legal pressure rather than by self-determination, and such pressure becomes necessary, in the main, when the patient's functioning in broad areas of social adaptation shows malignant trends, either in terms of harming himself or of harming others.

Considerable pilot work has been done with "community informant questionnaires," which were mailed to informants in the community at the time of the patient's admission to the hospital and again 3 months after he was discharged. The names and addresses of informants were furnished by the patient. This procedure is relatively inexpensive, it can be handled by clerical staff, and it requires no travel funds. The 3-month interval can be altered or repeated as desired. With patients in the resident cohort who have been in the hospital more than 1 year, only posthospital information was requested.

In one hospital, nearly 80 percent of the questionnaires requesting information about the prehospital adjustment of patients were completed and returned by community informants. For questionnaires requesting information on posthospital adjustment, the return rate was only about 70 percent.

The community informant questionnaires are so designed that they can also be used as interviewing schedules. The initial questions concern identifying characteristics of the informant. The questionnaire is also used to determine whether the patient has died in the community or whether he was institutionalized again since his release from the hospital. The latter information will be used to supplement the data collected at the hospital for level 2 of social restoration. The majority of the remaining questions elicit information in four areas of social adjustment: social and family relations, social productivity (work, school, and other socially useful behavior), self-management (personal care and conduct), and antisocial behavior. Some questions ask the informant to indicate whether the patient has been engaged in a particular activity, such as work, and if so, to what extent. Other questions are structured in terms of comparison of the patient's behavior with the behavior of his peers in the community; still others ask the informant to indicate the patient's behavior by means of simple scales. Ideally, the same informants should complete both the prehospital and posthospital forms for a patient, but pragmatic considerations may force us to depart from this ideal.

There are a number of problems in the questionnaire approach. One concerns the appraisal of prehospital adjustment. Is hospital performance best measured by using as a baseline the patient's adjustment just prior to admission to the hospital or should the baseline be the point of most profound social disorganization, a point which may occur at a time other than just prior to admission to an institution? For this study, information was sought on the patient's adjustment during the 3-month period prior to his hospitalization. This avoids asking the informant to decide when the patient was most disturbed and has the additional advantage of providing information about him during the period immediately preceding the hospital's "taking over" his treatment.

Furthermore, the questions about prehospital adjustment must be parallel, or equivalent in content, to the questions asked during the posthospital follow-up program. For example, a question about work adjustment is designed to obtain information regarding the patient's work history during the 3-month period prior to his admission to the hospital and during a 9-month period following his release.

Other methods of gathering community adjustment information are being readied for pilot study. The method or methods which provide the most accurate information at the least cost per unit will be used in the full-scale research.

For members of the admission cohort, level 3 of social restoration may be measured by computing for each adjustment area the proportion of released patients who display a prehospital-posthospital improvement in social adjustment. Thus, the social productivity of these patients can be classified on the basis of information from prehospital questionnaires. Using a scoring scheme developed by the medical audit staff, the entire admission cohort of a hospital can be classified into five categories, ranging from high adjustment to low adjustment.

The information obtained from the posthospital questionnaires for admission cohort patients released during the observation phase of the study will be similarly classified. The number of patients released with hospital approval whose posthospital adjustment classification is higher than their prehospital adjustment classification can then be counted, and a hospital level 3 score for social productivity can be computed by using the formula

$$\frac{R(s) \text{ improved}}{R(s)} \qquad [10]$$

where R (s) denotes the number of individuals in the group released with hospital approval who remain adjusting in the community at a specified time after release, and the numerator represents the number of such individuals who show a prehospital-posthospital improvement in social productivity. A similar proportion will be computed for each of the other three social adjustment areas.

Since prehospital information probably will not be obtained for resident cohort members, we must be content with a proportion such as

$$\frac{R(s) \, 1,2}{R(s)} \qquad [11]$$

where the numerator represents the number of R (s) individuals classified on the basis of posthospital information in the two top categories of an adjustment area. For the resident cohort, we cannot speak definitively about improvement in social adjustment.

Summary

Most people associated with psychiatric hospital work are eager to improve their performance. The usual dilemma is to know how. The Medical Audit Plan for Psychiatric Hospitals, a research program being carried on at the Veterans Administration Hospital, Perry Point, Md., is developing a set of goals for public psychiatric hospitals. The program is also attempting to establish measuring rods for determining how completely hospitals have achieved their objectives and to uncover the facets of hospital structure or programing which influence the degree to which objectives are achieved.

This paper discusses one objective of the program, social restoration, defines this objective, and describes a system for recording relevant hospital-patient events. It also considers characteristics for measuring these events, proposes indices for estimating hospital restoration results, and suggests similar treatment of other hospital objectives.

Application of this methodology is being planned for a series of State hospitals. If the approach proves practicable, and if it yields meaningful information about hospital organization, it should be possible to make program adjustments in psychiatric hospitals with the hope of improving end results of the hospital effort.

REFERENCES

1. Pollack, E. S., Person, P. H., Kramer, M., and Goldstein, H. Patterns of Retention, Release, and Death of First Admissions to State Mental Hospitals. PHS Pub. No. 672 (Public Health Monogr. No. 58). Washington: U.S. Government Printing Office, 1959.
2. Ninth Annual Conference of Mental Hospital Statisticians: Progress in Reporting Mental Hospital Statistics. Pub. Hlth. Rep. 74: 878-882, 1959.
3. Dorn, H. F. Methods of Analysis for Follow-up Studies. Human Biol. 22: 238-248, 1950.

This study was sponsored by the School of Hygiene and Public Health, Johns Hopkins University, and was supported by grants from the Veterans Administration and the National Institute of Mental Health, Public Health Service.

19

A Cumulative Register of Psychiatric Services in a Community

ELMER A. GARDNER, HAROLD C. MILES, HOWARD P. IKER and
JOHN ROMANO

THIS is the first report of a longitudinal study of the interaction between an entire large American community and, for practical purposes, all parts of an extensive, highly developed network of psychiatric services which serve that community.

The heart of the study is a register to which are reported contacts between psychiatric patients and the gamut of psychiatric services in the community. A general outline of the operation of the register will be given below under Method.[1]

The project arose from the perception of the principal investigators that this particular community and the unusual network of psychiatric services in it offer an opportunity to collect simultaneously longitudinal data about persons with diagnosed mental disorders and similar data about the operation of a wide range of psychiatric services. In the past, longitudinal data about either psychiatric patients or psychiatric services have been limited to a particular type of patient or a particular type of service. Because of the broad scope of the reporting sources and the longitudinal design of the register, the data from it will have unique value in advancing our knowledge about both patients and services. Kramer, Pollack, Locke, and Bahn have discussed in detail the need for data of this type.[2] The total value of the register will be realized only as subsidiary studies are developed which will use the data from it as baselines or points of departure. The initial body of information, in large measure, serves to develop hypotheses or to frame questions for more intensive studies.

As suggested above, the development of the project to be described in this paper and others which will follow was made possible by a particularly fortunate combination of circumstances which include the nature of the psychiatric services in the community and the nature of the community itself. The complete listing of the services involved will be given under Method. They include a comprehensive range of the usual services in unusual quantity. The state mental hospital which serves the area is located near the center of this community. The Department of Psychiatry of the University of Rochester provides an intellectually stimulating common meeting ground for the psychiatrists practicing in the community, as well as the facilities which they need in treating their patients. This study is a part of the extensive research program of the department through which the interest and cooperation of the psychiatrists in the community was elicited.

Demographic and geographic factors add to the attractiveness of the area as a site for epidemiological research. For this project the community is an entire county which, according to the 1960 census, has a population of 586,400—318,600 in the city of Rochester and 267,800 in the suburban and rural agricultural areas around it.

The combination of high-quality services readily available locally and the long distances which separate Monroe County from comparable services reduces the tendency for patients to seek help outside this community. A survey of the private psychiatric hospitals in the eastern part of the country during the early part of 1960 showed that they were caring for only eight residents of the county. The central office records of the New York State Department of Mental Hygiene are checked each year for residents of the county admitted to state hospitals other than the local Rochester State Hospital. By this method, 145 were found in other state hospitals during the early months of 1960 when the register was initiated. Most of the 145 represented patients who had been hospitalized for many years.

Each of the principal investigators brought to the project his own particular interests. Accordingly, each started with a set of broad goals and the sets of goals varied. Gradually, as they have worked together in setting up the data-gathering apparatus of the register, they have come to agree on a common set of broad purposes. It must be understood that a statement of these purposes is intended to encompass all the separate studies which may originate from the register.

The investigative goals will be listed under three general headings which overlap considerably: Clinical, Epidemiological, and Service Evaluation (Administrative).

Clinical Investigative Goals

We hope to contribute toward the improvement of our nosology. Nosological difficulties have plagued research in mental disorders for more than a century. Involved is the whole problem of the validity and stability of the diagnoses applied to mental disorders. Sometimes this problem is so annoying that therapists give up and take refuge in the attitude that diagnoses are, for the most part, unimportant and irrelevant to treatment. Nevertheless, classification always has been a necessity in scientific progress. The better we can define that which we observe or attempt to manipulate, the more effective will be our efforts to control the variables in research efforts and to communicate our observations to others. Intrinsic to the community in which this project is operating is a common phenomenon which offers an unusual opportunity to study the stability of psychiatric diagnoses. We have the impression that it is fairly common for a patient to have contact with several separate psychiatric agencies in the course of a few months, with each contact in enough depth to result in a diagnostic impression. He may contact the same agency twice in the process. Whether or not there is free communication among the agencies, each makes quite a separate diagnostic evaluation. With the longtitudinal data-collecting machinery of the register, this situation may help in studying the stability of existing diagnostic systems. Persistent interchangeability may suggest that some of our present diagnostic categories are not discrete entities, and particular patterns of change from one diagnosis to another may indicate which are related.

Our clinical investigative goals include a better understanding of the course of mental disorders. Some of the patients reported to the register receive treatment, others do not. The register itself will give much information about the course of specific disorders as varying treatments are attempted. It will remain, however, for subsequent follow-up studies—designed from the data in the register as a broad and firm foundation—to give a more complete picture of the functional and clinical status of carefully selected samples of patients who do not receive treatment or who receive treatment but then are lost to follow-up via the register.

Epidemiological Goals

Originally, the project was thought of as a study of the incidence and prevalence of mental disorders. It will make possible some comparisons of rates of diagnosed mental disorder in this community with rates of mental disorder uncovered in other communities by different methods. These comparisons may demonstrate the relationship between the total amount of mental disorder in a community which can be found by field survey and the amount which will be diagnosed by a network of services when the service available limits detection to a minimal degree. Again, the total epidemiological value of the register will be realized only if it can be used as the foundation for periodic surveys, as suggested by the recent publication of the Committee on Preventive Psychiatry of the Group for Advancement of Psychiatry.[8] The register will make a significant contribution to such surveys by permitting them to be focused on sample areas where a minimum of effort will permit the addition of data from the surveys to the basic data in the register to give highly reliable and easily repeated incidence and prevalence information.

The lack of a sociologist or a cultural anthropologist with the team of investigators will handicap the full exploitation of the data in the register. It is planned to correlate the available demographic data from the patient population with census data, but there are definite limitations to such an approach. Although the investigators have sought repeated consultation from sociologists in planning the research approach, it is evident that such help is needed on a regular basis.

Service Evaluation (Administrative) Goals

These goals enlarge those described under the heading Clinical Investigative Goals to include the whole community and the whole network of services. They seek to add together data about individual patients who have in common the one factor of having received service from one facility or one type of service. They have important implications for administrators responsible for program design, especially those people responsible for the increasing involvement of tax money in community mental health programs. The register itself will shed light on several important questions, such as, "Which types of service meet the needs of which types of patients in a decisive way?" The lack of further contact by a patient with other sources of service might suggest that his needs have been met by a given service. The converse of this question is, of course, "Which types of service furnished to which types of patient are followed, in significantly high ratios, by the appearance of these patients shortly thereafter in the case loads of agencies providing different types of service?" Answers to these questions will permit us to direct patients more efficiently to the services which are most likely to meet their needs, as suggested by criteria of diagnosis, age, and so on. Again, definitive answers to questions about the results of service can come only from follow-up studies of patients reported to the register, but these follow-up studies can be designed to produce more conclusive results with less effort by using the data in the register as the universe from which to select samples for intensive investigation of clinical and functional status.

The register will also give the people responsible for providing mental health services to a community an opportunity to study the impact of new services on the case loads of the individual agencies which contribute to the total network. It offers an opportunity to learn how to design community health programs on the basis of factual data rather than on the basis of "authoritative opinion."

Method

This is a study of psychiatric service and the individuals receiving this service. We have defined psychiatric service as that provided by psychiatrists in patient care and evaluation or similar service rendered by professional personnel in a facility where a psychiatrist has the ultimate responsibility for patient care. Such a definition obviously excludes many individuals with psychopathology who utilize other sources of help, but when we attempt to go beyond these limits we can find no line of demarcation. Furthermore, the variation of knowledge and psychiatric sophistication among the reporting individuals then precludes even a minimal comparability of reported data. The social workers in the psychiatric clinics, for example, have a diagnostic and therapeutic orientation which is comparable to that of the psychiatrists in the clinics, in contrast to the workers at the social service agencies who have no common orientation which they share with the psychiatric services. On occasion, the boundaries of that which constitutes psychiatric service are blurred, and individual judgments have to be made. Since we make no systematic effort to obtain reporting for epilepsy or mental retardation, we include these patients in the register only when there is an accompanying psychiatric diagnosis. These people are not cared for primarily by the psychiatric services in our community, and the additional reporting sources required to include them would overtax our capacity to maintain reliability of our data.

A wide variety of psychiatric services, both privately and publicly financed, providing evaluative and therapeutic services and representing almost the full range of psychiatric theory and practice report to the Cumulative Register Study. It is our impression that most major mental disorders are detected by this network of services. How distorted this impression is remains to be seen. Table 1 lists all these facilities with the number of hospital admissions and clinic visits for 1960 to present a picture of the volume of service which they provide. We chose to include the Canandaigua Veterans Hospital in the register although it is the only reporting source not located within the boundaries of Monroe County. It lies approximately nine miles outside the

TABLE 1. PSYCHIATRIC FACILITIES REPORTING
TO THE CUMULATIVE REGISTER STUDY

Outpatient Facilities
Patient and Collateral Visits in 1960

Adult Services

Psychiatric Outpatient Department of Strong Memorial Hospital*	13,410
Outpatient Department of Rochester State Hospital*	5,076
Alcoholism Clinic in Rochester General Hospital	4,103
Veterans Administration Mental Hygiene Clinic*	3,661

Children and Adolescents

Rochester Child Guidance Clinic	5,365
Psychiatric Outpatient Department of Strong Memorial Hospital—Child Psychiatry Division*	3,298
De Paul Clinic of Catholic Charities	1,669

Diagnostic and Emergency Service

Emergency Department of University Medical Center—Psychiatric Division*	1,801

Inpatient Facilities

Total Admissions
(Includes Out-of-County Residents)

	Admissions	Bed Capacity
University of Rochester Medical Center* (July 1, 1960 through June 30, 1961)	1,238	98
Monroe County Infirmary Psychiatric Unit (1960)	1,362	36
Rochester State Hospital (April 1, 1960, through March 31, 1961)*	1,295	3,500
Residential Treatment Center for Children (1960)	11	16
Canandaigua Veterans Administration Hospital (1960)*	489	1,700

*These facilities provide service, in varying proportions, to other areas in addition to Monroe County. This table is intended to indicate the size of the facilities reporting to the register and not to demonstrate the amount of service to Monroe County residents or the part these facilities play in the study.

county boundaries, admits an average of 25 patients from this county yearly, and maintains a close relationship with the Veterans Administration Clinic in Rochester.

Both the inpatient units and outpatient facilities have provided virtually complete reporting since the initiation of the study. Although the reporting from a given source and from the entire network of service may not be complete initially, omissions tend to be detected over a period of time. This results from the elaborate system of checks made possible by the relatively small area included in the study, the interrelatedness of the sources, and the multiple contacts reported.

There are currently 47 psychiatrists engaged at least part time in the private practice of psychiatry. Of these, four have not participated in the register at any time and two have been incomplete in their reporting. Although it is difficult to check, we doubt that the non-reporting psychiatrists contact even 10 per cent of the total number of individuals seen in private practice.

The group studied consists of all residents of Monroe County who receive psychiatric service from the facilities or practitioners reporting to the register. To determine residency, the address at the time of contact is used. Certain groups, such as students with a permanent residence out of the county or chronically institutionalized individuals, are included in the register, but they may be omitted from specific analyses when the address is used to evaluate the socioeconomic environment. For this purpose the address is allocated to a census tract, and 1960 census data can then be employed when needed.

We use a one-page reporting form and have found that the questions must be concise, readily answerable, and clinically oriented. The data requested consist of two types: (1) identifying and demographic, and (2) clinical. The former includes the following: name, maiden name, address, date of birth, race, sex, marital status, and, when possible, Social Security number. The clinical data obtained are limited to questions about prior psychiatric service, the current diagnostic impressions, dates of beginning and terminating the current episode of service, the type of service, and the type of treatment provided. Rather than jeopardize the collection of our basic data we have restricted the number and complexity of the questions asked. Because this is an ongoing project, we can elaborate upon our basic data with periodic sampling.

Identification occasionally has been a problem and will become increasingly more difficult as our file grows. A soundex system and a careful search for names which may be misspelled or mispronounced

TABLE 2. MONROE COUNTY RESIDENTS REPORTED
TO CUMULATIVE REGISTER AS RECEIVING PSYCHIATRIC
SERVICE ON JANUARY 1, 1960, BY SEX AND RACE

	Number	Rates per 1,000 Population*	Age-Adjusted to Total Monroe County Population*
Total	4,958	8.46	
Male	2,352	8.31	8.55
Female	2,606	8.59	7.80
White	4,773	8.50	8.37
Nonwhite	185	7.38	10.80
White male	2,254	8.32	8.48
Nonwhite male	98	7.97	11.01
White female	2,519	8.67	8.23
Nonwhite female	87	6.81	10.67

*Population as given by the 1960 census.

are used to minimize the duplications which can occur. Social Security numbers, when available, are helpful in the effort.

Multiple diagnostic impressions may be given for any patient, and our reporting sources are told to use their own diagnostic terminology. This flexibility minimizes the distortion which can occur if the reporting person must use a rigid and unfamiliar nosologic scheme. The diagnoses are coded according to the APA Nomenclature, and one of the authors examines all the reports to clarify the diagnosis when necessary. If the diagnosis is deferred or the patient is believed to be without mental disorder, this is recorded as such.

Ideally, we attempt to obtain complete reporting for all new and reopened cases. Because of the diversity of our reporting sources, the data-gathering operation varies with almost each service, and our basic reporting form is modified to facilitate reporting from facilities of different types. Inpatient units providing diagnostic or short-term service report at the time of discharge, whereas long-term units report at both the time of admission and release. Any change from inpatient to outpatient care is recorded as a discharge, even though this may not be recorded as such by the hospital. Here, as in several other instances, our coding permits differentiation of the subgroups—such as patients released to convalescent care—from the group coded primarily as discharges.

For outpatient care, both clinic and private practice, reports are completed within the period of the first few interviews. For diagnostic or consultative service only a single report is requested, but for those continuing in outpatient care, follow-up information is requested at three-to-six-month intervals.

To minimize interpretation by ourselves or the reporting sources, only contacts in which the patient is seen are recorded. The data of the initial patient visit is recorded as the date of beginning service except in child therapy, in which the initial visit by the parent may be used. Outpatient care is terminated when the patient has not been seen for a period of time reasonably indicative of termination, usually three months beyond the planned return appointment. The date of the last visit is recorded as the date of termination unless hospitalization interrupts the outpatient care; then the date of admission to the hospital is recorded as termination of outpatient service.

Although the operation of the register has been varied to suit each reporting source, the data from all sources are recorded in the same manner on reporting forms and then coded for IBM cards. Two IBM card files are maintained. One contains the name, other identifying information, and a serial number for the individual; the other contains the remaining data with only the serial number for identification. A data card is completed for each new period of service and for each follow-up form which indicates some change in the patient's status.

A system of monthly checks, using the tabulating equipment, has been instituted to locate misfiled and omitted data cards. Editing boards have been designed for the 101 Statistical Machine to locate errors involving mutually exclusive conditions, impossible assignment of code numbers, blank columns in fields which always must be punched, and so on. Our analyses have been confined to tabulating equipment and are largely cross-sectional. The expansion of the study and the planning for a variety of cohort analyses already have demonstrated the need for the transfer of the data to magnetic tape and computer programs. This change in systems is now partially completed.

TABLE 3. MONROE COUNTY RESIDENTS REPORTED
TO THE CUMULATIVE REGISTER AS BEGINNING AN
EPISODE OF PSYCHIATRIC SERVICE BETWEEN
JANUARY 1, 1960, AND DECEMBER 31, 1960, NOT
PREVIOUSLY REPORTED, BY SEX AND RACE

	Number	Rates per 1,000 Population*	Age-Adjusted to Total Monroe County Population*
Total	5,003	8.53	
Male	2,547	8.99	9.09
Female	2,456	8.10	7.93
White	4,748	8.46	8.39
Nonwhite	255	10.17	11.55
White male	2,409	8.90	8.96
Nonwhite male	138	11.23	12.63
White female	2,339	8.05	7.85
Nonwhite female	117	9.16	10.34

*Population as given by the 1960 census.

For follow-up study we have been able to learn about the loss of patients to the study by death or emigration from the county. The New York State Health Department has been sending us their IBM cards which record the deaths of all Monroe County residents, and this is collated with our files. We also have a systematic mechanism for learning when persons reported to the register move about within the county or move out of the county.

Discussion

The accompanying tables present the total figures from the first year of data collection. At the beginning of 1960, 8.5 individuals for every thousand in Monroe County were receiving psychiatric care and another 8.53 per thousand contacted psychiatric services during the year. Thus, 17.0 per thousand population or approximately one out of every 60 Monroe County residents received some type of psychiatric service in 1960.

In subsequent reports, we shall proceed with the examination of these initial data as well as periodic tabulation and analysis of the psychiatric service provided during a specified interval of time. Cohort follow-up may provide a more dynamic picture but must await a longer period of observation to provide reliable data. It is the breadth, completeness, and duration of this longitudinal view of individuals coming into contact with psychiatric resources that we believe will be the unique contribution of this study.

NOTES AND REFERENCES

1. If a more detailed description is desired, it can be obtained by writing to the authors.
2. Kramer, M., Pollack, E. S., Locke, B. Z., and Bahn, A. K. National Approach in the Evaluation of Community Mental Health Programs. A.J.P.H. 51: 969-979, 1961.
3. GAP Committee on Preventive Psychiatry. Problems of Estimating Changes in Frequency of Mental Disorders. Rep. No. 50. New York, N.Y., 1961.

This project was supported by grants from the National Institute of Mental Health and the Milbank Memorial Fund. A pilot study in 1959 was aided by funds from the Ford Foundation.

We regret that the limits of space preclude our listing all the many individuals contributing to the formulation and operation of the project. We should like to express our appreciation to Dr. Henry Brill, Mr. Robert Patton, and others in the New York State Department of Mental Hygiene for their constant support and frequent consultative help. Drs. Morton Kramer and Anita Bahn from the Biometrics Branch of the NIMH have made many invaluable suggestions in the development of the goals and methodology of the study. Dr. Christopher Terrence, director of the Rochester State Hospital, Dr. William Hart, director of the Monroe County Infirmary Psychiatric Unit, and Dr. Louis Lopez, director of the Canandaigua Veterans Hospital, have been readily available to aid in planning and sustaining the reporting from their facilities.

We particularly wish to express our indebtedness to the many psychiatrists, psychologists, and social workers whose cooperation make this project a reality. Those psychiatrists in private practice who have generously donated time from an already full schedule and active practice have especially provided a new body of knowledge in psychiatry.

Section IV

Examples of Program Evaluation

20

Evaluation of Public Health Nursing Services Through a Study of Patient Progress

MAUDE CONWAY BAILEY

EVALUATION of public health nursing services has been a subject of interest and concern to supervisory, consultant, and administrative nursing staffs of the South Carolina State Board of Health for many years. Therefore, it was not surprising that Miss Doris Roberts' report of a Study of Patient Progress was received with great enthusiasm and interest by the public health nurses who attended the meeting of the Southern Branch, APHA, in the spring of 1962. Two South Carolina nurses who attended Southern Branch were members of the program committee for the semiannual conference for public health nursing supervisors in South Carolina. Miss Roberts was invited to attend and interpret the method at the supervisors' conference on December 4 and 5, 1962. The public health nursing supervisors, state nursing staff, and the director of local health services were impressed with the patient progress method and decided that it would be used in selected counties if it met with the approval of the local health officers. The director of public health nursing and the director of local health services submitted the plan to the local health officers at their quarterly meeting in December, 1962, and it was approved.

The patient progress study approach is a method especially geared to program evaluation. It involves the identification of needs of patients which are assessed by public health nurses and the recording of changes identified in these needs within a three-month study period. In adapting the study to South Carolina, it was planned to have all counties with public health nursing supervisors and all their field staffs participate in the study. Actually, this was not possible in all areas, therefore in a few counties some selection of staff was necessary. A total of 17 counties with 86 staff nurses and 21 supervisors participated in the study. This represented all but one county with supervisors and 77 per cent of their total field staffs.

South Carolina's objectives in participating in the study were:

To ascertain the scope of services offered in local health departments.

To determine gaps or changing emphases in services.

To examine sources of referrals other than nursing.

To determine nurses' awareness of needs of patients.

To assess the role the nurse plays in case-finding.

To evaluate the effectiveness of nurses in getting patients under medical supervision.

To identify needs for services other than those provided by nurses.

To explore the possible effectiveness of public health nursing services.

Study guides, patient and family schedules were mimeographed and made available to the local health departments. The study began in all 17 counties between January 14 and February 13, 1963.

Because this was the first study of such magnitude and because the Public Health Service was ready to test portions of a guide to the study method which was being developed, we were able to obtain more consultant help from the Public Health Service than may otherwise have been available.

A consultant nurse, Division of Nursing, Public Health Service, spent a month in South Carolina during January and February assisting nursing supervisors in interpreting the study method to their respective staffs. In June she spent two weeks assisting the supervisors in editing and reviewing information recorded.

As might be expected, some of the study procedures and classifications had to be adapted to our policies and services in South Carolina. In addition, guidelines had to be developed to meet individual county differences as the study progressed. For example, although the aim was to have each nurse admit a total of 20 patients to the study, several had not achieved this quota at the end of two months. Rather than have the data-collecting phase extend over a long period, and since the patient group was over 1,200, it was arbitrarily decided to discontinue admitting patients at the end of two months. Each patient remained in the study for a period of three months unless discharged earlier. The study period had been completed for the majority of the patients in June. Tabulation of data was done by clerks in the participating health departments under the direction of a statistician,

Public Health Service, and a records consultant, South Carolina State Board of Health. By October all data had been tabulated.

Findings

On October 24 and 25, 1963, only ten months after initiation, findings of the study in the form of tables and graphs were ready for review, interpretation, and discussion at the supervisors conference. Those present for the conference were the participating supervising nurses, state nursing staff, nine health officers, three division directors, and representatives of the Public Health Service.

During the study period 1,227 patients from 776 families were admitted to the study in the 17 counties.

Of the 776 families, 575 or 74.1 per cent fell into the "one service" category consisting of 644 or 52.5 per cent of the 1,227 patients with the following distribution: 273 or 42.4 per cent health supervision, 280 or 43.5 per cent chronic disease, and 91 or 14.1 per cent communicable disease. Of the 776 families, 201 or 25.9 per cent fell into the "more than one service" category consisting of 583 or 47.5 per cent of the patients with the following distribution: 217 or 37.2 per cent health supervision, 252 or 43.2 per cent health supervision and morbidity, and 114 or 19.6 per cent morbidity.

The size of the families ranged from 115 with nine or more members to 36 with only one member. There were 532 or 69 per cent of the families with more than one patient and 244 or 31 per cent with only one patient per family.

One of the objectives of the study was to determine the source of referral of patients to public health nursing service. As seen in Figure 1, most of the new patients were referred by the public health nurse or health department clinics. It is gratifying to find that private physicians refer a large number of patients for public health nursing service. It was somewhat disappointing to note that so few referrals came from schools.

As might be expected, 636 or 51.8 per cent of all referrals were for health supervision, 400 or 32.6 per cent chronic disease, 169 or 13.8 per cent communicable disease, and 22 or 1.8 per cent all other disease categories.

The long-range care which is indicated for chronic or communicable disease and health supervision explains, in part, why so few patients were discharged by the end of three months.

The majority of the patients, 1,014 or 82.6 per cent were in the study for the full three-month period. There were 213 or 17.4 per cent

FIGURE 1. SOURCE OF REFERRAL OF PATIENTS

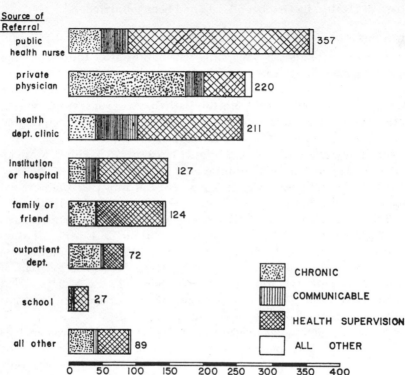

Number of patients.

of the patients discharged from nursing service prior to the end of the study. Of these, 128 were in the study for more than two months, but less than three months, and 85 were in the study less than two months.

Among the 1,227 patients, 15,002 needs were identified. These needs were related to the following conditions: 7,692 or 51.3 per cent to health supervision, 5,071 or 33.8 per cent to chronic disease, 1,972 or 13.1 per cent to communicable disease. All other conditions accounted for 267 or 1.8 per cent.

Identified needs according to type of service is presented in Figure 2. As can be seen, almost 50 per cent of all needs identified were directly related to nursing care. Immunizations and tests represented approximately 20 per cent of the needs identified, and medical care and social needs represented approximately 30 per cent. When one realizes that this represents an average of six nursing needs per patient and less

FIGURE 2. PATIENT NEEDS EVALUATED

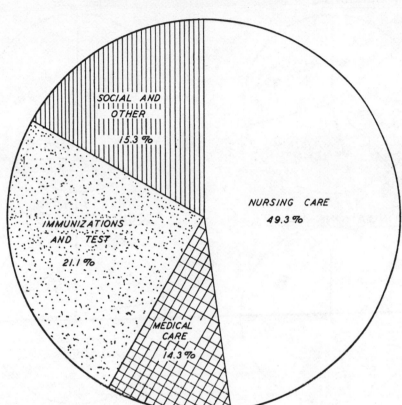

Total needs evaluated=15,002.

than two possible needs for medical attention, one must question whether it connotes comprehensive care.

In Figure 3, needs related to nursing, immunizations and tests, medical, social and other are further differentiated. As one would expect, 2,266 or 30.7 per cent of the nursing needs identified were for physical care. It is not surprising that 1,355 or 18.3 per cent of the needs were identified as behavior or emotional nor that 1,887 or 25.5 per cent were related to nutrition. Findings relative to medical and social needs were not unusual.

An objective of public health nursing is to teach patients or family members to care for their particular needs. In Figure 4 progress of

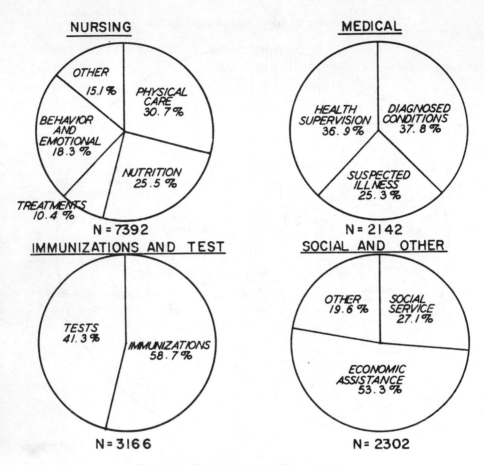

FIGURE 3. TYPE OF NEEDS EVALUATED

nursing care needs during the three-month study period is well demonstrated. Of the 6,574 needs initially identified as unmet, care for 5,201 or 79.1 per cent of these had been assumed by the family or else the condition had been corrected at the end of three months. At the end of the study period, the need continued for 977 or 14.9 per cent.

Needs of patients are not static as demonstrated in the difference at the end of the study of those initially classified as adequate. Most needs remained in the "adequate care" group, but some needs were unmet at the end of the study period.

One function of the public health nurse is to refer patients for medical supervision when needed as well as to urge patients to remain un-

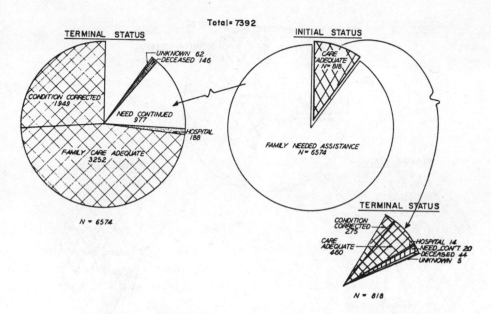

FIGURE 4. PROGRESS OF NURSING CARE NEEDS

der medical supervision as long as needed. Of the 2,142 medical needs initially identified, 1,035 or 48 per cent were under medical supervision (Figure 5).

It is of interest that 903 or 81.6 per cent of the 1,107 medical needs identified initially "not under care" were either corrected or else were under medical supervision at the end of three months. At the end of the study 190 or 17.1 per cent were still not under medical supervision.

In the initial identification of needs, 541 or 25.3 per cent of the medical needs were classified "suspected illness" (Figure 3). Of these, 141 or 26.1 per cent were under medical supervision initially. At the end of three months, 295 or 73.7 per cent of the 400 needs initially not under medical care were brought under medical care or else the condition had been corrected. The diagnosis was disproved in only 35 or 8.8 per cent of the "suspected illness" needs identified. The need continued for 88 or 22 per cent. Deceased, unknown, and hospitalized accounted for the remaining 4.3 per cent.

Immunizations and tests represented 21.1 per cent of all needs initially identified. At the end of three months most of these needs had been adequately satisfied.

Social and related needs accounted for 2,302 or 15.3 per cent of all

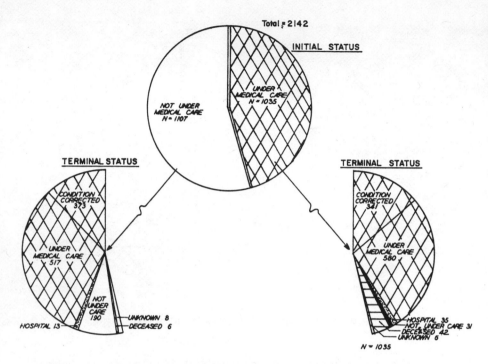

FIGURE 5. PROGRESS OF MEDICAL CARE NEEDS

needs initially identified. Of these, 1,742 or 75.7 per cent were not under care initially. As can be seen in Figure 6, 1,155 or 66.3 per cent of these needs had been eliminated or were under care by the end of the study. In 21.8 per cent service was not applied for, and the service was not available to meet the need for 162 or 9.3 per cent.

Chronically ill patients are often limited in the area of locomotion, bathing, dressing, and feeding. For the purpose of this study patients were rated on their limitation in the above-mentioned areas as shown in Figure 7. There were 440 chronically ill patients representing all disease categories in the study. Of these 266 or 60.5 per cent had no limitations in these areas during the entire study period. Limitations were present in 82 or 18.6 per cent which remained unchanged. In 57 or 12.9 per cent, there was improvement and in 12 or 2.7 per cent regression was noted.

Discussion

The findings of this study have been and will continue to be useful in many ways. From the standpoint of program, it is evident that pos-

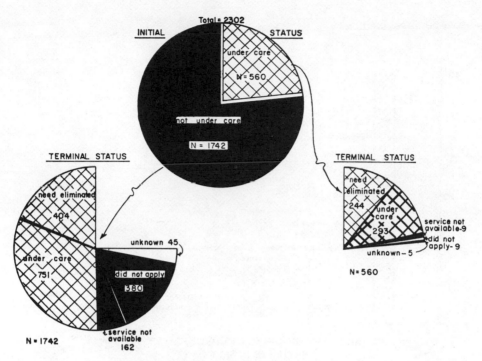

FIGURE 6. PROCESS OF SOCIAL SERVICE
AND RELATED NEEDS

sible disproportionate emphasis is being placed in certain service categories. Why is this? Is it because of a real need of both patients and
families or expressed demands of the community? Definite gaps in
service were noticeable in some agencies. We are interested in knowing the reasons for this. Are the reasons based on lack of need in a
community, hesitancy of health department personnel to initiate certain programs, indecision with regard to health department responsibility, or inertia? Regardless of the reason, these findings serve as a
basis for administrative guidance and consultation in terms of a balanced program with emphasis on service in all categories according to
need. Already personnel of the state office have met with the staffs
of several local health departments to analyze new data and to discuss
ways of improving the over-all program. This kind of analysis will be
done in the other counties.

Since the study was patient-centered, it was possible from the beginning for supervisors to spot strengths and weaknesses in nurses,
nurses who were sensitive to patient situations, and those who needed

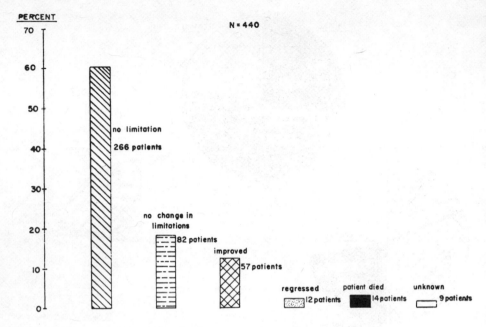

FIGURE 7. PROGRESS OF CHRONICALLY ILL
PATIENTS IN SELF-CARE

help in assessing needs of individuals and families. Of particular significance to supervisors was the difficulty encountered by some nurses in differentiating medical, social, and nursing needs. The trend to delegate more medical responsibility to nursing and the tendency of the nurse to think in terms of orders rather than patient and family needs are probably responsible for some of this difficulty. This method of assessing needs proved helpful in pointing up the importance of providing for guidance to the nurses in this area.

Supervisors and staff nurses felt that experience in determining elements of patient needs was valuable to the nurses in establishing priorities for service to patients in their respective districts. As supervisors worked with staff in the study, they also had time for self-analysis. Many realized some of their own inadequacies and shortcomings as supervisors. To the supervisors, the patient schedules proved to be an excellent supervisory tool—one which can be used to strengthen their own supervisory skills as well as the skills of the nurses working under their direction. They feel this method will be particularly helpful in orienting new nurses, in helping nurses who have difficulty in giving depth to nursing care, and in supervising care of certain patients who present many problems. Patient schedules are made available and are being used by supervisors for this purpose. The patient schedule has become part of the patient's record in two counties where the study method is being used for patients admitted to special stroke projects. This enhances the opportunity for continuous evaluation of the patient's progress, the effectiveness of the nurse's service, and the depth of the supervisory process.

The demonstration of strength and weakness in public health nursing performance points up needs in the area of depth in the supervisory process and justifies increased attention to inservice education for supervisors and staff nurses. It shows the need for employment of additional supervisors so that more time can be given to individual guidance of staff nurses in order to improve quality of service as well as to promote growth of the staff.

Health department personnel can use the study findings to interpret to medical societies and appropriating bodies the effectiveness of public health nursing services, the nurse's role in case-finding, her effectiveness in motivating patients to seek medical supervision and related services, the scope of the health department program and outstanding areas of need for service in various communities.

From an educational standpoint, the study has resulted in a request by the School of Nursing, University of South Carolina, to the Division of Nursing, Public Health Service, for an orientation of the entire faculty to the method of evaluating patient progress with the objective of incorporating this method throughout the entire student program. We feel this experience of student nurses will be reflected in service as they are employed in various public health agencies in South Carolina.

Recommendations

As a result of this experience we were able to make the following suggestions to the Public Health Service for incorporation into the guide for studying patient progress:

More time should be allocated for staff orientation. A minimum of five days is necessary for this activity. The amount of orientation necessary may represent a great deal of agency time, but supervisors feel time spent in interpretation and actual practice in assessing patient needs is of paramount importance and can be justified as inservice education.

As the study progressed it became evident that a nurse on the state level should have been assigned to this activity. It is almost impossible for interpretation to be uniform without one person to weigh decisions and to convey information to others. This is important, too, in terms of future plans for using the study method.

In the initial planning, arrangements should be made in terms of time and training for clerical staff to tabulate data.

Perhaps our original objectives for evaluating public health nursing services through a study of patient progress seemed ambitious. We believe they have all been met in some measure.

We realize that no one method is the complete answer to evaluation of public health nursing services. However, this method has proved to be of real value not only in the evaluation of the accomplishment of public health nurses' services, but it is already resulting in improved quality of services by the public health nurses in South Carolina.

This paper was presented before the Public Health Nursing and Mental Health Sections of the American Public Health Association at its annual meeting in Kansas City, Mo., November, 1963.

21

Evaluation of an Antismoking Program Among High School Students

MARY MONK, MATTHEW TAYBACK, and JOSEPH GORDON

WITHIN the past five years, as the evidence that cigarette smoking is a major cause of lung cancer has mounted, investigators have begun to examine more closely the smoking population and the smoking habit. These studies have included research into the number of people who smoke, why they smoke, and how they might be persuaded to stop. Such studies, of course, are of great interest to public health officials, educators and others who are concerned with the prevention of a habit, especially among young people, that contributes to some 40,000 lung cancer deaths a year in the United States alone.

There have been numerous investigations of the extent of smoking among high school students,[1] some indicating that nearly half may be regular smokers by the twelfth grade. One study of high school students[2] indicated that conformity to others and a desire to impress others were two main reasons the students gave for smoking; a lack of enjoyment and concern for health were the major reasons given for not beginning or for discontinuing smoking.

Attempts to reduce or prevent cigarette smoking among young people are increasing, but there is also a growing demand on the part of public health administrators and health educators to assess the success of these efforts. Programs to eliminate or reduce smoking are reported to have met with varying success. An evaluation of a program in Oregon in which three posters and pamphlets were distributed over the period of a school year[3] showed that the number of new smokers was significantly reduced by presenting evidence to high school students that smoking was related to lung cancer. A city-wide campaign in Edinburgh, with posters, meetings, and newspaper publicity pointing out the hazards of smoking, had little effect upon smoking among adults.[4]

The report of a three-year program in Winnipeg, Canada,[5] indicates that smoking markedly declined among high school students in an area where the "program was enthusiastically received and student participation was most active" (p. 56). There was only a slight reduction in smoking among high school boys in other areas, where the program was not presented.

The study reported here was jointly carried out by the Baltimore City Health Department, the Maryland Division of the American Cancer Society, the Baltimore City Department of Education, and the Johns Hopkins School of Hygiene. The objectives of the study were: (a) to design a program which would persuade high school students to stop or not to begin smoking cigarettes; (b) to evaluate the success of the program; and (c) to gain information helpful in deciding what the future program and materials in such an effort should be.

Program and Methods of Evaluation

Prior to inaugurating the program in September, 1963, approval was obtained from the school administrators to conduct the program and its evaluation. With the considered judgment of school officials, two comparable schools were selected—one, the experimental school in which the antismoking program would be held, and the other the control school with no program. Both schools were male senior high schools, each with approximately 3,000 students and each with a fairly large proportion of students in college preparatory courses. In September of 1963 all students in both schools filled out questionnaires in their home rooms to determine smoking habits at the beginning of the project. Questions dealt with current smoking habits, attitudes about smoking, age, kind of school course, parents' occupations and smoking habits, and in what activities the students participated. The questionnaires were anonymous.

The antismoking program was then instituted in the experimental school; except for completing the same questionnaire in May, 1964, there was no further activity conducted in the control school. Students in the experimental school had 26 exposures in the antismoking project over a period of seven months. Because most of the materials available presented the evidence concerning smoking and lung cancer and because the evidence was shown to be convincing in a previous study,[3] the program primarily concentrated on this theme. Within these limits the following campaign was conducted:

1. In September and April school-wide assemblies, mainly through the school's public address system to all home rooms, were held. Participants in the discussions were the school principal, the president of the student council, the commissioner of health, a scientist who had conducted research in cancer, and two

physicians specializing in cancer and chest surgery. In these programs there were discussions of the facts on smoking and lung cancer, the effects of smoking on the circulatory system, and a plea to students not to start smoking, or to give it up if they had.

2. Sixteen two-color 11″ x 14″ posters were placed on display in home rooms at semi-monthly intervals from October, 1963 to May, 1964. These posters were designed to appeal to teenagers.

3. Two letters by the commissioner of health were sent to all students at their homes, one in November, 1963, and the other in February, 1964. The first enclosed the New York State Department of Health leaflet, "Smoking—It's Up to You," and the second gave a brief summary of the Surgeon General's Report on Smoking and Health. [1]

4. A series of three articles appeared in the school newspaper, one in September, another in October, and a third in March. The articles reviewed some evidence about smoking and disease.

5. Two leaflets were distributed: "Shall I Smoke?", a publication of the American Cancer Society, was given to all students in October, and a new Health Department publication, "Why Buy a Pack of Trouble?", containing excerpts from the Surgeon General's Report, was given to all science students.

6. One large exhibit entitled "Why Buy a Pack of Trouble?" was placed on display in the gymnasium from March to the end of the school year.

Group discussions on smoking and health were held by the school physician or nurse with nearly all tenth-grade students in groups of six to eight boys. These were held in conjunction with routine physical examinations. In addition teachers were asked to discuss the evidence about smoking and lung cancer and initiate appropriate classroom projects. Teachers of science, physical education, English, and art received special teaching kits; films, tape recordings, and other materials were available.

In May, 1964, all students in both schools were again asked to fill out the same questionnaires they had answered the previous fall. Teachers in both schools completed forms indicating how many students had taken part in classroom discussions, or projects about the effects of cigarette smoking.

As a supplement to the written questionnaire, 95 students, representing all grades and courses in the experimental school, were interviewed in order to determine their reaction to the program and what they thought might be more effective in such a program. These interviews were held during school hours, in school, and were approximately 15 minutes long. The interviewers were from the Johns Hopkins School of Hygiene.

Results

The major results of the study are presented in terms of the total proportion of regular smokers in the two high schools for 10th, 11th, and 12th grades in the fall and in the spring. A regular smoker is defined as a boy who smokes at least one day a week. Since the two high schools were not identical with respect to the students attending them, the students in the courses at each school which were most similar are compared separately. These courses are identified as "college-prep." In the college-prep courses at both schools, 90 per cent to 97 per cent of the boys stated on the questionnaires that they plan to go to college. The occupations of the fathers of boys in these courses were also similar in the two schools. At the experimental school students in these courses represent about 65 per cent of the total student body; at the control school they represent about 85 per cent.

Further problems connected with the comparability of the schools, the validity of the questionnaire responses, and the use of a group rather than an individual measure of change, will be considered later in the discussion.

In the experimental school 90 per cent of the 3,748 enrolled students returned completed questionnaires in the fall of 1963. The percentage of students who were regular smokers was 37 in the 10th grade, 43 in the 11th, and 50 in the 12th grade (see Table 1). Among the students in the college-prep course the proportions were somewhat lower: 24 per cent were regular smokers in the 10th grade, 36 per cent in the 11th, and 44 per cent in the 12th.

In the spring of 1964, seven months after the first questionnaire and following the program described above, nearly 87 per cent of the enrolled students (3,390) filled out another questionnaire about their smoking habits and related information. At this time the proportion of regular smokers had increased among the 10th-grade students (Table 1), both in the total and college-prep groups. In the 11th and 12th grades the proportion of regular smokers decreased for both these groups. For all grades combined there was essentially no change in smoking, either in the total school or the college-prep course.

The comparable figures for the control school, where 95 per cent of the 2,218 enrolled students filled out questionnaires in the fall,

TABLE 1. PER CENT OF REGULAR SMOKERS IN
EXPERIMENTAL SCHOOL IN FALL AND SPRING,
BY GRADE FOR TOTAL AND COLLEGE-PREP COURSE

			Total		College Prep	
			%	No.	%	No.
Grade	10	Fall	36.7	(1,135)	24.5	(673)
		Spring	40.7	(989)	29.3	(593)
	11	Fall	42.6	(1,102)	36.0	(769)
		Spring	40.8	(961)	35.2	(676)
	12	Fall	49.7	(1,132)	44.0	(755)
		Spring	47.8	(988)	42.3	(652)
Total		Fall	43.0	(3,369)	35.2	(2,197)
		Spring	43.1	(2,938)	35.8	(1,921)

show that the percentages of regular smokers were 24, 33, and 41 in
the 10th, 11th, and 12th grades, respectively (Table 2). For the students
in the college prep course the corresponding percentages were 24, 29,
and 31.

In the spring, in the control school the number of smokers increased
in the 10th grade and decreased in the 11th and 12th (Table 2). These
changes from fall to spring, based on questionnaires filled out by 95

TABLE 2. PER CENT OF REGULAR SMOKERS IN
CONTROL SCHOOL IN FALL AND SPRING,
BY GRADE FOR TOTAL AND COLLEGE-PREP COURSE

			Total		College Prep	
			%	No.	%	No.
Grade	10	Fall	24.1	(721)	24.0	(716)
		Spring	27.7	(722)	27.1	(708)
	11	Fall	32.7	(683)	28.9	(591)
		Spring	30.9	(657)	25.7	(505)
	12	Fall	40.6	(705)	31.0	(494)
		Spring	37.1	(576)	27.9	(405)
Total		Fall	32.4	(2,109)	27.5	(1,801)
		Spring	31.6	(1,958)	26.9	(1,618)

per cent of the enrolled students (2,063), very closely parallel the changes in the experimental school. As was true in the experimental school, the change in smoking for all grades in the control school was negligible.

Although the total amount of smoking in the experimental school did not appear to be affected by the antismoking program, we considered it possible that certain groups within the school may have been more influenced than others. Consequently, we looked at changes in smoking among members of sports teams, and members of school clubs, who might be more concerned with activities in the school. There was little difference between the schools among these groups with respect to change in smoking habits (Table 3).

It also seemed possible that outside influences might interact with the antismoking program; who belonged to social clubs outside school; also among students whose parents smoked, as well as those whose parents did not smoke (Table 3). Very little change was noted in any

TABLE 3. PER CENT REGULAR SMOKERS AMONG
MEMBERS OF DIFFERENT GROUPS, BY SCHOOL, IN
FALL AND SPRING (COLLEGE-PREP COURSE ONLY)

	Per cent Regular Smokers			
	Experimental School		Control School	
	%	No.	%	No.
Members of sports teams				
Fall	32.8	(591)	24.7	(543)
Spring	30.9	(521)	24.1	(543)
Members of school clubs				
Fall	27.7	(873)	20.6	(793)
Spring	26.6	(750)	17.9	(711)
Members of outside social clubs				
Fall	40.4	(872)	36.1	(659)
Spring	39.8	(957)	34.2	(808)
Students both of whose parents smoke				
Fall	39.6	(722)	28.8	(607)
Spring	41.9	(583)	30.0	(507)
Students neither of whose parents smoke				
Fall	29.4	(541)	21.1	(466)
Spring	29.7	(558)	21.4	(495)

of these groups, although it is of interest that members of outside social groups are more likely to smoke than others, while members of school clubs and sports teams are less likely to do so. The expected relationship between student and parent smoking is also shown.

In the questionnaire we asked about attitudes toward smoking. Students checked whether they strongly or mildly agreed, were neutral, or mildly or strongly disagreed with eight statements about smoking. Since there were only small differences between grades, all grades were combined in the analysis. For four of these statements there was very little change in attitude in either school among college-prep students. For two statements—"When I have children I hope that they never smoke" and "There is nothing wrong with smoking"—students in both school changed their attitudes and were less favorable to smoking (Table 4). In the spring more smokers and nonsmokers agreed that they hoped their children would never smoke, although the differences were not significant for smokers in either school. More students in the spring disagreeed that there is nothing wrong with smoking, but the same proportions changed in both schools among both smokers and nonsmokers.

For two statements the desired change at the experimental school was greater than at the control school—"There is nothing wrong with smoking as long as a person smokes moderately" and "Smoking is dangerous to health." Only the change in attitude toward smoking as a health danger showed a significant difference between the schools, however. In the experimental school there was increasing agreement from fall to spring, while in the control school the change was negligible.

After the final questionnaires had been returned, 95 boys at the experimental school were interviewed. About 40 per cent of these boys were from the 10th grade, one-third from the 11th, and the remainder from the 12th; nearly one-half were from the college-prep course. Although the questionnaires in the fall and spring did not reveal it, on interview 22 of the 95 students stated they smoked less in the spring than they had in the fall; they were still, however, regular smokers. Altogether 44 per cent of the students interviewed were regular smokers.

One major objective of the interview was to determine if the information contained in the leaflets, letters, and assembly programs had been retained by the students. In answer to the question, "Do you think smoking affects health?", 94 out of 95 students said "Yes"; the 95th replied, "They say so." When asked how smoking affects health, 53 per cent of the students gave as their first response that it shortens the breath or "makes you short-winded" (Table 5). Significantly, this response was more likely to be given by smokers than nonsmokers. One of the main items in the program, however, was that cigarette smoking causes or is associated with lung cancer, and 16 per cent of the

TABLE 4. PER CENT OF STUDENTS AGREEING WITH
STATEMENTS ABOUT SMOKING, ACCORDING TO SMOKING
STATUS BY SCHOOL, IN FALL AND SPRING (COLLEGE-PREP COURSE ONLY)

	Per cent of Students Agreeing			
	Experimental School		Control School	
	%	No.	%	No.
Smokers				
Hope children never smoke				
Fall	59.0	(774)	57.5	(496)
Spring	61.6	(688)	62.3	(435)
Nothing wrong with smoking				
Fall	28.0		32.6	
Spring	21.9		25.7	
Smoking dangerous to health				
Fall	58.1		66.1	
Spring	67.7*		65.3*	
Nothing wrong with moderate smoking				
Fall	62.6		65.3	
Spring	50.6		56.5	
Nonsmokers				
Hope children never smoke				
Fall	76.9	(1,283)	83.4	(1,197)
Spring	82.4	(1,088)	86.8	(1,072)
Nothing wrong with smoking				
Fall	14.1		12.9	
Spring	10.1		8.0	
Smoking dangerous to health				
Fall	76.3		85.0	
Spring	81.5†		84.7†	
Nothing wrong with moderate smoking				
Fall	37.0		33.6	
Spring	26.7		26.0	

*Difference in change between schools significant at 0.01 level.
†Difference in change between schools significant at 0.02 level.

students mentioned this first as a way smoking affects health; an additional 5 per cent offered the information that "they" say smoking causes lung cancer. When all answers to the question were considered, one-third of the students replied that smoking causes lung cancer, and one-fifth that "they" say so. Three-quarters mentioned that it made you short-winded (Table 5).

Of interest to us also was what the students had noticed about the program. More than half of the students mentioned first that they had noticed the posters; 15 per cent first mentioned the questionnaires (Table 6). As the first response, other parts of the program were noted by 10 per cent or less of the boys. Reviewing all responses to the question about the program, we found that 80 per cent of the boys noticed the posters; slightly over half remembered the discussions over the public address system; and a little less than half recalled leaflets they had received, or mentioned the questionnaires. The letters mailed to the homes of the boys were remembered by about one out of four.

In the interview students were also asked what they thought might help cut down or keep students from smoking. A continuation of the program was most often mentioned as a way to cut down smoking; altogether 40 per cent of the boys mentioned this. There was also a large number of students, over 40 per cent, who felt that to prohibit

TABLE 5. PERCENT OF STUDENTS GIVING DIFFERENT
RESPONSES TO HOW SMOKING AFFECTS HEALTH

Effects on Health	First Response %	All Responses %
Shortens breath	53	74
Causes or is associated with lung cancer	16	33
They say causes cancer	5	22
Bad for lungs (no disease mentioned)	14	32
Others (shorten life, bad for TB, affects the brain, etc.)*	12	--
Total No. of students	95	95
Total No. of responses	95	236

* First response only.

TABLE 6. PER CENT OF STUDENTS MENTIONING
DIFFERENT PARTS OF ANTISMOKING PROGRAM

Part of Program	First Response %	All Responses %
Public address discussion	8	51
Leaflets	5	40
Posters	55	82
Letters to home	4	23
Questionnaires	15	41
Other*	12	--
Nothing*	1	--
No. of students	95	95
No. of responses	95	290

* First response only.

smoking on school grounds and to make cigarettes harder to buy (higher price or tax, no sale to minors) would be effective antismoking measures.

Methodologic Considerations

Before discussing the implications of this study, some problems concerning the validity and measures of effectiveness of the program must be considered. First, do the questionnaire answers about smoking reflect the actual behavior of the students? Second, was the control school similar enough to the experimental school to allow for an adequate evaluation of the antismoking program? Third, were the groups that were compared in the fall and spring the same groups; i.e., how much change in smoking might be the result of dropouts, transfers, and so forth, of students whose smoking habits differed from the majority in the group?

The validity of the data is supported by a number of facts: (a) there is an increase in the proportion of smokers from the 10th through the 12th grades, as expected on the basis of other studies and observations; (b) there is a greater amount of smoking among students in the nonacademic courses than in the college-prep courses. Other studies have also pointed out the increased smoking among students with low academic achievement, although the difference may disappear after students leave high school; (c) there is a positive correlation between parental and student smoking, and the relation between father's occupation and student's smoking is as expected. (Less smoking was found among sons of professional, managerial, and clerical workers than among those of craftsmen and semi- or unskilled workers.)

In addition to these expected relationships, which lend credence to the questionnaire information, it was the impression of school officials that there were somewhat more smokers at the experimental than at the control school.

This raises the question of the initial comparability of the schools. Although the proportions of smokers in the 10th grade college-prep courses were about the same at both, there were in the junior and senior classes more smokers in the experimental school (Tables 1 and 2). Despite this, however, we feel that these two schools were probably more similar than any other two high schools in the city. They were chosen because both admit students from all over the city for their college-prep courses, although in the control school the course tends to be more oriented toward mathematics and science, and a larger proportion of the total students are in the college-prep course than at the experimental school. As mentioned earlier, in the college-prep courses about the same proportion of boys intended to go on to college and the occupations of their fathers were similar in the two schools. The median ages of students were also the same.

Since the questionnaires were anonymous, it was not possible to determine individual changes in smoking from fall to spring; only group changes could be measured. A number of factors could affect the composition of these groups from fall to spring, and changes in the kind of students could affect the change that was observed in smoking. School dropouts, transfers, and absentees might have had an effect on group differences. We also learned in the spring that a small group of students had graduated from the control school in February—older students, presumably. Consequently, we looked at the median ages of students in each grade in the fall and in the spring. Theoretically, this age should have increased 7/12 of a year (or 0.58); actually, for the total number of students in the 10th and 11th grades it did advance nearly that much, but in the 12th grade the increase was somewhat less than expected, especially at the control school where there had been a February graduation. In the college-prep course the ages increased about as much as expected.

Occupations of fathers were also examined in both fall and the spring; again, the distribution of occupations was nearly the same at both seasons for the different classes at each school. From these comparisons we assumed that the change in the proportion of smokers from fall to spring primarily represented a change in smoking habits and not a change in the kind of student being questioned.

If, then, it is reasonable to assume that the results of the questionnaires reflect what happened to the smoking behavior of students in the two schools, what do they and the interview data suggest for further action in antismoking programs?

Discussion

Although the program at the experimental school seemed to have no effect on smoking, a number of questions arise about the program.

1. A program of only seven months' duration might not be expected to counteract all the prosmoking influences at work for the last 50 years. These influences have formed an attitude in the community and in the nation which, although it does not condone cigarette smoking among high school students, does not view it as a major problem. Consequently, any program which is confined to only one sphere of influence in a student's life may be expected to exert a small change within a short period of time.

2. The effort in promulgating traditional antismoking education methods was not great because the program was visualized as primarily consisting of hitherto untried, repetitious exposures to the health hazards of smoking as an adjunct to standard classroom procedures. Perhaps there should have been greater teacher and student participation. Less than half the teachers at the experimental school said they had discussed the effects of smoking, or had assigned some work to students based on the dangers of smoking. Among students only members of the school newspaper and the president of the student council were involved in the program. In the school in Winnipeg, where an antismoking program was successful, the teachers and students cooperated enthusiastically and their activity was judged to be the crucial factor.[5]

3. The program was carried on in a school where there was a sizable number of regular smokers to begin with, and habitual smokers are more likely to resist any antismoking education program.

For these reasons the results of the evaluation do not necessarily advise against continuation of antismoking programs. A more intensive effort, aimed at different kinds of students and continued for a longer time, would seem to be indicated.

The results do, however, suggest changes in future programs. One of the questions asked the students was when they began smoking. Over 95 per cent of the boys who had ever smoked regularly said they had first smoked before the age of 16. Other studies have also shown that during junior high school, when students are from 12 to 15 years old, the majority of smokers begin the habit. It seems advisable, therefore, that future programs concentrate on the upper elementary grades and junior high schools.

There are other findings in the study which suggest that the groups of students who smoke the most are the most difficult to reach through regular school activities. Students in the noncollege prep courses, and students who belong to social clubs outside school, smoke more than the students involved in school activities. How these students can be influenced is a question that concerns not only public health officials, but also educators. Possibly student leaders advocating against smoking might influence this group; on the other hand, they might antagonize it. Perhaps parents of the students not actively involved in school activities can influence their children about smoking. We have given this problem a great deal of consideration, but as yet are unable to propose any methods of dealing with it. In any event, the problem of how to approach this group will not be solved entirely by gaining the cooperation of teachers and student leaders, although their cooperation would undoubtedly increase the success of the program among a great number of students.

The questionnaires and interviews show that the major message, "smoking is dangerous to health," was adequately presented (see Tables 4 and 5), although more specific information concerning the relationship between smoking and lung cancer was apparently not as effectively conveyed (Table 5).

The interviews also suggest that the posters were effective in gaining the attention of students. Without further study, however, it is impossible to know what kinds of information, presented in what ways, would have the greatest effect on preventing students from smoking. Although more intensive classroom instruction among younger students than in this program might well result in a reduced number of smokers, the value of such programs is not known. In order to overcome attitudes and habits accepted in the whole community, a program in the schools alone would need to be very persuasive. Consequently, efforts to effect changes among other parts of the community, and evaluation of these efforts, are required.

Continued evaluation of antismoking programs, and research to determine factors most important in the development of smoking, should be supplemented by study of the reasons for resistance to such programs. There is little doubt that for some time efforts to reduce smoking will be primarily through education; the most effective use of various methods directed toward many different groups of people is not yet known.

Summary

1. The number of regular smokers was determined before and after an antismoking program was carried out in the school year, 1963-1964, in an all-boys' high school in Baltimore (the experimental school). The number of smokers in a comparable school without the program was determined at the same time.

2. In both schools the proportion of smokers increased slightly in the 10th grade and decreased in the 11th and 12th; the total change for all students and for those in comparable, college-prep courses at the two schools was negligible in both schools. Forty-three per cent of all students were smokers at the experimental school in the fall and in the spring; 32 per cent at the other school.

3. With respect to the statement that smoking is dangerous to health, students exposed to the program were more likely to believe this at the end of the year than at the beginning; students at the control school did not change their attitudes about the health dangers of smoking. There were no other significant changes in attitude between the schools.

4. In interviews with students at the experimental school, there was evidence that some parts of the program had not been as effective as others in terms of students' remembering the content or receiving the material.

5. Because the program was of limited duration and intensity, was carried out among students at an age when many had already begun smoking, and was countered by much prosmoking material, the following recommendations were suggested:

   (a) Programs should be initiated among elementary school and junior high school students where smoking is less well established.

   (b) Efforts should be developed to gain the involvement of all students in the program; the cooperation and interest of school administrators and teachers in the program should also be sought.

(c) Ways should be developed to change adult and community attitudes toward smoking.

(d) Research not only to evaluate these attempts, but also to determine motives for smoking and reasons for resistance to an antismoking program of this nature should be included.

REFERENCES

1. Smoking and Health: Report of the Advisory Committee to the Surgeon General of the Public Health Service. Washington: U. S. Department of Health, Education, and Welfare, 1964, Chap. 14.
2. Salber, E. J., Welsh, B., and Taylor, S. V. Reasons for Smoking Given by Secondary School Children. J. Health & Human Behavior, 4: 118-129, 1963.
3. Horn, D. Modifying Smoking Habits in High School Students. Children, 7: 63-65, 1960.
4. Cartwright, A., Martin, F. M., and Thomson, J. G. Efficacy of an Antismoking Campaign. Lancet 1: 327-329, 1960.
5. Morison, J. B., Medovy, H., and MacDonnell, G. T. Health Education and Cigarette Smoking. Canad. M. A. J. 91: 49-56, 1964.

This paper was presented before a joint session of the National Tuberculosis Association, the American Cancer Society, the American Heart Association, the Public Health Cancer Association of America, and the Epidemiology, Health Officers, Maternal and Child Health, and Social Health Sections of the American Public Health Association at the ninety-second annual meeting in New York, N.Y., October, 1964.

The study was supported in part by a grant from the American Cancer Society, Maryland Division, and by a General Research Support Grant from the National Institutes of Health to the Johns Hopkins School of Hygiene and Public Health. The computations were done in the computing center of the Johns Hopkins Medical Institutions which is supported by Research Grant FR-0004 from the National Institutes of Health.

22

Survey Evaluation of Three Poliomyelitis Immunization Campaigns

ROBERT E. SERFLING and IDA L. SHERMAN

IN the 7 years since the advent of Salk inactivated poliomyelitis vaccine and the more recent development of Sabin oral vaccine, city and county health officers have been challenged by the problem of measuring the effectiveness of communitywide immunization programs.

In many communities mass campaigns have been programed without adequate plans to assess their effectiveness. Evaluation of results has frequently been based on number of doses of vaccine used in the campaign without correction for wastage and other losses. Such losses, sometimes as high as 25 percent, may lead to overestimates of acceptance. In addition, a communitywide figure fails to reveal variations in participation by various segments of the community, as well as differences in response by age groups. To obtain this important information, counting participants through use of registration cards has frequently been attempted. Effective analysis of the cards has rarely, if ever, been accomplished. Deciphering the hastily completed clinic records, often illegible and frequently incomplete, is a discouraging task. The frustration and delay attending this procedure often results in postponement of analysis until interest wanes, and the project is then shelved.

A quite different and wholly practical method of evaluation is the sample survey.[1] This can be undertaken immediately after a program is completed. Preliminary results can be available within a week, and detailed final results, within a month. A few health department employees can collect the information in 2 or 3 days.

The survey technique was used to evaluate mass vaccination programs in Columbus and Atlanta, Ga., and in Syracuse, N.Y. These vaccination campaigns had been carried out in different "polio" climates: in Columbus, during a normal spring with no poliomyelitis reported in the community; in Atlanta, in early summer after 4 cases were reported from a circumscribed area of the city; and in Syracuse, during late summer after 20 poliomyelitis cases had occurred in the city and adjacent counties. The evaluation surveys were conducted by the respective city health departments, in cooperation with the Public Health Service's Communicable Disease Center, following distribution of the vaccine.

Surrounding counties were included in the Atlanta and Syracuse immunization programs, but the survey results presented here are confined to the cities. In all three programs, vaccine was distributed without charge, and extensive efforts were made to provide numerous distribution points at convenient locations.

In Columbus, an attempt was made to saturate the community with inactivated polio vaccine. Three injections were made available at monthly intervals during the spring of 1961, a time of normally low incidence of poliomyelitis. Mobile clinics using jet injectors distributed the vaccine during weekdays. The program engaged the attention of more than 20 persons for a period of more than 3 months and received maximum cooperation on the part of city and Public Health Service personnel. Columbus news, radio, and television facilities publicized the campaign widely, and the city government, civic leaders, and the Public Health Service participated enthusiastically.

In Atlanta, the appearance of four cases of type 3 poliomyelitis by early June 1961 forewarned of an epidemic, and type 3 oral vaccine was supplied by Dr. Albert B. Sabin for distribution to persons under 15 years of age. The program was conducted under the joint sponsorship of the State department of health and local health departments of the metropolitan area of Atlanta, and was directed primarily to the middle and lower socioeconomic population groups. There was reasonable spontaneity in participation at the clinics due to the publicity given the threatened epidemic. Organized clinics were held on weekdays, except for isolated instances in which a public health nurse distributed the vaccine at selected churches in the lower socioeconomic area.

An emergency program was initiated in Syracuse along with portions of Onondaga, Madison, and Oneida Counties after approximately 20 cases of paralytic poliomyelitis, including 12 in the city of Syracuse, had occurred in the area.[2] The vaccination program began on Wednesday, August 29, and continued through Friday, August 31. On the evening of August 28, newspapers in the city had carried an announcement of the death, due to poliomyelitis, of a 32-year-old, unvaccinated white male in nearby Oneida County.

Methods

The Communicable Disease Center developed a quota sampling survey technique in 1958 for use in ascertaining the need for selective local immunization programs.[1] The technique was used in some 125 leading cities of the United States. It was specifically directed toward obtaining an estimate of the proportions vaccinated, by age groups, in demarked socioeconomic areas of the city. The primary objective was to provide comparisons of vaccination levels within the cities and thus detect "soft spots" requiring remedial action. As mass immunization progressed, estimates of total doses distributed in the city became of interest, and more generalized sampling procedures became necessary.

An area probability sampling scheme employing city blocks as primary sampling units was used in the three surveys. The blocks were allocated to census tracts in proportion to the population density within the tract. Within blocks, a systematic random sample of one-fourth of the housing units was selected. Table 1 presents data on sample size, city population, and completion of interviews at housing units selected for the sample.

TABLE 1. SURVEY DATA

	Columbus, Ga.	Atlanta, Ga.	Syracuse, N.Y.
Date of survey, 1961	June	July	November
City population, 1960	116,779	[1]446,123	216,038
Number blocks visited	174	169	56
Approximate number blocks in city	1,470	[1]4,380	1,990
Number housing units visited	1,371	1,080	576
Number occupied housing units	1,261	956	550
Number interviews completed	1,177	891	528
Percent completed	93. 3	93. 2	96. 0
Number interviews completed–			
On first visit	896	684	372
By telephone	175	143	140
On revisit	106	64	16
Number occupied housing units not interviewed:			
Not reached	67	60	9
Refusal	2	4	10
Other reason[2]	15	1	3

[1] Fulton County only, excluding business area.
[2] Families on vacation, illness in family, and other.

To study response in the various socioeconomic areas of the three cities, census tracts were ordered by socioeconomic rank and then grouped by quartiles. One-fourth of the tracts were classified as upper, one-half as middle, and one-fourth as lower socioeconomic areas. Procedures for classifying the tracts in the three cities differed somewhat since the completed 1960 census tract data were not available when the surveys were made. In Atlanta, advance copies of tables from the 1960 census tract data[3] were used. In Syracuse, 1960 city-block statistics[4] were used with some adjustments for correspondence with previous sociological studies by Dr. Charles V. Willie, department of sociology, University of Syracuse, which were described during personal discussions. In Columbus, the Hollingshead two-factor index of social position[5] was computed for each survey family, and average values were calculated for each census tract after the survey was completed. Interviewing in Columbus and Atlanta was done by Communicable Disease Center staff members, augmented by local health department personnel, and in Syracuse entirely by health department nurses and sanitarians.

To illustrate the work and time required to plan and conduct a survey of this type, initial planning in Syracuse required 1 week and was carried out by two consultant statisticians from the Communicable Disease Center. Fieldwork was completed in 3 days by four teams, each consisting of two health department nurses. One or two nurses worked each evening on telephone callbacks, and two sanitarians revisited families who could not be reached by telephone.

Results

Tables 2, 3, and 4 show survey data for each city, including status with respect to inactivated poliomyelitis vaccination before the mass immunization campaign. For Columbus, the data show the percentage of persons with three or more inactivated polio vaccine injections before and at the close of the campaign. The data for Atlanta show the percentage of persons under 15 years of age who obtained a single dose of type 3 oral vaccine, and for Syracuse, the percentage of persons who obtained a single dose of type 1 oral vaccine. The results are summarized in the chart.

In Columbus, a small increase occurred in the percentage of preschool children under 5 with three or more injections. However, in the middle and lower socioeconomic groups the response was not sufficiently great to raise the proportion with three or more doses to that of children in the upper socioeconomic groups.

In Atlanta and Syracuse, a much better response to the single-dose oral vaccine program was observed among preschool children in the

TABLE 2. VACCINATION STATUS BEFORE AND AFTER INACTIVATED VACCINE PROGRAM, COLUMBUS, GA., APRIL-MAY 1961

| Age group | Socioeconomic group | Number persons in sample | Percent with indicated number of doses | | | | | |
| | | | 0 | | 1 or 2 | | 3 or more | |
			Before	After	Before	After	Before	After
Under 5[1]	Upper	147	8.9	5.4	21.1	17.7	70.1	76.9
	Middle	229	17.9	10.9	17.5	20.5	64.6	68.5
	Lower	215	28.4	15.8	25.1	27.0	46.5	57.2
5–14	Upper	268	.8	.8	4.1	2.6	95.1	96.6
	Middle	345	3.8	.9	7.0	7.2	89.3	91.9
	Lower	371	8.6	1.3	12.4	7.3	79.0	91.4
15–39	Upper	393	25.2	12.5	10.9	12.2	63.9	75.3
	Middle	605	28.4	16.4	13.1	14.9	58.5	68.8
	Lower	519	54.9	26.2	9.4	18.9	35.6	54.9
40 and over	Upper	256	78.9	64.9	5.5	10.5	15.6	24.6
	Middle	380	88.4	69.5	3.9	8.4	7.6	22.1
	Lower	492	94.3	63.2	1.8	10.6	3.9	26.2

[1]Excluding 21 infants under 3 months.

TABLE 3. VACCINATION STATUS BEFORE AND AFTER ORAL VACCINE PROGRAM,[1] ATLANTA, GA., JUNE 1961

Age group	Socioeconomic group	Number persons in sample	Percent giving history of 3 or more doses of inactivated vaccine	Percent receiving type 3 oral vaccine during program	Percent with neither inactivated nor oral polio vaccine
Under 5[2]	Upper	25	76.0	72.0	4.0
	Middle	174	50.2	77.6	12.1
	Lower	82	30.1	76.2	15.9
5–14	Upper	71	97.1	53.9	0
	Middle	395	72.1	78.4	4.8
	Lower	184	41.8	75.9	10.3

[1] Oral vaccine limited to children under 15.
[2] Excluding 13 infants under 3 months.

TABLE 4. VACCINATION STATUS BEFORE AND AFTER ORAL
VACCINE PROGRAM, SYRACUSE, N.Y., AUGUST 1961

Age group	Socioeconomic group	Number persons in sample	Percent giving history of 3 or more doses of inactivated vaccine	Percent receiving type 1 oral vaccine during program	Percent with neither inactivated nor oral vaccine
	Upper	32	71.9	100.0	0
Under 5[1]	Middle	100	71.0	91.0	3.0
	Lower	60	50.0	88.3	1.7
	Upper	62	100.0	93.5	0
5–14	Middle	162	89.5	92.6	2.5
	Lower	113	65.5	96.5	.9
	Upper	95	81.0	85.3	5.3
15–39	Middle	278	57.2	83.5	8.6
	Lower	149	42.3	81.9	12.8
	Upper	147	7.5	30.6	67.3
40 and over	Middle	365	7.1	35.1	63.0
	Lower	171	6.4	40.4	58.5

[1] Excluding 8 infants under 3 months.

middle and lower socioeconomic groups. Prior differences in immunization levels by socioeconomic groups were not reflected in the percentages receiving the single dose. The percentages, however, were higher in Syracuse than in Atlanta.

Discussion

The results of the three surveys provided the respective health departments with crucial information on response by age and socioeconomic area for subsequent intensified, localized programs within the cities.

The surveys allow one obvious conclusion: The threat of a poliomyelitis epidemic is a powerful stimulus to participation in a mass immunization program. Best response was in Syracuse, where an epidemic of poliomyelitis type 1 was threatening. Next best response was in Atlanta, where the appearance of a few cases in a localized sector of the city apparently aroused interest in the distribution of type 3 oral vaccine. Poorest response was in Columbus, where no cases of poliomyelitis had occurred for 18 months.

The best prior inactivated poliomyelitis vaccine coverage was in the upper socioeconomic segments of all three cities. In the oral programs,

RESULTS OF IMMUNIZATION CAMPAIGNS IN THREE CITIES

as measured by sample surveys

COLUMBUS, GA. THREE DOSES OF INACTIVATED POLIOMYELITIS VACCINE, April-May 1961

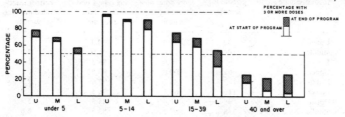

ATLANTA, GA. SINGLE DOSE OF TYPE III ORAL POLIOMYELITIS VACCINE, June 1961

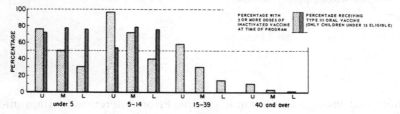

SYRACUSE, N. Y. SINGLE DOSE OF TYPE I ORAL POLIOMYELITIS VACCINE, August 1961

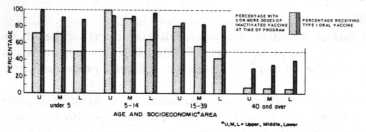

This graph is a slight modification of the one published in PUBLIC HEALTH REPORTS.

differences by socioeconomic level generally were negligible, except for
lower response by the upper socioeconomic children of school age in
Atlanta. In Atlanta's program, pediatricians frequently did not recommend oral vaccine for children who had been well immunized with
inactivated vaccine. No attempt was made by the health department
to "sell" the program to the pediatricians, since the objective of the

campaign was to reach those segments of the population more closely associated with the area in which the few cases of poliomyelitis had occurred.

Another factor to be considered in comparing the oral and inactivated vaccine programs is that the oral programs involved only one dose. The falloff in three-dose programs, with either inactivated or oral vaccine, requiring successive visits to clinics is greater in the lower socioeconomic areas.

Eight months after the type 3 campaign in Atlanta, types 1 and 2 oral vaccines were distributed, 1 month apart, to the entire population throughout the city. Special programs were centered in certain low socioeconomic census tracts. In one study, handbills were left at each household informing the residents that a mobile van would be in the area the following day to distribute oral type 1 vaccine. The van arrived at the designated times and places and distributed the vaccine to all persons who appeared. A subsequent survey showed that, for children under 5 years of age, response was poorest among those who had not previously received any inactivated poliomyelitis vaccine (table 5). In view of the ease of obtaining the oral vaccine, the low response among previously unvaccinated children was disturbing.

In Syracuse, where each case of poliomyelitis occurring in the community was reported in the daily newspapers, a barrage of publicity opened the vaccination program. Location was announced of the 20 schools throughout the city which would serve as distribution points, as well as the centrally located city health department. At the end of the first day it was noted that response lagged at the clinics in the poorer sections of the city in comparison with attendance at clinics elsewhere in the community. Intensified publicity continued. News of the clinics spread from employers to employees in the shops and factories and from housewife to housewife, and interest was stirred by newspaper announcements.

TABLE 5. NUMBER AND PERCENTAGE OF CHILDREN
RECEIVING TYPE 1 ORAL VACCINE, ATLANTA, GA.

Number of inactivated polio vaccine doses	Number of children in sample	Number receiving oral vaccine	Percent receiving oral vaccine
0.	118	64	54.2
1–2.	86	73	84.9
3 or more.	59	44	74.6

Surveys conducted at the close of the immunization programs revealed the effectiveness of the campaigns and eliminated the necessity of analyzing voluminous individual registration records. In some instances where the clinics were swamped by persons seeking the vaccine, individual registration was abandoned in order to meet the demand.

In a mass immunization program where attendance is necessary at three successive clinics held a month apart to acquire three doses of oral or inactivated polio vaccine, analysis of registration records becomes increasingly complex and may exceed the capabilities and facilities of local health departments. Simple tallies by observers who record the number of persons attending by broad age groups may serve as guides for intensifying effort in local areas during the campaign but are of little value in estimating the immunization levels of the population after the campaign.

Summary

Three surveys of immunization levels after mass distribution of poliomyelitis vaccine indicate that estimates by age, socioeconomic area, and number of doses can be obtained rapidly and economically. In the situations described, the threat of an epidemic proved to be a more effective stimulus than the intensive efforts by health department personnel and other civic agencies in a nonepidemic period.

REFERENCES

1. Serfling, R. E., Cornell, R. G., and Sherman, I. L. The CDC Quota Sampling Technic with Results of 1959 Poliomyelitis Vaccination Surveys. Am. J. Publ. Hlth. 50: 1847-1857, 1960.
2. U.S. Communicable Disease Center: Poliomyelitis Surveillance Report No. 249. Atlanta, Ga., 1962.
3. U.S. Bureau of the Census: Advance Table PH-1: Population and Housing Characteristics, 1960. U.S. Government Printing Office, Washington, 1962.
4. U.S. Bureau of the Census: Census of Housing: 1960. Series HC (3)-287. U.S. Government Printing Office, Washington, 1962.
5. Hollingshead, A. B. Two-Factor Index of Social Position. Privately printed, New Haven, 1957.

Dana Quade, Ph.D., Paul Levy, M.S., and Jesse Arnold, A.B., Epidemic Intelligence Service statisticians, Statistics Section, assisted with technical direction of the surveys. Sara Wingo, statistical assistant, supervised tabulation of the data.

Cooperating in these studies were J. F. Hackney, M.D., the late James A. Thrash, M.D. and D. E. Bigwood, M.D., health officers of Atlanta and Columbus, Ga., and Syracuse, N.Y., respectively.

23

Evaluation of a Poison Center

G. L. ROBB, H. S. ELWOOD, and R. J. HAGGERTY

THE increase in the number of poison information centers in the United States since the establishment of the first one in Chicago in 1953 has been remarkable. In April, 1961, nearly 450 such centers— either poison information or poison control centers[1]—were in operation.[2] If numbers are any criterion of success, the poison center idea would seem to qualify. When success comes so quickly and easily, however, it may be pertinent to ask several questions: Are poison centers doing enough to justify this great expenditure of time and money? How do parents and physicians who use such centers feel about them? What is the role of such centers in the fields of treatment and prevention, respectively? Should they function more widely in the prevention of accidents in general?

The Boston Poison Information Center is operated on a 24-hour basis, offering telephone consultation to physicians and the public. It is staffed by a pediatric resident in at least his third year of training, who also carries heavy duties as the admitting officer and resident-in-charge of the Medical Emergency Clinic of the hospital. The usual resources—card file, library, reprint collection, local consultants, and telephone calls to manufacturers—are used to identify poisons and aid in recommending appropriate therapy. A full-time medical secretary is available to assist him.

This center, like many in the country, grew very rapidly from an average of 20 calls per month in 1954—its first year—to nearly 500 calls per month in 1960. Because of the problems in management arising from this growth, we were forced to re-examine our organization in an effort to decide how to provide optimal service. The fact that life-threatening poisonings were occupying only a small part of the center's activities was apparent when a review of the 1959 statistics showed that of a total of 4,336 calls only six had involved subsequent deaths, three of which were adult suicide victims. This study was designed to find out what the center was accomplishing. While it is only concerned with the Boston Poison Information Center, the results

point up some general aspects of poison center operations that may
be of value to others.

Methods

The present study was conducted by the authors during the summer of 1959 by mailing separately designed questionnaires to each of
the following groups:

1. Parents who had consulted the center during the previous
    seven months for children 15 years old or under.

    Inquiries concerning adult or animal poisonings and several
    other miscellaneous categories were excluded both on the basis
    of their heterogeneity and because of our particular pediatric
    interest.
2. Physicians who had consulted the center during the previous
    12 months.
3. All residents who had served in the center since its inception.

Follow-up questionnaires were sent to all in each group who did
not respond to the first mailing. Data were tabulated and analyzed
by hand sorting.

Results

Parents' Questionnaires

Of the 2,876 calls to the center during the first seven months of 1959,
946 were excluded because they concerned adults or animals, represented professional inquiries unrelated to poisoning episodes, or were
incompletely or illegibly recorded. Questionnaires were sent to the
remaining 1,930 parents. Of these, 959 did not reply, or they were
returned unopened. Several of the families had moved and left no
forwarding address, and 66 questionnaires were returned after the
analysis was completed. There remained 800 returned questionnaires
pertaining to 819 poison ingestions; some of the calls concerned two
or more children in the same family. Comparison of the ages of the
children (Figure 1) and the types of poison ingested in the respondent and nonrespondent groups revealed marked similarities, but no
further information concerning possible differences between these
two groups was available. Of the questionnaires returned, 61 percent
concerned boys—a nearly universal finding of male preponderance of
poisonings.[3] In 70 percent of the 800 poisoning episodes reported,
the parents had called the center directly; in 30 percent their physicians had called.

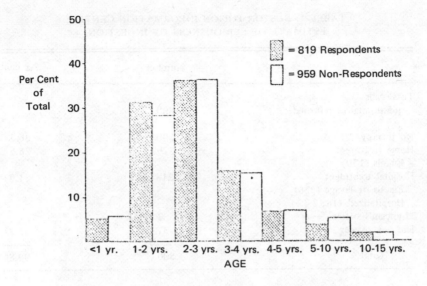

FIGURE 1. BOSTON POISON INFORMATION CENTER,
AGE OF RESPONDENTS AND NONRESPONDENTS

As a measure of how serious these ingestions were, one question ascertained the treatment given. Of the 800 poison inquiries, only 18, or 2.2 percent of the cases, required hospitalization. There were no deaths in this group, and fully 36.3 per cent required no therapy at all (Table 1). Thus, with rare exceptions, the majority of calls did not represent serious, life-threatening episodes, but rather concern and uncertainty upon the part of parents and physicians.

The first question asked of the parents was "How did you know of the center?" Although there had been no systematic advertising to the public, all local newspapers, one television, and several radio stations had run feature stories or programs on its activities, and the telephone number had been listed on the first page of the telephone directory along with police and fire department numbers. Table 2 lists the various sources from which parents learned of the center. Surprising to us was the frequency of personal contact—physicians 29.1 percent, friends 20.2 percent—as opposed to radio, television, the telephone directory, and even the newspapers. Hospitals and pharmacists accounted for 107 ot the 193 instances listed as learning from "other" sources, indicating another important personal contact.

In order to obtain opinions concerning the practical functioning of the center, the parents were asked a series of questions beginning

TABLE 1. BOSTON POISON INFORMATION CENTER,
ESTIMATE OF SERIOUSNESS OF INGESTION

	Number	Per cent
Total calls—		
questionnaires returned	800	
No therapy	290	36.3
Home treatment	229	28.6
Emesis (139)		
Hospital treatment	218	31.0
Emesis or lavage (226)		
Hospitalized (18; 2.2%)		
Physician's office	2	
Did not answer	31	3.9
Total	800	99.8

TABLE 2. BOSTON POISON INFORMATION CENTER,
PARENTS' SOURCE OF KNOWLEDGE OF CENTER

	Number	Per cent
Physician	262	29.1
Friends	182	20.2
Newspaper	111	12.3
Telephone book	56	6.2
Radio-TV	25	2.8
Other	193	21.4
No answer	71	7.9
Total	900*	99.9

* Some gave more than one source.

with "Was there a delay in obtaining the information you needed from the center?" Twenty-eight percent answered "yes." In response to the following question, "How do you feel your case was handled by the poison center?," only 2.9 percent of the 70 percent who had called the center directly were displeased with the service (Table 3). All but one among this 2.9 percent had listed "delay" as their only criticism, indicating that dissatisfaction was usually associated with delay, but delay did not of itself usually lead to dissatisfaction. When the generally high parental opinion of the center (Table 3) is coupled with the paucity of serious ingestions (Table 1), it is apparent that the majority received a great deal of satisfaction from merely being reassured or advised to carry out simple home treatment.

This center had not instructed the residents answering calls to give parents information pertaining to the prevention of poisoning. It was of interest, then, to hear many of these physicians giving such warnings at the time of the initial call. The question was therefore asked of the parents, "Did anyone at the center give you instructions regarding the handling and safe storage of dangerous substances in the home?" Seventeen percent answered "yes," and of these, 85 percent felt this information would help prevent other poisonings. As another example of the effect of personal contact in health education, 85 per cent of the parents who had received preventive advice had told their friends of these instructions.

Finally, we wished to ascertain the subsequent accident experience of these children to determine if any of the center's present activities could have played a role in the prevention of additional mishaps. Of the 819 children reported to have had poison ingestions, 52 had experienced subsequent poisonings in the next 1 to 12 months. Six of these were in families who remembered having received preventive information at the time of their first contact with the center. Thus, 11.6 percent of the repeater group received preventive information compared to 17 percent of the total. While the trend of these percentages suggests that such advice may be effective, the numbers are

TABLE 3. BOSTON POISON INFORMATION CENTER,
SATISFACTION WITH SERVICE

	Parents	Physicians
	n=559*	n=446
	Per cent	Per cent
Very satisfied	71.9	69.2
Satisfied	19.0	12.1
Dissatisfied	2.9	1.7
Did not answer	6.2	17.0
	100.0	100.0

*Only parents with direct contact with center.

small and the difference not very large. An additional 104 families had experienced other accidents requiring "medical treatment" or "hospitalization" during this period.

Since Dietrich has proposed conditioning children to associate accidents with unpleasant experiences in an effort to prevent recurrences, we attempted to ascertain whether or not these children had been "more careful," "less careful," or "the same" since the accident, and to correlate this behavior with the method of therapy and whether or not the incident was remembered.[4] There was little correlation of subsequent behavior with the therapy used; emesis or lavage were only slightly more likely to be followed by more careful behavior (23.2 percent) than no therapy at all (16 percent). However, when one correlated memory of the accident with subsequent behavior, there was a trend for those who remembered to be more careful (Table 4). As would be expected, children over three years of age were more likely both to remember and to be more careful subsequently. The complex reasons why one child remembers and another does not are certainly not clear from our analysis and were not touched upon in the questionnaire, but it does seem apparent that one goal of such centers should be to find out how to help the child remember the accident. In part, this supports Dietrich's theory of the importance of education in accident prevention.

At the time the study was conducted, the center was in serious

TABLE 4. BOSTON POISON INFORMATION CENTER,
BEHAVIOR FOLLOWING INGESTION

| | | Per cent | | |
		More Careful	Less Careful	Same
All Ages				
Remembers accident	(n=146)	55.4	0.7	43.9
Does not remember	(n=213)	11.5	0	88.5
Under 3 Years of Age				
Remembers accident	(n=77)	39.0	1.3	57.7
Does not remember	(n=214)	8.9	0	91.1
Over 3 Years of Age				
Remembers accident	(n=69)	73.8	0	26.2
Does not remember	(n=29)	31.0	0	69.0

financial difficulty. The question was asked, "Which of the following would you favor as a source of further financial aid?" Fifty percent thought that Community Chest or Health Department funds should be used, while nearly 50 percent suggested charges or donations from those receiving services—an interesting and very even split between the two opposing general philosophies of payment for medical services.

There were a good many unsolicited comments on the center, the majority of which indicated a desire to have more provided in the way of educational material—booklets, radio and television programs, lectures, and accident prevention as a universal health unit practice.

Physicians' Questionnaires

Of 623 physicians who consulted the center during the one year prior to this study, 446 returned questionnaires—a creditable 71.6 percent.

When the center first began operation, a notice was printed in the "New England Journal of Medicine." Bimonthly case reports of interesting poisonings have been presented in this Journal since 1956. Members of the two local pediatric organizations were sent a booklet written by the center personnel, and 12 to 15 talks to professional groups were given by the director each year.[5] It was felt important, then, to determine which of these methods of informing physicians of the center's operations was most effective. As with the parents, the superiority of personal contact was clear (Table 5). "Colleagues"

TABLE 5. BOSTON POISON INFORMATION CENTER,
PHYSICIANS' SOURCE OF INFORMATION

	Number	Per cent
Colleagues	182	37.9
New England J. Med.	103	21.5
Newspaper	27	5.6
Other medical literature	13	2.7
Telephone directory	13	2.7
Radio-TV	5	1.0
Other sources (most "just knew")	137	28.5
	480*	99.9

*Some gave more than one source.

were the single most frequent source of information, with professional literature second, and newspapers, radio, and television very poor thirds.

Physicians' opinions of the service very nearly paralleled the parents, with only 1.7 percent indicating dissatisfaction (Table 3). An attempt was made, using a checklist, to determine the quality of the center's many functions (Table 6). Of the three general areas ques-

TABLE 6. BOSTON POISON INFORMATION CENTER,
PHYSICIAN RATING OF SERVICES (N=446)

| | Per cent | | | | | |
	Excellent	Good	Fair	Poor	Did Not Answer	Total
Information: Accuracy	72.5	8.5	0.7	0	18.3	100
Conciseness	65.5	9.4	2.0	0	23.1	100
Clarity	65.0	11.6	1.3	0	22.1	100
Practicability	61.2	12.7	1.3	0.2	25.6	100
Did in Prevention: Effectiveness	47.2	8.1	2.0	0.2	42.5	100
Practicability	43.1	8.1	2.2	0.2	46.2	100
Public Relations: Promptness	72.4	7.8	2.1	1.5	16.2	100
Courtesy	75.5	4.3	0.4	0	19.8	100

tioned—specific information, public relations, and preventive suggestions—specific information was checked most often as excellent, with no one stating that this was poor. In the area of public relations, courtesy scored high, promptness less so. Aids in prevention, while not a formal part of the residents' duties, were most often left unanswered, but when checked were rated excellent by a large majority (Table 6), an indication that this was less often performed rather than being performed poorly when done.

In contrast to the parent group, in which one quarter felt there was a delay in obtaining information, only 2.5 percent of the physicians reported such a delay (Table 7). An explanation for this difference could not be ascertained from the questionnaires. The reasons may have included more rapid response by residents to requests from consulting physicians, a greater appreciation by the latter of the residents' many other duties, or a knowledge of the rare need for immedi-

TABLE 7. BOSTON POISON INFORMATION CENTER,
DELAY IN OBTAINING INFORMATION

	Parents n=559 Per cent	Physicians n=446 Per cent
Yes	28.3	2.5
No	67.6	83.7
Did not answer	4.1	13.7
	100.0	99.9

ate answers in the effective management of most patients. The number of times each physician had used the center was tabulated. Seventy-five percent had used it 1 to 5 times, 14.8 percent 6 to 10 times, and 10 percent more than 10 times. Of those who had used it more than 3 times, 92.2 percent were very satisfied and found it "very useful," while of those who had only used the center 1 to 3 times, 82.4 percent found it "very useful."

Several specific complaints were made, no one of which occurred more than 11 times. These involved difficulty in establishing telephone contact, too many "peripheral" questions before information was given, and impractical therapeutic advice, e.g., lavage too often recommended for small, nontoxic amounts. It was gratifying to find so few complaints considering the pressure under which the residents worked, but enough criticisms were recorded to indicate specific areas of need for improvement. A large number of physicians spontaneously added comments such as, "enthusiastically in favor of this service to the community."

Because of complex medicolegal considerations, information was given only to physicians during the first several years of the center's operation. For several reasons, notably that many families either did not have physicians or occasionally could not reach them during an emergency, this policy was changed in 1956 to include the acceptance of calls directly from parents. It was reassuring to learn that only 4.3 percent of the physicians disagreed with this policy.

A final question sought to determine physicians' opinions of the best way to finance the center. Less than 20 percent felt that some official agency should pay for this service, with the majority favoring fees or donations from the patients served. Pharmaceutical concerns, medical foundations, or a medical society were the next most frequent suggestions. Thus physicians, much more often than parents, felt that families served should pay for the service. Donations have subsequently been solicited from users with only minimal results. In 1960, $507.50 was received out of a total operating expense of $8,770.50.

Residents' Questionnaires

Twenty-five of the 38 residents who had worked in the center from 1954 through 1959 returned completed questionnaires (66 percent). They were asked several questions about their experiences while taking "poison calls" and their attitude toward these. Twenty-three of these 25 (92 percent) answered "yes" to the question, "Has this experience been of value to you in your management of patients who have ingested a poison?" Both negative answers came from residents who have been subsequently engaged in a laboratory subspecialty of pediatrics. Many were enthusiastic, giving such comments as "this is invaluable training for a resident . . . essential to any well-planned rotation."

Each resident covering this service had the experience of managing acute poison crises in families. We were interested in determining whether or not this would help the pediatrician-in-training to manage crises in general. Sixty-four percent felt that it had been helpful, but many added that this was also a function of their whole hospital experience. They were then asked whether or not "this experience helped prepare you for educating parents in the prevention of accidents in general and poisons specifically." Eighty percent answered "yes," and many added strong statements such as "I am now very pill, bottle, cupboard and out-of-toddler's reach conscious." Although most of these residents were not yet in practice when the questionnaire was sent—some being in military service or in subspecialty training—we were interested to know how many had been called upon to talk to parent groups about poisonings and had found their experience with the center useful in this setting. Thirty-six percent had given such talks, and those who had done so had found the experience in the center most valuable.

Since one of the reasons for undertaking this study was the crisis presented by the increasing load of calls, the residents were asked if these calls had interfered with their other duties. While only 44 percent answered "yes," almost all of this group had worked in the center during 1958-1959, the year when the volume of calls increased to approximately 500 per month.

One of the possible solutions we had considered to provide for this increased load was to have a nonmedical person screen all calls. Another was to require all parents to call their local physician first, the center thus receiving only physicians' calls. In response to requests for opinions of these possibilities, the residents were nearly equally split on both questions, 60 percent favoring the handling of all calls by a physician and 56 percent stating that the center should receive calls directly from parents as well as physicians. Strong opinions were expressed on both sides, indicating that there was no clear mandate for either course.

Discussion

Questionnaires were the sole method used for data collection in this study. That this method can only measure objective data and conscious attitudes is well known. The low number of respondents, in spite of a follow-up letter to all (41.4 percent of parents, 71.6 percent of physicians, and 66 percent of residents) was disappointing and casts a certain amount of doubt upon the results as they pertain to the entire group, for it is well known that people who answer questionnaires are likely to have quite different opinions from those who do not. The similarity of the age of the children of the responders and the nonresponders and the fact that their ingestions were of the same type and severity suggests that the groups may not have been too dissimilar. All that we can claim, however, is to have sampled the opinion of the responders.

From the data obtained it is clear that this poison center, and probably most others, is not dealing primarily with life-threatening poisonings. Neither parents nor physicians can be expected to know the ingredients and toxicity of the myriad of new products to which children may be exposed. That this poison center is generally answering a need in a satisfactory manner seems clear when only 2.9 percent of parents and 1.7 percent of the physicians expressed dissatisfaction with the center's services. The reason for dissatisfaction most frequently given by both parents and physicians was the delay in obtaining information. A few others in both groups felt that too many "unnecessary" questions were asked. At moments of such crises, parents, particularly, cannot be blamed for their annoyance at having to answer questions about age, sex, address, telephone number, circumstances of the accident and other facts, but realization of this reaction can help the person asking these questions in handling such annoyances at the time.

If saving lives is a rare function of poison centers, and this seems clear, can the "entry" they provide into families at times of emotional crises be utilized for prevention? Although no absolute answer can be given, there are two results which suggest that this may be the case. While 17 percent of the total group received preventive advice, only 11.6 percent of those who experienced subsequent poisonings had received such information. Children who remembered the incident, for whatever reason, seemed to have learned to be more careful, although this was also a function of age—older children remembering more often and being more careful thereafter.

Following this study, we embarked upon a program of referral of all families using the center to their local health departments for a public health nurse home visit. Since then, the studies of McInnes and Bissell[6] and Wehrle, et al., [7] have shown that such referral is a poor case-finding method in terms of locating families with increased risk of subsequent accidents. Our impressions support this. Wehrle's data[7] show that while most families which have had one poisoning episode are unlikely to have a second, and are not particularly different from the general population, those which have had repeated ingestions are distinguished by several criteria of family dysfunction. Since this study was conducted, we have attempted to get information on these criteria, including lack of immunizations among the children, repeated accidents or poisonings in the family, chronic unattended health problems and family instability; but this effort proved unsuccessful, for the required information was too extensive and often too emotionally laden to be obtained at the time of the initial telephone call. It seems that the follow-up of a limited number of families who use the poison center is best left to the district health nurse who frequently knows of families with repeated accidents and other health problems, but has previously lacked a clear reason for a home visit. Such visits utilize the accident crisis as the basis for beginning intervention, for at such a time motivation for changing behavior is likely to be higher and the results more satisfactory.[8]

The fact that both parents and physicians learned of the center more often by personal contact than by the formal communication media (with the exception of a number of physicians who had read of the center in professional publications) lends further support to using this indirect means of health education. Those parents who did receive advice on accident prevention were very apt to pass it on to friends. Properly handled, we believe such an educational function is most vital to the nature of all similar centers, particularly as a part of their role in comprehensive community prevention programs. In an attempt to further this end we now mail a prevention pamphlet to all parents who have used the center.

The considerable role such centers can play in medical education is indicated by the residents' replies. Aside from the need to have a physician available to answer telephone calls, and there was considerable difference of opinion among the former residents over this "need," most of them learned a good deal about the importance of poisonings and accidents from this first-hand experience. Many have since used it in preventive services to individual families and parent groups. The value of this teaching was of such priority at this center that the problem of an overwhelming number of calls was solved by dividing the load between the four pediatric teaching hospital services in Boston,[9] each service being responsible for the calls for a period in each day. This has been eminently successful in keeping the load to a workable level, and, more important, in extending this learning experience to approximately 24 additional residents per year. If, as demonstrated in this study, patients often learn of the poison center, and presumably about poisons and accidents, from their physicians, the long-range educational effect of this teaching of pediatric residents should be quite extensive.

It has been suggested that poison information centers, as institutions experienced in the management of one type of accident crisis, might logically be expanded to give first-aid advice for other accidents. While this possibility has not, as yet, been fully explored, we feel that medicolegal problems would arise more frequently, that nonpoisoning accidents can usually be handled without the necessity of access to a large body of technical information, and that the optimal initial management of the injured person is likely to be by his own physician. It would seem that poison information centers would serve the public best by continuing to provide accurate information regarding poisonings and by actively participating in an organized community-wide, accident prevention program.

Conclusions

On the basis of an evaluation of the Boston Poison Information Center, we must conclude that such centers are probably saving few lives, but that their activities have met with satisfied acceptance by both the public and physicians. The function of personal contact in broadening both patients' and physicians' knowledge of this health resource, combined with the long-term effects of teaching residents the importance and handling of poisonings, emphasizes the increasing role these centers can play in accident prevention. It does not seem wise to broaden their scope to include the management of all acute accidents, but they should have a close relationship with other community-based accident prevention programs.

NOTES AND REFERENCES

1. A distinction is made in this paper between these two types: "information" centers provide information only—usually by telephone; "control" centers also provide patient care.
2. U.S. Department of Health, Education, and Welfare. Directory of Poison Control Centers. Washington: Public Health Service, Division of Accident Prevention, National Clearinghouse for Poison Control Centers, 1961.
3. Cann, H., Iskrant, A. P., and Neyman, D. S. Epidemiologic Aspects of Poisoning Accidents. A.J.P.H. 50: 1914-1924, 1960.
4. Dietrich, H. F. Accidents, Childhood's Greatest Physical Threat, Are Preventable. J.A.M.A. 144: 1175-1179, 1950.
5. Procedure Book for the Management of Childhood Poisonings. Boston: Boston Poison Information Center, 1956.
6. McInnes, R. S., and Bissell, D. M. Accidental Poisoning as a Casefinding Procedure. Publ. Hlth. Rep. 75: 853-858, 1960.
7. Wehrle, P. F., DeFreest, L., Penhollow, J., and Harris, V. G. The Epidemiology of Accidental Poisoning in an Urban Population. III. The Repeater Problem in Accidental Poisoning. Pediatrics, 27: 614-620, 1961.
8. Caplan, G. Initial Exploration. In Prevention of Mental Disorders in Children. New York: Basic Books, 1961, chapter I.
9. Massachusetts General Hospital, Boston Floating Hospital, Boston City Hospital, and Children's Hospital Medical Center.

24

Use of Death Rates in Evaluating Multiple Screening

CHARLES M. WYLIE

ILLNESS can be controlled or cured only when the patient or his physician recognizes the need for treatment. The physician's help is usually sought, however, only when symptoms or signs occur that are not culturally accepted as normal. Since much long-term illness passes through a prolonged asymptomatic phase, there is a great unmet need for medical treatment in the population of the United States. Multiple screening has been devised to separate off persons with this need, without requiring the total adult population to be examined periodically by physicians.

Multiple screening uses two or more tests to sort out persons who probably have abnormalities from those who probably do not. The immediate aim of multiple screening is to refer for medical care those who have positive test results. Its ultimate aim is to reduce illness, disability, and death in the population by the early detection and treatment of disease.

Even when multiple screening is completely effective in detecting disease in the early stages, screenees will continue to die for various reasons. Screening tests do not cover all asymptomatic disease, and medical care is not sufficiently advanced to control all diagnosed conditions. Moreover, some conditions existing in the positive screenees may not be diagnosed, and new conditions may arise after screening, to remain undetected for some time.

Since persons with positive screening tests have more disease than those with negative test results, we may expect that death rates also will differ in these two groups. Unless medical care is much more effective than is currently assumed, persons with positive tests will have the higher death rates. Therefore, death rates may form a useful basis for evaluating screening tests, the more effective test separating off groups with high death rates.

The purpose of this paper is to present mortality figures for 2,298 residents of Baltimore who took multiple screening tests in 1954, to compare death rates in persons with positive and with negative test results, and to describe methods for using death figures to evaluate multiple screening.

Background

In the last 3 months of 1954, the Commission of Chronic Illness invited 6,967 selected residents of Baltimore, aged 17 years and older, to attend a clinic for multiple screening. The residents were part of a random sample of the city population who had been reported free from serious health problems on household interview some months previously.[1]

Of those invited, 2,023 came for screening. An additional 275 persons, who desired to attend the clinic after reading newspaper descriptions of the project, took the tests. Of the total screened, 35 percent were under 35 years of age, 39 percent were between 35 and 49 years, and 26 percent were 50 years of age and older. Seventy-nine percent were white, and 45 percent were males.

For descriptive purposes, the screening tests may be divided into two groups: (a) major tests, in which persons were referred to their physicians if the abnormal result was previously unknown; and (b) minor tests, for which no referrals were made. Major tests consisted of blood pressure measurement, six-lead electrocardiogram, 70-mm. chest X-ray, blood and urine sugar tests 1 hour after a glucose drink, hemoglobin level, urine albumin, serologic test for syphilis (STS), and two questions about discomfort on exertion. The minor tests included hearing, vision, dental examinations, and height and weight measurement.[2]

The followup procedures, to determine the status of each person on December 31, 1959, have been fully described elsewhere.[3] By searching the latest available city and suburban directories for Baltimore and its surrounding area, we obtained for a part of the study group more recent addresses and telephone numbers than appeared in our records. We then mailed a mimeographed letter and a questionnaire to each individual; 52 percent completed and returned the questionnaire. For an additional 23 percent, answers were obtained by telephone. Finally, we searched the 1955-59 death certificate files for the names of all persons who had not been contacted by letter or telephone and to confirm deaths reported in the returned questionnaires.

The follow-up program clarified the current status of 2,031 screenees. For 267 individuals, 12 percent of all screenees, information was incomplete. We believed that they were not then resident in the Baltimore metropolitan area, and we knew that they had not died in Maryland in the 5 years following screening. In this paper, all of this group are assumed to be alive.

Mortality

Table 1 distributes the 2,298 persons and the 105 known deaths by age when screened and by the group test results. In each age range, death rates were markedly higher for persons with positive major tests than for persons with positive minor tests or with no positive tests. Since those with positive major tests included the greater proportion of older persons, we have made some adjustment for age to describe the overall mortality experience (footnote 2, table 1). The age-adjusted death rate for persons with positive major tests was twice that for persons with minor positive results and 18 times higher than for those with negative results.

TABLE 1. NUMBER PERSONS SCREENED IN 1954, NUMBER DYING DURING 1955-59, AND NUMBER OF DEATHS PER 1,000 SCREENEES FOR EACH TEST GROUP, BY AGE IN 1954

Test results	All ages			Under 35			35-49			50 and over			Age–adjusted death, rate per 1,000[2]
	Screened[1]	Deaths	Deaths per 1,000	Screened	Deaths	Deaths per 1,000	Screened	Deaths	Deaths per 1,000	Screened	Deaths	Deaths per 1,000	
All tests	2,298	105	45.7	790	5	6.3	862	20	23.2	631	80	126.8	52.1
Positive:													
Major	964	78	80.9	165	2	12.1	373	12	32.2	417	64	153.5	65.9
Minor	719	24	33.3	178	1	5.6	327	7	21.4	209	16	76.0	34.5
Negative	615	3	4.9	447	2	4.5	162	1	6.2	5	0	.0	3.6

[1]Includes 15 persons of unknown age.

[2]Calculated by the direct method for a population containing equal numbers of persons under age 35, 35-49, and 50 years and over.

The distribution of causes of death differed considerably between screenees with and screenees without positive major tests. Table 2 shows that 78 of the 105 deaths (74 percent) occurred in persons with positive tests results; 43 of the 50 deaths from cardiovascular causes (86 percent) occurred in that group. Crude death rates for the various disease classes were higher for persons with positive tests, but not signi-

TABLE 2. NUMBER OF DEATHS AND CRUDE DEATH
RATE IN SCREENEES BY MAJOR TEST RESULT,
ACCORDING TO CAUSE OF DEATH, 1955-59

Cause of death[1]	Number of deaths with major test—		Crude death rate per 1,000 with major test	
	Positive	Negative	Positive	Negative
All causes	78	27	73.3	21.9
Hypertensive heart disease (440-447)	10	3	9.4	2.4
Vascular lesions affecting central nervous system (330-334)	5	0	4.7	.0
Other cardiovascular disease (400-434, 450-468)	28	4	26.3	3.2
Malignant neoplasms (140-205)	12	10	11.3	8.1
Other	23	10	21.6	8.1

[1] Figures in parentheses refer to International List numbers.

ficantly so for neoplasms, for which there was no specific screening
test.

Some persons, including a few who eventually died, did not take
the complete series of tests. Known diabetics, for example, were not
asked to take the blood and urine sugar tests, and, due to mechanical
failure, some 400 chest X-rays were unsatisfactory. Table 3 shows the
number of persons who completed each test and the number who later
died, correlated with age and with test result. The findings for the
hearing, vision, and dental examinations were not analyzed.

For all tests except hemoglobin level, persons with positive test results had higher death rates than those with negative tests. This finding was consistent in all age groups for the chest X-ray and electrocardiogram. The higher death rates for those with positive height and
weight tests occurred only among persons under 50 years of age. In
the remaining tests, the higher death rates for positives occurred
in the older groups. In the 34 screenees with positive hemoglobin
tests, no deaths occurred. As we would expect, mortality was higher
among the older screenees, whether test results were positive or negative.

TABLE 3. NUMBER PERSONS SCREENED IN 1954, NÚMBER DYING
DURING 1955-59, AND DEATHS PER 1,000 SCREENEES FOR
EACH TEST, BY AGE IN 1954

Test result	All ages			Under 35			35-49			50 and over		
	Screened	Deaths	Deaths per 1,000	Screened	Deaths	Deaths per 1,000	Screened	Deaths	Deaths per 1,000	Screened	Deaths	Deaths per 1,000
Chest X-ray:												
Positive	394	49	124.4	60	2	33.3	106	4	37.7	228	43	188.6
Negative	1,642	39	23.8	669	3	4.5	665	13	19.5	308	23	74.7
Electrocardiogram:												
Positive	315	51	161.9	42	1	23.8	86	3	34.9	187	47	251.3
Negative	1,977	54	27.3	748	4	5.4	775	17	21.9	454	33	72.7
Blood pressure:												
Positive	167	25	149.7	13	0	.0	59	4	67.8	95	21	221.0
Negative	2,125	80	37.6	777	5	6.4	802	16	20.0	546	59	108.1
Questionnaire:[1]												
Positive	147	24	163.3	14	1	71.4	44	1	22.7	89	22	247.1
Negative	2,014	73	36.2	739	3	4.1	766	18	23.5	496	52	104.8
Blood sugar:[2]												
Positive	80	12	150.0	11	0	.0	26	1	38.5	43	11	255.8
Negative	2,187	92	42.1	773	5	6.5	828	19	22.9	586	68	116.0
Urine sugar:[2]												
Positive	62	11	177.4	14	0	.0	19	0	.0	29	11	379.3
Negative	2,141	93	43.4	725	5	6.9	810	19	23.5	606	69	113.9
Urine albumin:												
Positive	97	20	206.2	33	0	.0	24	3	125.0	40	17	425.0
Negative	2,111	84	39.8	709	5	7.1	804	16	19.9	598	63	105.4
Serologic test for syphilis:												
Positive	49	5	102.0	6	0	.0	21	1	47.6	22	4	181.8
Negative	2,163	97	44.8	759	5	6.6	813	19	23.4	591	73	123.5
Hemoglobin:												
Positive	34	0	.0	20	0	.0	11	0	.0	3	0	.0
Negative	2,213	103	46.5	759	5	6.6	834	20	24.0	620	78	125.8
Height and weight:[3]												
Positive	581	37	63.7	126	2	15.9	223	7	31.4	232	28	120.7
Negative	1,712	67	39.1	664	3	4.5	636	12	18.9	412	52	126.2

[1] Symptoms of cardiac disease.
[2] 1 hour after drinking 50 gm. of glucose.
[3] 30 percent or more above central weight for persons of medium frame, according to
Metropolitan Life Insurance Co. tables.

Indices of Effectiveness

Most studies of multiple screening have measured test performance by effectiveness in separating off persons with specific diseases. In this study, we desired to evaluate each test by its efficiency in separating off those who died in the 5 years following screening.

Table 4, based on figures in table 3, presents five indices which have some value in measuring this performance. Death sensitivity, the percentage of all dead persons classified as positive by each test, is listed in column A. This index can be considered only along with death specificity, which is the percentage of all 5-year survivors classified as negative by each test (column B). Four tests—urine sugar, STS, hemoglobin, and height and weight—give poor results when these indices are considered jointly.

Column C shows the age-adjusted death rates for persons with posi-

TABLE 4. INDICES OF SCREENING EFFECTIVENESS BASED ON
DEATHS OF SCREENEES DURING 1955-59

Test	Death sensitivity[1] (A)	Death specificity[2] (B)	Age-adjusted death rates per 1,000		Age-adjusted mortality ratio[3] (E)	Average rank (F)
			Positive (C)	Negative (D)		
Chest X-ray	55.7	82.3	86.6	32.9	2.6	4
Electrocardiogram	48.6	87.9	103.3	33.3	3.1	2
Blood pressure	23.8	93.5	96.3	44.8	2.1	6
Questionnaire[4]	24.7	94.0	113.7	44.1	2.6	3
Blood sugar[5]	11.5	96.9	98.1	48.5	2.0	7
Urine sugar[5]	10.6	97.6	126.4	48.1	2.6	5
Urine albumin	19.2	96.3	183.3	44.1	4.2	1
Serologic test for syphilis	4.9	97.9	76.5	51.2	1.5	8
Hemoglobin	.0	98.4	.0	52.1	.0	10
Height and weight[6]	35.6	75.1	56.0	49.9	1.1	9

[1] Deaths classified positive / All deaths x 100

[2] 5-year survivors classified negative / All 5-year survivors x 100

[3] Death rate in positives/death rate in negatives.

[4] For symptoms of cardiovascular disease.

[5] 1 hour after drinking 50 gm. of glucose.

[6] 30 percent or more above central weight for persons of medium frame, according to Metropolitan Life Insurance Co. tables.

tive tests. Tests with the highest rates are the urine albumin, urine sugar, questionnaire, and electrocardiogram. The death rate in positives is an inadequate sole criterion for measuring test performance, since it gives a high rank to the urine sugar test, previously evaluated as poor.

Age-adjusted death rates in persons with negative tests are given in column D. The lower this death rate, the more effective was the test. Ranking high in efficiency are the chest X-ray and electrocardiogram, while in lowest ranks are the STS and hemoglobin tests. The death rate in the negatives is a criterion which correlates fairly closely with the joint consideration of sensitivity and specificity.

Finally, column E gives the mortality ratio, the death rate in positives divided by the death rate in negatives. The urine albumin, electrocardiogram, and chest X-ray tests rank high, and the STS, hemoglobin, and height and weight tests rank low by this criterion.

At present, we can say only that each criterion contributes something to the evaluation of the tests; none seems outstandingly good or bad, and none is adequate for sole consideration. We have therefore produced an average ranking for each test (column F), giving equal weight to each of the five indices. This average ranking suggests that the STS, hemoglobin, and height and weight tests performed so poorly in separating off high mortality groups that they might well be abandoned. Highly effective were the urine albumin, electrocardiogram, chest X-ray, and questionnaire.

Discussion

As a method of evaluating multiple screening tests, the use of diagnoses made as a result of screening has many defects. In few studies are persons with negative tests examined to determine whether test results are false negatives, and there is considerable evidence that many examinations do not provide sufficient information for making a diagnosis. Medical schools do not stress the diagnosis of asymptomatic disease; therefore, many general practitioners have difficulty in deciding what labels to attach to conditions found in asymptomatic patients with positive diagnostic tests. For example, some physicians may make a diagnosis of heart disease based only on an electrocardiographic abnormality found on screening; other physicians might make a negative diagnosis on the basis of the same finding.

In contrast to medical diagnoses, deaths do not depend on evaluation by physicians. Since groups with high death rates need medical care more urgently than groups with low death rates, screening tests perform a useful function if they refer high mortality groups for medical care. The use of death rates to evaluate screening test performance has, therefore, some validity.

The degree of validity is not perfect, however. Some screening tests aim at conditions which rarely cause death; the hemoglobin level for anemias and intraocular pressure for glaucoma are examples of this group. Mortality studies can underevaluate the success of such tests. Also, some screening tests, such as the chest X-ray for tuberculosis, detect conditions for which medical care is highly effective. A comparison of death rates in persons with both positive and negative test results would again underevaluate the effectiveness of such tests. However, the majority of tests are probably treated fairly by mortality data, since the conditions detected are frequent causes of death and are only moderately affected by presently available medical knowledge.

Should each test be evaluated only in terms of deaths from conditions which should be detected by the test? The answer is probably "No." If the electrocardiogram, for example, successfully separates off persons with noncardiovascular disease as well as cardiovascular cases, that test should be given due credit for this additional yield. Furthermore, a test such as height and weight, not aimed at a particular disease condition, can be evaluated only in terms of deaths from all causes. This is probably the optimum procedure for all tests.

One pioneering study of multiple screening has published mortality data.[4] Many of the tests used in that study of longshoremen in San Francisco were similar to the tests used in Baltimore. Despite the great differences in the populations tested, the ranking of the effectiveness of the tests is similar. An unexpected finding, both in Baltimore and in San Francisco, has been the superior performance of the urine albumin test. Albuminuria in older groups of the asymptomatic population seems to have a prognosis more grave than was previously suspected.

This follow-up study in Baltimore suffers from the defect of incomplete information for 12 percent of all screenees. The 267 incompletely traced persons included more persons in the younger age groups, more nonwhites, and more persons with negative tests than those whose current status is accurately known. This defect has probably had little effect on death figures for each test and for the ranking of tests, but it may have produced an artificially low death rate among screenees with negative tests. Thus, the annual crude death rate per 1,000 persons with all tests negative was 1.2 in Baltimore, compared with 4.3 for longshoremen in San Francisco where losses to follow-up were less severe.

The second major problem in the Baltimore study is the relatively small number of persons screened, and the small number of deaths on which the analysis must be based. Age groups had, therefore, to be broad in this presentation, and even the "age-adjusted" death rates were rather crude adjustments.

Finally, we would briefly mention one theoretical problem involved in using death rates to evaluate screening test performance. A screening test, able to separate off an older group of positives, will produce a group with a higher mortality because of age alone. Only when death rates are compared for positive and negative groups of similar age range will the effectiveness of a test in screening for disease be determined. The age-adjusted mortality ratio discussed in this paper minimizes the effect of separating off the older age groups.

Are we being unfair to the test in making this age adjustment, however? Should a test be given credit for screening for both age and disease, since both conditions result in greater need for medical care? We believe that the answer to both questions is "No," but realize that opinions will differ.

Summary and Conclusions

To evaluate the effectiveness of multiple screening, this study has used 5-year mortality figures for 2,298 residents of Baltimore who took multiple screening tests in 1954. The study has shown that screening tests separate off high mortality groups who can reasonably be given priority in medical care. This finding gives a sound basis for multiple screening and weakens the contention that all adults should be seen periodically by physicians, not just those with positive screening tests.

Five indices which use death rates in evaluating screening tests have been presented. Each index has good and bad points, and no one index is adequate to form the sole basis for evaluation. The indices suggest that tests with adequate performance were 70-mm. chest X-ray, six-lead electrocardiogram, blood pressure measurement, questionnaire for symptoms of cardiovascular disease, blood and urine sugar, and urine albumin. Tests with poor performance were the serologic test for syphilis, hemoglobin level, and height and weight test.

Little is known of how much persons with positive screening test results are benefited by the early detection of their diseases. It is possible that multiple screening may fail in its ultimate aim to reduce illness, disability, and death in the population, because medical care may not control the diagnosed conditions. Only when the benefits of early detection are clearly established can multiple screening be encouraged widely in the United States.

REFERENCES

1. Commission on Chronic Illness. Chronic Illness in a Large City. Cambridge: Harvard Univ. Press, 1957.
2. Roberts, D. W., and Wylie, C. M. Multiple Screening in the Baltimore Study of Chronic Illness. J.A.M.A. 161: 1442-1446, 1956.
3. Wylie, C. M. Participation in a Multiple Screening Clinic with Five-year Followup. Pub. Health Rep. 76: 596-602, 1961.
4. Buechley, R. W., Drake, R. M., and Breslow, L. Height, Weight, and Mortality in a Population of Longshoremen. J. Chronic Dis. 7: 363-378, 1958.

Rose Mary Jacobs and Janet Hare contributed significantly to the study. The study was financed in part by Grant IG-6791A from the National Institutes of Health, Public Health Service.

25

Followup Study of Narcotic Drug Addicts After Hospitalization

G. HALSEY HUNT and MAURICE E. ODOROFF

A FEW studies have attempted to evaluate systematically the status of patients at varying lengths of time after hospital treatment for drug addiction.[1-3] These have been based either upon a questionnaire sent to discharged patients or upon the records of patients readmitted to a Federal narcotic treatment hospital. In a recent study[4] the major source of the information was a team of 4 parole officers who supervised 346 former addicts on parole from New York State correctional institutions.

In the present study the data were gathered by a field team which attempted to make contact with all addict patients discharged from the U.S. Public Health Service Hospital at Lexington, Ky., during the period from July 17, 1952, to December 31, 1955, who gave a home address in any part of New York City. Followup contacts on all patients not classified as readdicted were continued during the calendar year 1956, and the study was terminated on December 31, 1956. At that time the National Institute of Mental Health, Public Health Service, took over the followup team as part of their New York Demonstration Center and has continued certain studies of selected groups of former addict patients.

Purpose of Study

The original primary goal of the study was to arrive at some estimate of the value of hospital treatment of narcotic drug addicts in preventing their relapse into a state of readdiction. In addition it was hoped that the rate of readdiction could be correlated with pertinent demographic characteristics and with various aspects of the patients' hospital experience.

Before these more fundamental determinations could be made, it was necessary to find out, first, whether contact could be achieved and maintained with persons who had been treated for narcotic drug addiction after they had been discharged from the hospital and had returned to their own community, and second, if contact could be achieved, to find out whether one could determine with reasonable certainty whether or not the former patients had become readdicted to narcotic drugs.

The study was undertaken to try to get answers to three questions.

1. Can contact be achieved with addict patients discharged from the Public Health Service Hospital at Lexington to New York City?

2. If so, can it be determined with reasonable certainty which patients remain abstinent and which become readdicted?

3. If the first two questions can be answered affirmatively, what are the gross readdiction rates at various times following discharge, and what relationships, if any, can be found between relapse rates and such factors as age, sex, ethnic group, social status, and length of hospital stay?

Principles of Treatment

The Public Health Service first began work with the problem of narcotic drug addiction in 1923 when Dr. Lawrence Kolb, a Service officer trained as a psychiatrist, conducted a survey of the prevalence of addiction in the United States. Kolb's studies produced the first reasonably valid estimate of the amount of addiction in the United States, an estimated 110,000 addicts.[5] In subsequent clinical and psychiatric investigations at the Hygienic Laboratory (now the National Institutes of Health) and among Federal prisoners, he studied the physiology and psychology of narcotic drug abuse. His work became the foundation for the currently accepted medical approach to the treatment of narcotic drug addiction which identifies the addict as a mentally ill person in need of medical treatment, notwithstanding his tendency to engage in criminal acts.

The work of Treadway, Kolb, and Himmelsbach[6-8] led to formulation of a hospital regimen for narcotic drug addiction which includes (a) provision for the withdrawal of the addicting drug in a secure environment, (b) continued psychiatric treatment, and (c) rehabilitation through an opportunity for the patient to work and learn a trade.

The medical and social aspects of narcotic drug addiction were recognized by Congress when it authorized, in 1929, the construction of two Public Health Service Hospitals for the purpose of confining and treating persons who had committed offenses against Federal law and who were addicted to narcotic drugs. The hospital at Lexington was opened in 1935 and a similar hospital in Fort Worth, Tex., in 1938. To the extent space was available, the Service was authorized to treat addicts who were willing to enter the hospital voluntarily for treatment.

In addition, facilities were provided for conducting research into the properties and effects of addicting drugs and effective methods of treatment and rehabilitation.

The treatment program at Lexington assumes that narcotic drug addiction is primarily a symptom of emotional disturbance or functional inadequacy and that addiction has two separate aspects, physical dependence and psychological dependence. Physical dependence is easily treated by withdrawal of the addicting drug in a controlled drug-free environment. Psychological dependence is more difficult to treat since it involves a basic functional inadequacy of the individual. Treatment aims at gaining patient acceptance of the desirability of living without drugs and at helping him to meet stress without recourse to drugs. Thus, psychological therapy and work therapy are used in rehabilitating the patient following relief from physical dependence on drugs.

The recommended length of stay for voluntary patients has tended to decrease over the years. For the first few years of operation of the hospital at Lexington, a period of 9 to 12 months was considered the optimum length of stay for these patients. The recommended period was later reduced to 6 months, and still later to 4½ months. These changes grew partly out of the need to reduce overcrowding and partly from the difficulty of demonstrating that the more prolonged periods of hospitalization added significantly to the value of treatment.

A more detailed discussion of the treatment program at Lexington is given by Lowry.[9]

Method of Study

The group studied consisted of all the patients discharged from the Public Health Service Hospital at Lexington during the period from July 17, 1952, to December 31, 1955, who (a) had been hospitalized with a diagnosis of narcotic drug addiction, (b) were reported by the hospital as having completed the withdrawal period, and (c) gave a home address in any part of New York City. Patients who were hospitalized more than once during the period of the study are included in the tabulations only for the first posthospitalization period, although some of them were seen by the followup team after their second or subsequent discharges.

In any future studies, consideration should be given to defining "completion of withdrawal" with precision. This was not done in the present study, and it is probable that some of the patients who left the hospital against medical advice did so within a few days after receiving the last dose of narcotic drug, with no opportunity to receive any benefits accruing from additional hospitalization. Patients who stayed 30 days or longer may be presumed to have become free of clinical signs of abstinence.

Followup contacts were continued until the study was terminated on December 31, 1956, so that each patient was followed for a minimum of 1 year after discharge or until he was determined to have become readdicted, whichever happened first. The maximum period of followup for abstinent patients, therefore, varied from 1 year to nearly 4½ years. Since 87.3 percent of the patients were classified as readdicted within 12 months after discharge, any bias introduced by the unequal period of followup tends to favor the abstinent group. If each "abstinent" patient had been followed for 4½ years, the proportion remaining abstinent for that length of time would in all probability have been smaller than the results reported here.

Followup Procedure

The full-time followup team established in New York consisted of two psychiatric social workers and one public health nurse. The senior psychiatric social worker and the public health nurse had been members of the staff of the hospital at Lexington. Early in the study the senior psychiatric social worker resigned, the second social worker became chief of the team for the remainder of the study, and another male psychiatric social worker was added to the staff.

At the time of discharge of every patient meeting the criteria for inclusion in the study, the hospital mailed to the followup team the name and address of the patient, of any known relatives and friends, and a résumé of available social information concerning the patient.

The followup team sent a letter to each discharged patient informing him that the team was aware that he had returned home and telling him that they were interested in helping him. If no response was received, a second letter was sent indicating regret that the patient had not as yet had an opportunity to respond and emphasizing the interest of the followup team in seeing him. Different kinds of letters to meet a variety of needs were devised and duplicated. The duplicated letters preserved as personal a tone as possible and were uniformly worded around an offer to help the patient with his problem.

Extreme care was taken to observe confidentiality. Envelopes gave only a post office box number and letters made no mention of hospitalization. If the patient did not respond to either letter, or if letters were returned marked "unknown at this address," the team cautiously proceeded to get in touch with members of the family, asking only for the patient's address. In telephone contacts the patient or member of his family were encouraged to come to the office for an interview, although as much information as possible was elicited during the telephone conversation. If both the patients and those having knowledge of them failed to respond, an attempt was made to locate the patients through direct visits. If patients or their families could not be located or refused to respond, information was sought from the New York City police files, files of the Federal Bureau of Narcotics, or the New York City Social Service Exchange. All these organizations accepted the need for complete confidentiality of information.

There were 1,912 patients referred to the New York followup team, and the team was successful in achieving some degree of contact with 1,881, or 98.4 percent. The first question, therefore, was answered in the affirmative: the followup team could achieve and maintain substantial contact with a larger proportion of addict patients following their discharge from the hospital.

Determination of Readdiction

The determination of readdiction, however, proved to be much more difficult. In planning the study, it had been assumed that the patients would be either fully abstinent or fully readdicted, and that the only problem would be that of determining the presence or absence of full-blown readdiction. Since all patients in the study had, by definition, been fully addicted at least once, it was thought that any return to the use of drugs would lead to rapid reestablishment of addiction. In the early stages of the study, the followup team classified a number of patients as readdicted when they had satisfied themselves that a patient had taken as little as a single injection of heroin.

It was later found that this assumption was incorrect, and that occasionally some patients would take one, two, or even more, injections of heroin during the readjustment period immediately after discharge from the hospital or during later periods of special stress, but then cease the use of drugs before readdiction had become established. Based on such evidence, a distinction was made between irregular use and readdiction.

Readdiction was defined for the purpose of this study as the use of a narcotic drug in the amount of at least one injection per day for a period of 2 weeks. Any use of drugs less frequently than once a day or for a period of less than 2 weeks was classified as irregular use. From the medical point of view physical dependence is necessary for a diagnosis of drug addiction, and it is unlikely that one daily injection of a narcotic drug for a 2-week period would result in significant physical dependence. The definition adopted is therefore a probabilistic one. It assumes that although the daily injection of a single dose of a narcotic drug for a 2-week period does not induce addiction in most persons previously not addicted, such doses taken voluntarily by one previously addicted make it highly probable that he is, or will become, readdicted.

Patients were therefore classified in accordance with these definitions.

● *Abstinent.* The patient is not taking any narcotic drugs at the time of observation and has not taken any since the previous observation.

● *Irregular use.* The patient is using, or has used, narcotic drugs to some extent since the previous observation, but has not taken as much as one injection per day for a period of 2 weeks.

● *Readdicted.* The patient is using, or has used, narcotic drugs to the extent of at least one injection per day for a period of 2 weeks.

Since the followup team could not ascertain under controlled conditions the number of doses a patient took in a given period of time, it was necessary for them to seek criteria which would permit a reasonably accurate determination. During the early years of the study various attempts were made to develop schemes for translating bits and pieces of information about individual patients into an objective rating scale. Efforts were made, for example, to devise a series of relative weights to be given to information received from a patient, his family, law enforcement agencies, and physicians, with the thought that the sources of information could be arrayed in a series with consistently increasing validity. All of these attempts proved fruitless and were abandoned.

The procedure finally adopted was developed on the basis of the followup team's experience that sufficient information could be obtained in almost all cases to warrant a considered conclusion that a given patient was either abstinent or addicted. The interviewers became adept in identifying and evaluating individual bits of evidence and in validating them by checking police, hospital, and social agency files.

Objective corroborative evidence of readdiction was obtained from these outside sources for substantial numbers of patients. Many patients (469 of the 1,881 followed) were arrested for narcotic offenses. A number of these showed overt withdrawal symptoms after a few hours in jail. Others approached physicians to obtain drugs and were reported as drug users under the New York law. Many patients who became readdicted (249) applied for hospitalization either in New York City or at the Lexington hospital.

The criteria finally adopted for determining readdiction, therefore, were based on (a) a series of clues stemming from the awareness of the interviewers of the signs and symptoms of readdiction, (b) objective verification from social agencies, police, and health department files, and (c) admission to the hospital at Lexington or the Riverside Hospital in New York. While absolute evidence of readdiction was available for only a fraction of the patients, for most, the team was able to come to a firm conclusion about the presence or absence of readdiction. During the final year of the study, the chief of the followup team reviewed the records of all patients and was responsible for determining the final classification of each patient in the study. If there were any doubts about the diagnosis of readdiction, the patient was classified as an irregular user or as abstinent.

It is recognized that a more objective measure of readdiction would have been desirable, but the experience of the team during this study with many of the same patients leads to the belief that any errors in classification of patients were not of sufficient magnitude to affect the conclusions seriously.

Findings of Study

There were 1,912 patients referred to the New York City followup team. Some degree of contact was achieved with 1,881 or 98.4 percent. Table 1 is a comparison of the patients referred for study and those subsequently followed, grouped by voluntary and nonvoluntary status, sex, and age, and classified by ethnic group.

The team was unable to locate 31 patients, only one of whom was a nonvoluntary patient. Following is the distribution by sex and ethnic group of the remaining 30 voluntary patients who could not be followed. The male to female ratio for the total group referred is nearly four to one; a disproportionate number of females could not be followed ($P < 0.01$).

Race	Male	Female
White	5	7
Negro	6	6
Puerto Rican	2	0
Chinese and others	4	0
Total	17	13

TABLE 1. PATIENTS WITH NEW YORK CITY ADDRESSES
DISCHARGED FROM THE PUBLIC HEALTH SERVICE HOSPITAL, LEXINGTON,
KY., BETWEEN JULY 17, 1952, AND DEC. 31, 1955,
REFERRED FOR STUDY AND SUBSEQUENTLY FOLLOWED

Status, sex, and age (years)	Referred					Followed				
	Total	White	Negro	Puerto Rican	Chinese and other	Total	White	Negro	Puerto Rican	Chinese and other
All patients ..	1,912	721	948	187	56	1,881	709	935	185	52
Voluntary	1,533	655	669	156	53	1,503	643	657	154	49
Male	1,176	479	517	128	52	1,159	474	511	126	48
Under 30	774	260	398	114	2	770	260	396	112	2
Over 30	402	219	119	14	50	389	214	115	14	46
Female	357	176	152	28	1	344	169	146	28	1
Under 30	197	58	117	21	1	193	58	113	21	1
Over 30	160	118	35	7	0	151	111	33	7	0
Nonvoluntary	[1]379	66	279	31	3	[2]378	66	278	31	3
Male	338	56	249	30	3	337	56	248	30	3
Under 30	269	42	204	23	0	268	42	203	23	0
Over 30	69	14	45	7	3	69	14	45	7	3
Female	41	10	30	1	0	41	10	30	1	0
Under 30	35	9	26	0	0	35	9	26	0	0
Over 30	6	1	4	1	0	6	1	4	1	0

[1] 310 prisoners, 69 probationers.
[2] 309 prisoners, 69 probationers.

Comparison With Other Discharged Patients

The New York City group followed differed significantly as a sample in a number of characteristics from all patients discharged from Lexington during the last full fiscal year of the study. The New York City group had higher proportions of nonvoluntary patients, of men, of Negroes, and of patients under 30 years of age ($P < 0.01$ for each). The proportion in each of these classifications for all discharged patients and for patients followed are summarized.

	Patients followed (percent)	All patients discharged (percent)
Nonvoluntary	20.1	15.8
Males	79.5	75.2
Negroes	49.7	42.5
Under 30 years	67.3	47.6

Characteristics of the Study Group

Among the patients admitted voluntarily, the group followed had about equal proportions of whites (42.8 percent) and Negroes (43.7

percent); the Puerto Ricans comprised 10 percent and the Chinese about 3 percent. About three out of every four patients in the New York group were men, and two-thirds of these were under 30 years of age. The voluntary patients were predominantly young men; about one-third were white and one-half Negro.

The nonvoluntary patients in the group followed (309 prisoners, 69 probationers) were 73.5 percent Negro, 17.5 percent white, 8.2 percent Puerto Rican, and less than 1 percent Chinese and other. Two-thirds of the nonvoluntary patients were male Negroes and 81.9 percent of these were under 30 years of age. The nonvoluntary patients were predominantly young, male, and Negro.

Readdiction Rates After Discharge

The addiction status at the end of the followup period for the study group is found in Table 2. Out of 1,881 patients followed, 1,694 (90.1 percent) were judged by the study's criteria to be readdicted, 124 (6.6 percent) abstinent, and 63 (3.3 percent) used narcotics irregularly or their addiction status could not be determined.

The rapidity with which patients resumed the use of narcotic drugs after discharge was striking. Within 6 months after referral, 5 out of 6 patients had resumed the use of narcotic drugs (83.3 percent of all patients, or 92.5 percent of those who became readdicted during the course of the study). By 2 years after referral, 9 out of 10 had resumed the use of narcotic drugs (Table 3). Patients who were classified as readdicted by the study's criteria were no longer included in the tabulations once they were so classified so that, in effect, we followed to the end of the study only the patients who remained completely abstinent after referral.

Variations in Relapse Rates

Table 4 presents data on the 1,694 patients who became readdicted, the 124 abstinent patients, and the 63 patients using narcotics irregularly or for whom use could not be determined classified by ethnic group, type of admission (voluntary and nonvoluntary), sex, and age.

Age proved to be the principal significant variable in the determination of rates of readdiction, with men 30 years of age and older having generally lower readdiction rates than those under 30. Age had no significant effect among female voluntary patients. There were so few female nonvoluntary patients that no significant comparison with respect to age could be made. Comparisons of types of admission,

TABLE 2. READDICTION STATUS OF ALL PATIENTS AT COMPLETION OF FOLLOWUP PERIOD

Status	Total Patients		White		Negro		Puerto Rican		Chinese and other	
	Number	Percent	Number	Percent	Number	Percent	Number	Percent	Number	Percent
All patients	1,881	100.0	709	100.0	935	100.0	185	100.0	52	100.0
Readdicted	1,694	90.1	630	88.9	848	90.7	173	93.5	43	82.7
Abstinent	124	6.6	53	7.5	55	5.9	8	4.3	8	15.4
Irregular or undetermined	63	3.3	26	3.6	32	3.4	4	2.2	1	1.9

TABLE 3. CUMULATIVE NUMBER AND PERCENT OF PATIENTS RESUMING THE USE OF NARCOTIC DRUGS AT VARIOUS TIMES AFTER REFERRAL

Months after referral	Cumulative number	Cumulative percent
Under 6	1,567	83.3
6-12	1,642	87.3
13-18	1,671	88.8
19-24	1,679	89.2
25 or more	1,694	90.1

length of stay, sex, and ethnic group, data permitting, thus take the variable of age into consideration. In addition, readdiction rates were significantly lower for:

1. The nonvoluntary group of patients aged 30 or more as compared with their voluntary counterparts.

2. The white nonvoluntary group less than 30 years of age as compared with their Negro counterparts.

3. Patients under 30 years of age staying in the hospital 31 days or more as compared with those staying 30 days or less.

Ethnic group and sex produced no significant differences among the voluntary patients or among the nonvoluntary except for the single significant difference in readdiction rates between young white and Negro men. The readdiction rates for these groups were 78.6 and 93.1 percent respectively (df = 2; x^2 = 12.7467; $P < 0.01$).

Age. The readdiction rate for all men 30 years of age or older, 85.1 percent, is significantly lower than that for all men under 30 years, 92.6 percent (Table 5). This holds both for voluntary male patients under 30, with a readdiction rate of 93.5 percent, and for those over 30, with a rate of 87.4 percent (df = 2; x^2 = 12.6870; $P < 0.01$), and for nonvoluntary male patients under 30, with a rate of 89.9 percent, and over 30, with a rate of 72.5 percent (df = 2; x^2 = 15.4798; $P < 0.01$).

The difference between the readdiction rates for the younger and older voluntary male patients is, however, due to the difference between the readdiction rates for younger (93.8 percent) and older (85.5 percent) voluntary white male patients (Table 6). The difference between the readdiction rates for the younger and older nonvoluntary male patients is due to the difference between the readdiction rates for younger (93.1 percent) and older (73.3 percent) Negro male patients (Table 7). Being over 30 years of age increases a patient's chance of remaining abstinent for both voluntary white and nonvoluntary Negro male patients.

Type of admission. The readdiction rate for all nonvoluntary patients (85.7 percent) is lower than the rate for voluntary patients (91.2 percent). Inasmuch as all but 8 nonvoluntary patients had a length of stay of 121 or more days, the comparison is limited to patients with a similar length of stay (Table 8). For those under age 30, the readdiction rates are 90.5 percent for voluntary patients and 90.2 percent for nonvoluntary patients, rates which proved not to be statistically significant (df = 2; x^2 = 0.2023; $P = 0.92$ +). For those aged 30 or more years, the readdiction rates were 88.8 percent for the

TABLE 4. RATES FOR PATIENTS WHO WERE READDICTED, ABSTINENT, OR
IRREGULAR USERS BY STATUS, SEX, AND AGE, CLASSIFIED BY ETHNIC GROUP

Status, sex, and age (years)	Total patients		White		Negro		Puerto Rican		Chinese and other	
	Num-ber	Per-cent	Num-ber	Per-cent	Num-ber	Per-cent	Num-ber	Per-cent	Num-ber	Per-cent
					Readdicted					
Total	1,694	90.1	630	88.9	848	90.7	173	93.5	43	82.7
Voluntary	1,370	91.2	578	89.9	603	91.8	147	95.4	42	85.7
Male	1,060	91.4	427	90.1	469	91.8	123	97.6	41	85.4
Under 30	720	93.5	244	93.8	366	92.4	109	97.3	1	—
Over 30	340	87.4	183	85.5	103	89.6	14	—	40	86.9
Female	310	90.1	151	89.3	134	91.8	24	85.7	1	—
Under 30	174	90.1	50	86.2	104	92.0	19	90.4	1	—
Over 30	136	90.1	101	91.0	30	90.9	5	—	0	—
Nonvoluntary[1]	324	85.7	52	78.8	245	88.1	26	83.9	1	—
Male	291	86.4	43	76.8	222	89.5	25	83.3	1	—
Under 30	241	89.9	33	78.6	189	93.1	19	82.6	0	—
Over 30	50	72.4	10	71.4	33	73.3	6	85.7	1	—
Female	33	80.4	9	90.0	23	76.7	1	—	0	—
Under 30	29	82.9	8	88.9	21	80.8	0	—	0	—
Over 30	4	—	1	—	2	—	1	—	0	—
					Abstinent					
Total	124	6.6	53	7.5	55	5.9	8	4.3	8	15.4
Voluntary	83	5.5	42	6.5	30	4.6	5	3.2	6	12.2
Males	62	5.3	29	6.1	25	4.9	2	1.6	6	12.5
Under 30	30	3.9	9	3.5	18	4.5	2	1.8	1	—
Over 30	32	8.2	20	9.3	7	6.1	0	—	5	10.9
Females	21	6.1	13	7.7	5	3.4	3	10.7	0	—
Under 30	12	6.2	7	12.1	4	3.5	1	4.8	0	—
Over 30	9	6.0	6	5.4	1	3.0	2	—	0	—
Nonvoluntary[2]	41	10.9	11	16.7	25	9.0	3	9.7	2	—
Males	34	10.1	11	19.6	18	7.3	3	10.0	2	—
Under 30	19	7.1	8	19.0	8	3.9	3	13.0	0	—
Over 30	15	21.7	3	21.4	10	22.2	0	—	2	—
Females	7	17.1	0	—	7	23.3	0	—	0	—
Under 30	5	14.3	0	—	5	19.2	0	—	0	—
Over 30	2	—	0	—	2	—	0	—	0	—

TABLE 4. RATES FOR PATIENTS WHO WERE READDICTED, ABSTINENT, OR IRREGULAR USERS BY STATUS, SEX, AND AGE, CLASSIFIED BY ETHNIC GROUP

Status, sex, and age (years)	Total patients		White		Negro		Puerto Rican		Chinese and other	
	Number	Percent	Number	Percent	Number	Percent	Number	Percent	Number	Percent
	Irregular users or use undetermined									
Total	63	3.3	26	3.6	32	3.4	4	2.2	1	1.9
Voluntary	50	3.3	23	3.6	24	3.7	2	—	1	—
Male	37	3.2	18	3.8	17	3.3	1	—	1	—
Under 30	20	2.6	7	2.7	12	3.0	1	—	0	—
Over 30	17	4.4	11	5.1	5	4.3	0	—	1	—
Female	13	3.8	5	3.0	7	4.8	1	—	0	—
Under 30	7	3.6	1	—	5	4.4	1	—	0	—
Over 30	6	4.0	4	3.6	2	6.0	0	—	0	—
Nonvoluntary[3]	13	3.4	3	4.5	8	2.9	2	—	0	—
Male	12	3.6	2	—	8	3.2	2	—	0	—
Under 30	8	3.0	1	—	6	3.0	1	—	0	—
Over 30	4	5.8	1	—	2	—	1	—	0	—
Female	1	—	1	—	0	—	0	—	0	—
Under 30	1	—	1	—	0	—	0	—	0	—
Over 30	0	—	0	—	0	—	0	—	0	—
All patients	1,881	100	709	100	935	100	185	100	52	100

[1] 265 prisoners, 59 probationers. [2] 34 prisoners, 7 probationers. [3] 10 prisoners, 3 probationers.

TABLE 5. READDICTION RATES OF MALE PATIENTS, BY AGE

Readdiction status	Under 30 years		Over 30 years		Total	
	Number	Percent	Number	Percent	Number	Percent
Readdicted	961	92.6	390	85.1	1,351	90.3
Abstinent	49	4.7	47	10.3	96	6.4
Irregular or undetermined	28	2.7	21	4.6	49	3.3

Note: df=2; x^2=20.5888; $P<0.01$.

TABLE 6. READDICTION RATES OF VOLUNTARY WHITE
MALE PATIENTS, BY AGE

Readdiction status	Voluntary white males under 30 years		Voluntary white males over 30 years		Total	
	Number	Percent	Number	Percent	Number	Percent
Readdicted	244	93.8	183	85.5	427	90.1
Abstinent	9	3.5	20	9.3	29	6.1
Irregular or undetermined	7	2.7	11	5.2	18	3.8

Note: df=2; x^2=9.4206; P<0.01.

TABLE 7. READDICTION RATES OF NONVOLUNTARY NEGRO MALE
PATIENTS, BY AGE

Readdiction status	Nonvoluntary Negro males under 30		Nonvoluntary Negro males over 30		Total	
	Number	Percent	Number	Percent	Number	Percent
Readdicted	189	93.1	33	73.3	222	89.5
Abstinent	8	3.9	10	22.2	18	7.3
Irregular or undetermined	6	3.0	2	4.5	8	3.2

Note: df=2; x^2=19.0969; P<0.01.

voluntary group and 69.3 percent for the nonvoluntary group. The voluntary group had a statistically significant higher rate of readdiction (df = 2; x^2 = 15.8410; $P < 0.01$). Of the total group of 910 patients with a length of stay of 121 or more days, 540 were voluntary patients and only 370 nonvoluntary. Furthermore, the readdiction rates are nearly the same for the younger and older groups of voluntary patients, 90.5 percent and 88.8 percent, so that if these groups are combined and tested against the rate of readdiction of 90.2 percent for nonvoluntary patients under 30 years of age, the difference between the rates is not statistically significant (df = 2; x^2 = 0.2440; $P = 0.90-$). Thus it becomes clear that it is the reduced rate of readdiction in the nonvoluntary group of patients aged 30 years or more

TABLE 8. READDICTION RATES BY LENGTH OF HOSPITAL STAY,
TYPE OF ADMISSION, AND AGE

Length of hospital stay and age	Followed	Readdicted		Abstinent		Irregular	
		Number	Percent	Number	Percent	Number	Percent
		All patients					
Total	1,881	1,694	90.1	124	6.6	63	3.3
Under 31 days	633	590	93.2	25	3.9	18	2.9
Under 30 years	423	405	95.7	10	2.4	8	1.9
Over 30 years	210	185	88.1	15	7.1	10	4.8
31-60 days	204	180	88.2	14	6.9	10	4.9
Under 30 years	127	113	89.0	6	4.7	8	6.3
Over 30 years	77	67	87.0	8	10.4	2	2.6
61-120 days	134	121	90.3	6	4.5	7	5.2
Under 30 years	94	85	90.4	6	6.4	3	3.2
Over 30 years	40	36	90.0	0	—	4	10.0
121 days or more	910	803	88.2	79	8.7	28	3.1
Under 30 years	621	561	90.3	44	7.1	16	2.6
Over 30 years	289	242	83.7	35	12.1	12	4.2
		Voluntary patients					
Total	1,503	1,370	91.2	83	5.5	50	3.3
Under 31 days	633	590	93.2	25	3.9	18	2.9
Under 30 years	423	405	95.7	10	2.4	8	1.9
Over 30 years	210	185	88.1	15	7.1	10	4.8
31-60 days	202	179	88.6	14	6.9	9	4.5
Under 30 years	125	112	89.6	6	4.8	7	5.6
Over 30 years	77	67	87.0	8	10.4	2	2.6
61-120 days	128	116	90.6	5	3.9	7	5.5
Under 30 years	89	81	91.0	5	5.6	3	3.4
Over 30 years	39	35	89.7	0	—	4	10.3
121 days or more	540	485	89.9	39	7.2	16	3.0
Under 30 years	326	295	90.5	22	6.7	9	2.8
Over 30 years	214	190	88.8	17	7.9	7	3.3
		Nonvoluntary patients					
Total	378	324	85.7	41	10.9	13	3.4
Under 31 days	0	0	—	0	—	0	—
Under 30 years	0	0	—	0	—	0	—
Over 30 years	0	0	—	0	—	0	—
31-60 days	2	1	—	0	—	1	—
Under 30 years	2	1	—	0	—	1	—
Over 30 years	0	0	—	0	—	0	—
61-120 days	6	5	83.3	1	—	0	—
Under 30 years	5	4	—	1	—	0	—
Over 30 years	1	1	—	0	—	0	—
121 days or more	370	318	85.7	40	10.8	12	3.5
Under 30 years	295	266	90.2	22	7.5	7	2.3
Over 30 years	75	52	69.3	18	24.0	5	6.7

which accounts for the difference between the rates for the voluntary and nonvoluntary groups.

Length of stay. The relationship between the readdiction rate and length of hospital stay is a particularly important consideration. Studies conducted by the Public Health Service[10] indicate that signs of withdrawal disappear in 7 to 14 days after patients are withdrawn from narcotics but that physiological readjustment, as determined by laboratory tests, is seldom complete in less than 120 days. The recommended minimum length of stay at Lexington for voluntary patients is 145 days, but only 16.2 percent of all patients followed stayed 146 days or more (Table 9). Of the voluntary patients only 21, or 1.4 percent, stayed as long as 146 days, while 74.9 percent of the nonvoluntary patients stayed 146 days or more.

TABLE 9. PATIENTS STAYING MORE THAN 145 DAYS

Length of stay	Total		Voluntary		Nonvoluntary	
	Number	Percent	Number	Percent	Number	Percent
All patients	1,881	100.0	1,503	100.9	378	100.0
145 days or less	1,577	83.8	1,482	98.6	95	25.1
146 days or more	304	16.2	21	1.4	283	74.9

If length of stay has an effect on readdiction rates, then patients staying increasingly longer periods should have a significantly lower rate of readdiction than those staying for relatively shorter periods. Table 8 indicates only 8 nonvoluntary patients stayed less than 121 days. Since age also has an effect on readdiction rates, the problem is to determine whether there is any connection between readdiction rates and length of stay for voluntary patients with age held constant. Tests of the effect of length of stay on readdiction rates are therefore restricted to voluntary patients. In Table 8 patients are classified by age and period of stay: under 31 days, 31-60 days, 61-120 days, and 121 days and over.

The readdiction rates for voluntary patients over 30 years of age were not significantly different for length of stay, even with the inclusion of patients staying in the hospital less than 31 days (Table 10).

The readdiction rates for voluntary patients under 30 years of age

TABLE 10. READDICTION RATES FOR VOLUNTARY PATIENTS
OVER 30 YEARS, BY LENGTH OF STAY

Readdiction status	Under 31 days		31-120 days		121 days or more		Total	
	Number	Percent	Number	Percent	Number	Percent	Number	Percent
Readdicted	185	88.1	102	87.9	190	88.8	477	88.3
Abstinent	15	7.1	8	6.9	17	7.9	40	7.4
Irregular or undetermined .	10	4.8	6	5.2	7	3.3	23	4.3

Note: df=4; x^2=1.0077; P=0.90+.

were consistently lower and significant for patients staying 31 days or more than for those staying less than 31 days (Table 11).

When the effect of patients staying under 31 days is removed, however, the readdiction rates for the three remaining periods (31-60, 61-120, and 121 or more days) are not significantly different (Table 12).

Episodes of Hospitalization

The effect on readdiction rates of the number of episodes of hospitalization was explored. In order to minimize the effect of length of stay, age, and type of admission on readdiction rates by the number of episodes of hospitalization, the data in Table 13 are so classified. Comparison between the readdiction rates for one and for two or more episodes of hospitalization proved significant ($P < .05$) only for nonvoluntary patients under 30 years of age staying 31 days or more. This group had a higher readdiction rate after the first episode of hospitalization than after two or more. Table 14 is an analysis of various comparisons.

Summary and Conclusions

This is a report of a field followup study of 1,912 addict patients living in New York City who were discharged from the U.S. Public Health Service Hospital at Lexington, Ky., between July 1952 and December 1955.

The study was undertaken to try to get answers to three questions:

1. Can contact be achieved with addict patients discharged from the Public Health Service Hospital at Lexington to New York City?

2. If so, can it be determined with reasonable certainty which patients remain abstinent and which become readdicted?

3. If the first two questions can be answered in the affirmative, what

TABLE 11. READDICTION RATES FOR VOLUNTARY PATIENTS
UNDER 30 YEARS, BY LENGTH OF STAY

Readdiction status	Under 31 days		31-60 days		61-120 days		121 days or more		Total	
	Number	Percent	Number	Percent	Number	Percent	Number	Percent	Number	Percent
Readdicted	405	95.7	112	89.6	81	91.0	295	90.5	893	92.7
Abstinent	10	2.4	6	4.8	5	5.6	22	6.7	43	4.5
Irregular or undetermined	8	1.9	7	5.6	3	3.4	9	2.8	27	2.8

Note: df=6; x^2=14.3290; $P<0.05$.

TABLE 12. READDICTION RATES FOR VOLUNTARY PATIENTS
UNDER 30 YEARS, BY LENGTH OF STAY OVER 30 DAYS

Readdiction status	31-60 days		61-120 days		121 days or more		Total	
	Number	Percent	Number	Percent	Number	Percent	Number	Percent
Readdicted	112	89.6	81	91.0	295	90.5	488	90.4
Abstinent	6	4.8	5	5.6	22	6.7	33	6.1
Irregular or undetermined	7	5.6	3	3.4	9	2.8	19	3.5

Note: df=4; x^2=2.9508; P=0.60+.

are the gross readdiction rates at various times following discharge, and what relationships, if any, can be found between relapse rates and such factors as age, sex, ethnic group, social status, and length of hospital stay?

The first question was answered affirmatively. The followup team, composed of two psychiatric social workers and one public health nurse, was able to achieve some degree of contact with 1,881 or 98.4 percent. The second question proved more difficult to answer, and no objective evaluation scale could be found. However, as the followup team increased rapport with the patient group, as the team gained more experience in evaluating the information they received from and about patients, and as confirmatory evidence piled up (such as the return of a patient to Lexington or his conviction in a local court) they were able to make the judgment with increasing confidence that individual patients either were abstinent or had resumed the use of drugs. Their final judgment, while subjective, is thought to have a high degree of validity.

The principal findings of the study were that more than 90 percent of the patients followed became readdicted, and more than 90 percent of those who became readdicted did so within 6 months after discharge from the hospital.

Age proved to be the principal significant variable in the determination of rates of readdiction, with men over 30 years of age having generally lower readdiction rates than those under 30. Age had no significant effect among female voluntary patients. There were so few female nonvoluntary patients that no significant comparisons, with respect to age, could be made. Comparisons of types of admission, length of stay, ethnic group, and sex, data permitting, thus take the variable of age into consideration.

In addition, significantly lower readdiction rates were found for (a) the nonvoluntary group of patients aged 30 or more as compared with their voluntary counterparts, (b) the white nonvoluntary group less than 30 years of age as compared with their Negro counterparts, and (c) patients under 30 years of age staying in the hospital 31 days or more as compared with those staying 30 days or less. Ethnic group and sex produced no significant differences among the voluntary patients nor among the nonvoluntary except for the single significant difference in readdiction rates between young (under 30) white and Negro men.

No improvement in readdiction rates was demonstrated for prolonged hospitalization in excess of 30 days.

TABLE 13. READDICTION RATES BY NUMBER OF EPISODES OF HOSPITALIZATION, TYPE OF ADMISSION, LENGTH OF STAY, AND AGE

Length of hospital stay, and age	Followed	Readdicted		Abstinent		Irregular	
		Number	Percent	Number	Percent	Number	Percent
	All patients						
Total	1,881	1,694	90.1	124	6.6	63	3.3
One episode	1,416	1,269	89.6	96	6.8	51	3.6
Under 31 days	517	480	92.8	22	4.3	15	2.9
Under 30 years	374	357	95.5	9	2.4	8	2.1
Over 30 years	143	123	86.0	13	9.1	7	4.9
More than 31 days	899	789	87.8	74	8.2	36	4.0
Under 30 years	683	617	90.3	44	6.5	22	3.2
Over 30 years	216	172	79.6	30	13.9	14	6.5
Two or more episodes	465	425	01.4	28	6.0	12	2.6
Under 31 days	116	110	94.8	3	2.6	3	2.6
Under 30 years	48	48	100.0	0	———	0	———
Over 30 years	68	62	91.2	3	4.4	3	4.4
More than 31 days	349	315	90.2	25	7.2	9	2.6
Under 30 years	160	142	88.8	13	8.1	5	3.1
Over 30 years	189	173	91.5	12	6.4	4	2.1
	Voluntary patients						
Total	1,503	1,370	91.2	83	5.5	50	3.3
One episode	1,096	992	90.5	65	5.9	39	3.6
Under 31 days	517	480	92.8	22	4.3	15	2.9
Under 30 years	374	357	95.5	9	2.4	8	2.1
Over 30 years	143	123	86.0	13	9.1	7	4.9
More than 31 days	579	512	88.4	43	7.4	24	4.2
Under 30 years	425	383	90.1	27	6.4	15	3.5
Over 30 years	154	129	83.8	16	10.4	9	5.8
Two or more episodes	407	378	92.9	18	4.4	11	2.7
Under 31 days	116	110	94.8	3	2.6	3	2.6
Under 30 years	48	48	100.0	0	———	0	———
Over 30 years	68	62	91.2	3	4.4	3	4.4
More than 31 days	291	268	92.1	15	5.2	8	2.7
Under 30 years	115	106	92.2	5	4.3	4	3.5
Over 30 years	176	162	92.0	10	5.7	4	2.3

TABLE 13. READDICTION RATES BY NUMBER OF EPISODES OF HOSPITALIZATION, TYPE OF ADMISSION, LENGTH OF STAY, AND AGE

Length of hospital stay, and age	Followed	Readdicted		Abstinent		Irregular	
		Number	Percent	Number	Percent	Number	Percent
		Nonvoluntary patients					
Total	378	324	85.7	41	10.9	13	3.4
One episode.	320	277	86.6	31	9.7	12	3.7
Under 31 days	0	0	-------	0	-------	0	-----
Under 30 years	0	0	-------	0	-------	0	-------
Over 30 years	0	0	-------	0	-------	0	-------
More than 31 days	320	277	86.6	31	9.7	12	3.7
Under 30 years	258	234	90.7	17	6.6	7	2.7
Over 30 years	62	43	69.4	14	22.6	5	8.0
Two or more episodes.	58	47	81.0	10	17.3	1	1.7
Under 31 days	0	0	-------	0	-----	0	-----
Under 30 years	0	0	-------	0	-----	0	-----
Over 30 years	0	0	-------	0	-----	0	-----
More than 31 days	58	47	81.0	10	17.3	1	1.7
Under 30 years	45	36	80.0	8	17.8	1	2.2
Over 30 years	13	11	84.6	2	15.4	0	-------

TABLE 14. COMPUTATIONS OF SIGNIFICANCE OF VARIOUS
RELATIONSHIPS SHOWN IN TABLE 13

Patient and stay	Degrees of freedom*	Chi-square	Significance: probability is
Voluntary:			
Under 30 days	2	0.3784	0.80+
Under 30 years of age	2	.5797	.70+
Over 30 years of age	2	1.0072	.50+
31 days or more	2	2.8134	.20+
Under 30 years of age	2	.7238	.70
Over 30 years of age	2	4.7687	.09
Nonvoluntary:			
31 days or more	2	2.8885	.20+
Under 30 years of age	2	6.4459	.05
Over 30 years of age	2	.5854	.70+

The findings of this study confirm Lowry's conclusion that: "Hospital treatment can start a patient on the way to recovery but it cannot provide a lifelong immunity that protects the patient against relapse. Hospital treatment can initiate rehabilitation but it must be completed after the patient returns to the community."

Aftercare is not available in most communities to which discharged addict patients go, and where some aftercare facilities exist, as in New York City, they are not adequate for the needs.

It is recommended that further studies be undertaken to secure additional knowledge of the long-term careers of addicted persons and of the dynamics of addiction and readdiction and to determine the effects of various kinds of treatment, including the planned variation of length of hospital stay. Improvements in method would involve (a) the development of more objective means of determining readdiction, (b) careful recording of the various therapeutic methods used for individual patients during hospitalization and the use of specifically controlled methods of treatment with types of patients selected randomly, and (c) the development of better data on the personal characteristics of patients and their social backgrounds, and the kinds and amounts of aftercare available to these patients.

REFERENCES

1. Pescor, M. J. A Statistical Analysis of the Clinical Records of Hospitalized Drug Addicts. Pub. Hlth. Rep., Supp. No. 143, 1943.
2. Pescor, M. J. Follow-up Study of Treated Narcotic Drug Addicts. Pub. Hlth. Rep., Supp. No. 170, 1943.
3. Knight, R. G., and Prout, C. T. A Study of Results in Hospital Treatment of Drug Addictions. Am. J. Psychiat. 108: 303-308, 1959-62.
4. Diskind, M. H. New Horizons in the Treatment of Narcotic Addiction. Federal Probation, 24: 56-63, 1960.
5. Kolb, L., and DuMez, A. G. The Prevalence and Trend of Drug Addiction in the United States and Factors Influencing It. Pub. Hlth. Rep. 39: 1179-1204, 1924.
6. Treadway, W. L. Drug Addiction and Measures for Its Prevention in the United States. J.A.M.A. 99: 372-379, 1932.
7. Kolb, L. Clinical Studies of Drug Addiction: The Struggle for Cure and the Conscious Reasons for Relapse. J. Nerv. Ment. Dis. 66: 22-43, 1927.
8. Kolb, L., and Himmelsbach, C. K. Clinical Studies of Drug Addiction. III, A Critical Review of the Withdrawal Treatment with Method of Evaluating Abstinence Syndromes. Am. J. Psychiat. 94: 759-799.
9. Lowry, J. V. Hospital Treatment of the Narcotic Addict. Federal Probation, 20: 42-51, 1956.
10. Himmelsbach, C. K. Clinical Studies of Drug Addiction. Physical Dependence, Withdrawal and Recovery. Arch. Int. Med. 69: 766-772, 1942.

Several members of the staff of the Bureau of Medical Services, Public Health Service, participated in planning and carrying out the study under Dr. Hunt's general direction. The principal staff members with their positions during the period of the study were Robert W. Barclay, program analysis and reports officer, Bureau of Medical Services; Leon Brill, chief, New York followup team; Dr. Kenneth L. Chapman, medical officer in charge, U.S. Public Health Service Hospital, Lexington, Ky.; Mary C. Gillis, chief, Social Service Branch, Division of Hospitals; Dr. Clifton K. Himmelsbach, chief, Division of Hospitals; Helen D. McGuire, chief, Medical Records Branch, Division of Hospitals; Joseph S. Murtaugh, chief Operating Reports, Analysis, and Procedures Branch, Division of Administrative Management; and Frances C. Nemec, chief medical record librarian, U.S. Public Health Service Hospital, Lexington, Ky.

Members of the New York followup team, in addition to Mr. Brill, were Mary McGovern, R.N., Harold J. O'Keefe, and Benjamin L. Zinda.

26

Patient Experience in Psychiatric Units of General and State Mental Hospitals

ELMER A. GARDNER, ANITA K. BAHN, and HAROLD C. MILES

THE area of community mental health and the organization of community mental health services has become a focal point in psychiatry. Problems concerned with the development of mental health centers, the role of psychiatric units in general hospitals as an integral part of such centers, and the gradual reduction in the size of public mental hospitals dominate current thinking and planning. Such planning, however, requires a careful evaluation of our present services and a projection of our future needs based on well-documented data.

In 1961, Forstenzer emphasized the "need to develop a working partnership between community services and the State hospital systems."[1] He feared "the risk of solidifying two separate and distinct programs, both operating at less than optimal levels, each handicapping the other, and each presumably concerned with different portions of the range of mental illnesses and possibly with different segments of the total population." Dorken, in discussing community mental health,[2] pointed out the need for proper survey data to know the extent of actual problems requiring attention and whether a particular mental health service is needed. He noted that the mental health centers in Minnesota were dealing with a population largely different from that of mental hospitals, and that they were reaching a segment of the community not previously reached. Schulberg presented the advantages and disadvantages of service by general hospital units as a core of community psychiatric services.[3] The general hospital tends to be treatment oriented and may not provide an adequate program of public health and preventive measures. Perhaps more important, there has been little or no research to determine the efficacy of general hospital units, their strengths and weaknesses.

In the planning of mental health services, particularly hospital beds, there has been a tendency to confuse demand with use and to consider one type of service in isolation from the others. Baldwin noted the "urgent necessity for detailed examination at an operational level, of the working of the present system, so that effects of planned changes may be measured, and adjustments made to accord more clearly with need as estimates become available."[4]

In considering the development of future health services, the role of the general hospital unit versus the public mental hospital, and the relationship between these and other services, the following questions may be posed:

1. How are these facilities (general hospital unit and public mental hospital) now used? Who uses these facilities? Do they serve similar or different segments of the population?

2. What is the subsequent psychiatric experience of patients hospitalized at either of these facilities? In what way does hospitalization in a public mental hospital or general hospital unit affect the course of a patient's disorder? What is the interaction, if any, between these facilities and between the hospital units and other community services?

While some of the answers cannot be obtained solely from descriptive data, the following data shed some light on these questions.

Background

For our study, a statistical comparison was made of first admissions (patients never before admitted to any psychiatric inpatient unit) during 1960 to the psychiatric services of Strong Memorial Hospital and to Rochester State Hospital. The physical and administrative characteristics of these two facilities (in 1960) are briefly described below.

Strong Memorial Hospital is a general hospital of 700 beds, owned and operated by the University of Rochester. Rochester Municipal Hospital, which the university operates, is so much a part of the same hospital complex that the whole is commonly referred to as the University Medical Center. (On July 1, 1963, the university purchased Municipal Hospital from the city of Rochester.) The psychiatric inpatient services comprise three floors for adults with a total of 86 beds and a children's unit of 12 beds. These 98 beds constitute 14 percent of all the hospital's beds. During 1960, 1,250 persons were admitted to the psychiatric services, of whom two-thirds were Monroe County residents. The bed occupancy averaged about 90 percent, with an average patient stay of 28-30 days. All the admissions were voluntary, though many might best be termed semi-voluntary. The cost per diem ranged from $30.30 to $42.10, with an average of $38.10. Most of this cost was paid by Blue Cross insurance coverage, which provided 30 days per admission for psychiatric hospitalization with renewal of the coverage after 90 days out of the hospital.

As this is a university teaching hospital, all patients are seen by third-year medical students and members of the psychiatric house staff. Approximately 40 percent of the patients are under private psychiatric care. Patients who are not under private care are cared for by the psychiatric residents, with supervision by the senior full-time faculty.

There is a daily average of six residents and interns, three or four medical students, a clinical director, psychologist, and psychiatric social worker for each of the three adult inpatient services (34, 28, and 24 beds, respectively). The children's unit (12 beds) has a daily average of three house officers and one or two medical students. In addition, senior faculty members provide considerable supervision by frequent case conferences or rounds. The daily average of 23 registered and practical nurses and 31 nursing assistants provides patient: staff ratios of 3.3:1 and 2.5:1, respectively. However, the teaching functions of the services insure an abundance of personnel and an intensity of care, which cannot be characterized adequately by patient: staff ratios or other figures.

There are active occupational and recreational therapy programs. The treatment orientation can be characterized best as eclectic. It ranges from intensive psychotherapy to drugs and electroconvulsive therapy (ECT). Although occasional patients are in a modified day or night care program, there are no specific units designated for such care. The services are oriented toward acute, short-term care, with an occasional patient remaining several months to years.

Rochester State Hospital, located within the city limits of Rochester in contrast to the isolation of most public mental hospitals, serves five counties and has 3,260 beds. Its bed occupancy during 1960 was 99 percent. Of 1,121 admissions, 808, or 72 percent, were from Monroe County. Twenty-seven percent of the admissions were voluntary. The per diem cost was $5.18, and a large portion of this was paid from state taxes. During 1960 there was a daily average of 108 registered and practical nurses, 555 nursing attendants, and 27 psychiatrists, 9 of whom were residents. This gave a ratio of 30 resident patients per nurse, 6 for each attendant, and 120 per psychiatrist. The hospital has a variety of services, ranging from the acute or reception units to those caring for the elderly demented patients, with a wide range of patient: staff ratios.

The state hospital has fairly active occupational and recreational programs but the treatment is, of necessity, less intensive than at the University Medical Center and more reliance is placed on drug therapy. Less ECT is used at the state hospital. The average stay on the reception service was 49 days during 1960, and 48 percent of the patients were released to convalescent care. Ten percent of the patients released from the hospital are placed in the family care program. There are small day and night care units which do not, as yet, play a major role in the hospital's services.

Both of these facilities nominally admit patients with almost any type of disorder, limited only by the number of beds available. The University Medical Center, however, does not function as a legal detention unit and, thus, rarely admits a patient under court jurisdiction or a person on convalescent care from the state hospital. This limitation necessarily precludes the admission of patients with some types or degrees of disorder. As we note later in this paper, there must be still other selective processes operating either in the referring sources or the hospitals, or both, despite the stated admission policies.

Method

A psychiatric case register was established for Monroe County, N.Y., on January 1, 1960. Virtually all admissions to psychiatric services (inpatient, clinic, emergency, and private practice) are reported to the central register. Records of deaths of all Monroe County residents, provided by the New York State Department of Health, are matched with this case register. Finally, we attempt to determine the migration of patients within and out of the county, and we have been partially successful in this.

A more complete description of the reporting and register operation has been published.[5] From such a cumulative case register it is possible to select a variety of cohorts and statistically observe their subsequent psychiatric experience over a period of time.

Characteristics of First Admissions

In 1960, there were about 800 admissions from Monroe County to the University Medical Center (UMC) and about an equal number to Rochester State Hospital (RSH). However, a much larger number, 511 compared with 318, of the admissions to UMC were first admissions (Table 1). Conversely, many more "chronic" patients were admitted to RSH. Some clues as to how this large pool of chronic readmissions to RSH is built up will be elucidated later by following all first admissions over a 2-year period.

TABLE 1. FIRST ADMISSION RATES [1] BY AGE, SEX, AND
DIAGNOSIS, INPATIENT SERVICES OF UNIVERSITY MEDICAL CENTER AND
ROCHESTER STATE HOSPITAL, MONROE COUNTY RESIDENTS, 1960

Age and sex	University Medical Center									
	All diagnoses		Schizophrenic reaction		Affective psychosis		Chronic brain syndrome		Other diagnoses [2]	
	Number	Rate	Number	Rate	Number	Rate	Number	Rate	Number	Rate
Both sexes [3]	511	87.2	148	25.2	89	15.2	34	5.8	240	40.9
Under 25	108	44.6	38	15.7	1	.4	0	.0	69	28.5
25-44	204	129.7	90	57.5	11	7.0	1	.6	102	65.2
45-64	144	116.3	19	15.2	55	44.1	13	10.4	57	45.7
65 and over	55	87.2	1	1.6	22	34.9	20	31.7	12	19.0
Males	203	72.3	56	19.6	30	11.0	14	5.3	103	36.5
Under 25	51	42.3	23	19.1	0	.0	0	.0	28	23.2
25-44	72	95.6	27	35.8	3	4.0	0	.0	42	55.8
45-64	56	93.5	6	10.0	18	30.1	7	11.7	25	41.7
65 and over	24	88.2	0	.0	9	33.1	7	25.7	8	29.4
Females	308	101.0	92	30.4	59	19.0	20	6.2	137	45.4
Under 25	57	46.9	15	12.4	1	.8	0	.0	41	33.8
25-44	132	162.6	63	77.6	8	9.9	1	1.2	60	73.9
45-64	88	135.9	13	20.1	37	57.1	6	9.3	32	49.4
65 and over	31	86.4	1	2.8	13	36.2	13	36.2	4	11.1

TABLE 1. FIRST ADMISSION RATES [1] BY AGE, SEX, AND
DIAGNOSIS, INPATIENT SERVICES OF UNIVERSITY MEDICAL CENTER AND
ROCHESTER STATE HOSPITAL, MONROE COUNTY RESIDENTS, 1960

						Rochester State Hospital			
Both sexes[3]	318	54.2	57	9.7	14	2.4	210	35.8	37	6.3
Under 25	22	9.1	10	4.1	0	.0	0	.0	12	5.0
25-44	52	33.2	27	17.9	1	.6	5	3.2	19	12.1
45-64	61	48.9	18	14.4	12	9.6	25	20.1	6	4.8
65 and over	183	290.0	2	3.2	1	1.6	180	285.2	0	.0
Males	142	53.3	29	10.2	2	.8	85	33.2	26	9.1
Under 25	13	10.8	5	4.1	0	.0	0	.0	8	6.6
25-44	31	41.2	16	21.2	0	.0	2	2.7	13	17.3
45-64	23	38.4	8	13.4	1	1.7	9	15.0	5	8.3
65 and over	75	275.6	0	.0	1	3.7	74	271.9	0	.0
Females	176	54.8	28	9.2	12	3.9	125	38.0	11	3.7
Under 25	9	7.4	5	4.1	0	.0	0	.0	4	3.3
25-44	21	25.9	11	13.6	1	1.2	.3	3.7	6	7.4
45-64	38	58.7	10	15.4	11	17.0	16	24.7	1	1.5
65 and over	108	300.9	2	5.6	0	.0	106	295.3	0	.0

[1] Rate per 100,000 population.
[2] Includes personality disorder, neurotic reaction, situational reaction, and psychophysiological disorder.
[3] Age-adjusted to Monroe County population, 1960 census.

A comparison of the rates of first admissions is shown by patient characteristics in Table 1 and Figure 1. Before age 65 first admission rates in both urban and nonurban areas were much higher for the University Medical Center (Fig. 1) while after age 65, rates were much higher for the State hospital.

Corresponding to this change in relative rates after age 65, and the fact that admissions of older persons are almost entirely accounted for by patients with chronic brain syndrome, the rate for chronic brain syndrome patients to UMC was relatively small (Table 1). In

FIGURE 1. FIRST ADMISSION RATES, BY AGE AND
AREA OF RESIDENCE: INPATIENT SERVICES OF UNIVERSITY
MEDICAL CENTER AND ROCHESTER STATE HOSPITAL, MONROE
COUNTY RESIDENTS, 1960

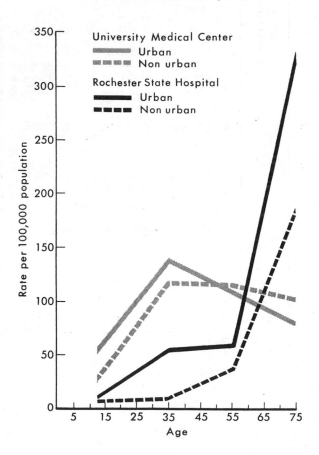

contrast, first admission rates for schizophrenic reactions were higher to UMC than to RSH up to age 45, and rates for affective psychosis were higher to UMC at all ages. Rate of admission to UMC for other diagnoses was also high.

Two-thirds of all first admissions to RSH were patients with chronic brain syndrome, while one-half of all first admissions to UMC were patients with personality disorder or neurotic reaction (Fig. 2). About 60 percent of the first admissions to RSH were 65 years and over; 60 percent to UMC were under 45 years of age.

More females than males were admitted to both hospitals, but the rates were not higher for females in all age groups (Table1). Unlike

FIGURE 2. FIRST ADMISSION COHORTS, BY DIAGNOSTIC
CATEGORIES: INPATIENT SERVICES OF UNIVERSITY MEDICAL
CENTER AND ROCHESTER STATE HOSPITAL, MONROE COUNTY
RESIDENTS, 1960

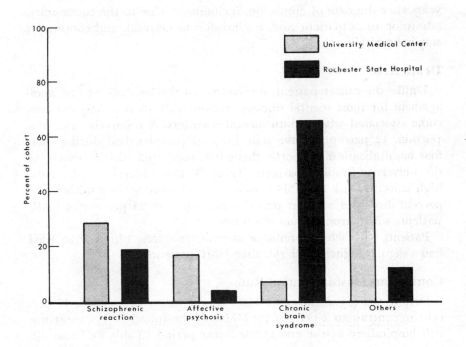

most public mental hospitals,[6] in the Rochester State Hospital the age-adjusted first admission rate for females was as high as that for males. The most plausible, though not proved, explanation of this phenomenon may be the existence of an observation unit in the county infirmary to which many younger urban males, including a number of alcohol addicts and prisoners, are admitted, rather than to RSH. Nevertheless, proportionally more of the RSH than UMC admissions came from the urban area (Table 2), largely reflecting the funneling of older, urban patients with chronic brain syndrome to RSH (Fig. 2).

In summary, the marked difference between these two hospital cohorts, particularly in the diagnostic and age profiles, emphasizes the selectivity of admissions and the need to consider this in any cohort follow-up comparison.

Cohort Experience

The fate of a cohort of mental patients over a long period of time may be described in a number of ways because of the dynamic character of these disorders. We compared only the most important features in the psychiatric experience of our two cohorts during the first 2 years after the date of admission, including release to the community, admission to outpatient care, readmission to hospital, and continuous stay in hospital.

Death Rate

Unlike the cancer patient, survival is not the keystone of case management for most mental diseases, although death is a frequent outcome associated with certain mental disorders. A relatively high proportion, 42 percent, of the state hospital patients died during their first hospitalization or shortly thereafter, compared with 5 percent of the university hospital patients (Table 3). This difference reflects the high mortality risk for RSH patients with chronic brain syndrome: 60 percent died over a 2-year period compared with 24 percent of UMC patients with chronic brain syndrome.

Patients with schizophrenic or affective reactions admitted to RSH had a slightly higher death rate than UMC patients.

Continuous Hospitalization Rate

Despite the higher hospital death rate, a larger proportion, 17 percent in contrast to 2 percent for UMC, of the initial RSH cohort was still hospitalized at the end of the 2-year period (Table 3). These dif-

TABLE 2. PERCENTAGE DISTRIBUTION OF FIRST ADMISSION
COHORTS BY SEX, AGE, AND AREA OF RESIDENCE, INPATIENT
SERVICES OF UNIVERSITY MEDICAL CENTER AND ROCHESTER STATE
HOSPITAL, MONROE COUNTY RESIDENTS, 1960

Patient character- istics	University Medical Center					Rochester State Hospital				
	All diag- noses (N=511)	Schizo- phrenic reaction (N=148)	Affec- tive psy- chosis (N=89)	Chronic brain syndrome (N=34)	Other diag- noses[1] (N=240)	All diag- noses (N=318)	Schizo- phrenic reaction (N=57)	Affec- tive psy- chosis (N=14)	Chronic brain syndrome (N=210)	Other diag- noses[1] (N=37)
Total cohort	100.0	100.0	100.0	100.0	100.0	100.0	100.0	100.0	100.0	100.0
Male	39.7	37.8	33.7	41.2	43.3	44.7	50.9	14.3	40.5	70.3
Female	60.3	62.2	66.3	58.8	56.7	55.3	49.1	85.7	59.5	29.7
Under 25	21.1	25.0	1.1	.0	29.2	6.9	17.5	.0	.0	32.4
25-44	39.7	61.5	11.2	2.9	42.0	16.4	47.4	7.1	2.4	51.4
45-64	28.4	12.8	63.0	38.2	23.8	19.2	31.6	85.7	11.9	16.2
65 and over	10.8	.7	24.7	58.8	5.0	57.5	3.5	7.1	85.7	.0
Urban area	58.7	60.8	55.1	73.5	56.7	77.7	78.9	64.3	79.5	70.3
Nonurban area	41.3	39.2	44.9	26.5	43.3	22.3	21.1	35.7	20.5	29.7

[1]Includes personality disorder, neurotic reaction, situational reaction, and psychophysiological disorder.

TABLE 3. STATUS OF FIRST ADMISSION COHORTS AT
END OF 2-YEAR FOLLOW-UP, INPATIENT SERVICES OF UNIVERSITY
MEDICAL CENTER AND ROCHESTER STATE HOSPITAL, MONROE
COUNTY RESIDENTS, 1960-62

Status	University Medical Center									
	All diagnoses		Schizophrenic reaction		Affective psychosis		Chronic brain syndrome		Other diagnoses [1]	
	Number	Percent	Number	Percent	Number	Percent	Number	Percent	Number	Percent
Total cohort	511	100.0	148	100.0	89	100.0	34	100.0	240	100.0
Died in hospital	9	1.8	0	.0	0	.0	5	14.7	4	1.7
Continuously in hospital during 2 years	12	2.3	5	3.4	1	1.1	4	11.8	2	.8
Released to community	490	95.9	143	96.6	88	98.9	25	73.5	234	97.5
Total released	490	100.0	143	100.0	88	100.0	25	100.0	234	100.0
Died while in community	17	3.5	2	1.4	3	3.4	3	12.0	9	3.8
Moved from county	16	3.3	4	2.8	0	.0	0	.0	12	5.1
Lost to followup	16	3.3	10	7.0	0	.0	2	8.0	4	1.7
Received subsequent psychiatric inpatient care	107	21.8	45	31.5	18	20.5	2	8.0	42	17.9
Readmitted: in hospital at end of 2 years	25	5.1	11	7.7	10	11.4	0	.0	4	1.7
One readmission: in community at end of 2 years	56	11.4	23	16.1	6	6.8	2	8.0	25	10.7
More than one readmission: in community at end of 2 years	26	5.3	11	7.7	2	2.3	0	.0	13	5.5
Remained in community without further psychiatric inpatient care	334	68.2	82	57.3	67	76.1	18	72.0	167	71.5
Outpatient psychiatric care only	163	33.3	44	30.8	35	39.8	7	28.0	77	32.9
No psychiatric care	171	34.9	38	26.5	32	36.3	11	44.0	90	38.6

TABLE 3. STATUS OF FIRST ADMISSION COHORTS AT
END OF 2-YEAR FOLLOW-UP, INPATIENT SERVICES OF UNIVERSITY
MEDICAL CENTER AND ROCHESTER STATE HOSPITAL, MONROE
COUNTY RESIDENTS, 1960-62

Status	All diagnoses		Rochester State Hospital							
			Schizophrenic reaction		Affective psychosis		Chronic brain syndrome		Other diagnoses[1]	
	Number	Percent	Number	Percent	Number	Percent	Number	Percent	Number	Percent
Total cohort	318	100.0	57	100.0	14	100.0	210	100.0	37	100.0
Died in hospital	125	39.3	2	3.5	1	7.1	122	58.1	0	.0
Continuously in hospital during 2 years	54	17.0	6	10.5	0	.0	47	22.4	1	2.7
Released to community	139	43.7	49	86.0	13	92.9	41	19.5	36	97.3
Total released	139	100.0	49	100.0	13	100.0	41	100.0	36	100.0
Died while in community	8	5.8	0	.0	2	15.4	6	14.6	0	.0
Moved from county	2	1.4	0	.0	0	.0	1	2.4	1	2.8
Lost to followup	7	5.0	0	.0	1	7.7	1	2.4	5	13.9
Received subsequent psychiatric inpatient care	33	23.7	10	20.4	2	15.4	10	24.4	11	30.5
Readmitted: in hospital at end of 2 years	14	10.1	7	14.3	0	.0	4	9.8	3	8.3
One readmission: in community at end of 2 years	12	8.6	2	4.1	2	15.4	3	7.3	5	13.9
More than one readmission: in community at end of 2 years	7	5.0	1	2.0	0	.0	3	7.3	3	8.3
Remained in community without further psychiatric inpatient care	89	64.0	39	79.6	8	61.5	23	56.2	19	52.8
Outpatient psychiatric care only	43	30.9	15	30.6	8	61.5	14	34.2	6	16.7
No psychiatric care	46	33.1	24	49.0	0	.0	9	22.0	13	36.1

[1] Includes personality disorder, neurotic reaction, situational reaction, and psychophysiological disorder.

ferences between the two hospital cohorts reflected the high retention rate for the RSH patients with chronic brain syndrome who remained alive; more than half had not left the hospital during the 2-
year period. The experience of the UMC patients with chronic brain
syndrome differed; only 14 percent of those surviving had not left a
hospital (in this analysis, direct transfer from the university hospital
to the state hospital was considered as one period of continuous hospitalization). The probable explanation is that UMC patients were
younger, and often their chronic brain damage was due to alcohol or
trauma rather than arteriosclerosis.

First Release Rate

The cumulative first release rate for all RSH patients at the end of
the 2-year period was only 44 percent, again reflecting the low release
rate of the chronic brain syndrome patients (20 percent). For RSH
patients with functional psychosis (schizophrenic reaction plus affective psychosis), however, the release rate was 90 percent. The 2-year
first release rate was 97 percent or more for each diagnostic group of
UMC patients, except for patients with chronic brain syndrome (74
percent).

The difference between the hospitals in the 2-year release rates for
functional psychosis is not remarkable. However, the rate of release
for various intervals within the 2-year period is considerably different.
UMC patients were released much earlier, as shown in Figure 3.

Readmission Rate

The rate of readmission during the 2-year period was not greatly
different for the two cohorts; overall between one-fourth to one-fifth
of the released patients returned to a hospital (Table 3).

The return rate was somewhat higher for the UMC than for the
RSH schizophrenic patients (32 percent compared with 20 percent).
If an RSH schizophrenic patient returned, however, he was more likely to remain in the hospital. Related to this, a higher proportion of
the UMC patients had more than one readmission.

Any comparison of the readmission rates during the observation period could be biased if the time of first release and, therefore, of the
remaining "readmission exposure time" is not taken into account.
However, this does not appear to be a significant factor here since all
schizophrenic patients discharged from UMC and 41 of 49 released
from RSH within the 2-year period were released within the first 6
months. Five of 41 (12 percent) of the RSH schizophrenic patients

FIGURE 3. CUMULATIVE PERCENTAGE OF PATIENTS RELEASED
WITH SCHIZOPHRENIC REACTION OR AFFECTIVE PSYCHOSIS: INPATIENT
SERVICES OF UNIVERSITY MEDICAL CENTER AND ROCHESTER STATE
HOSPITAL, MONROE COUNTY RESIDENTS, 1960

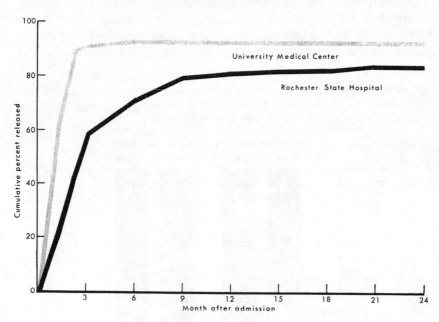

released within 6 months were readmitted. Five of the eight (63 percent) released after 6 months were readmitted during the 2-year period.

Of the released RSH patients with a diagnosis of personality disorder or neurosis, 30 percent returned to the hospital compared with
18 percent for the UMC patients. Many of this RSH group are alcohol
addicts who return for brief admissions. The return rate was also
greater for patients with chronic brain syndrome from RSH (24 percent) than from UMC (8 percent), but the difference is not statistically significant. The numbers involved are small.

With readmission there was a "drift" of patients from UMC to

RSH. This was most marked for the schizophrenic group (Fig. 4). For the UMC schizophrenic patients, 67 percent of their first readmissions were at UMC and the other 33 percent at RSH. In contrast, for the second readmission only 15 percent entered UMC and 85 percent were admitted to RSH. More than half of the latter group had been in UMC for their first readmission. Stated another way, of the 30 schizophrenic patients readmitted to UMC once, 20 percent were readmitted

FIGURE 4. READMISSION OF FIRST ADMISSION COHORTS WITH SCHIZOPHRENIC REACTION: INPATIENT SERVICES OF UNIVERSITY MEDICAL CENTER AND ROCHESTER STATE HOSPITAL, MONROE COUNTY RESIDENTS, 1960

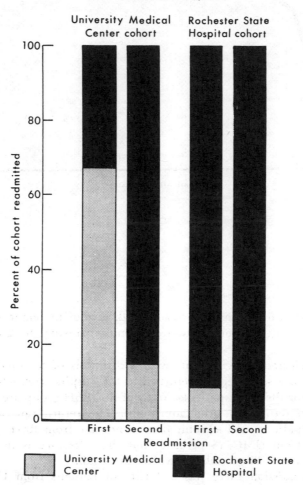

the second time to UMC. Twenty-seven percent of the group, however, were readmitted the second time to RSH. The same tendency, though to a lesser degree, was noted for other diagnostic groups; while only 33 percent of the first readmissions were to RSH, this proportion increased to 48 percent for the second readmission.

Our findings on readmission rates are not significantly changed when the numbers who died in the community, moved from the county, or were lost to follow-up are excluded from the analyses.

Total Time in Hospital

RSH patients who were still alive and under observation at the end of 2 years had spent 45 percent of the 2-year period in the hospital in contrast to an average of only 9 percent for UMC patients (Table 4).

For RSH patients with chronic brain syndrome, the hospital days accounted for an average of 72 percent of the total time, and for schizophrenic patients 29 percent. The corresponding figures for UMC patients were 19 percent and 14 percent. Sixty-five percent of those from RSH with chronic brain syndrome and 13 percent of those with schizophrenia spent more than three-fourths of their time in the hospital. The proportions for UMC were 14 percent and 4 percent, respectively.

Fourteen of the UMC schizophrenic patients but none of the RSH schizophrenic patients had moved from the county or were lost to follow-up. We know that these 14 patients were not readmitted to a New York State mental institution during this time. Even if we make the unlikely assumption that these patients spent more than 25 percent of the 2-year period in a mental hospital out of this state, the difference between these two groups in total time under inpatient care would still be significant.

Other Psychiatric Care

About one-half of all released patients subsequently received outpatient psychiatric care from either a clinic or a private psychiatrist. About one-third received such care without further hospitalization (Table 3). The rate of rehospitalization for schizophrenic patients who received outpatient care was 38 percent and for those who did not the rate was 23 percent. These rates were about the same for both hospitals. It appears that outpatient care did not reduce the rate of readmission for the schizophrenic patients. We can, however, draw no firm conclusions from these data because there are many variables which may affect the rates of rehospitalization besides outpatient treatment or the lack of it. These variables deserve careful study, but they are beyond the scope of this paper. Furthermore, the data from at least the next year (1961) of the operation of the register are needed to provide large enough groups of patients to make possible the study of several variables. We should like to consider: (a) the prognosis at the time of discharge of those who had posthospital outpatient follow-up compared with that of those who did not; (b) the type and intensity of the outpatient care; (c) geographic variables: distance of residence from the hospital as a determinant of follow-up; (d) the needs of families, some of them detrimental to the patients' welfare, as they act to force a patient into outpatient follow-up and later back into the hospital, making this group have higher rehospitalization rates; and (e) the ability of the therapists in the follow-up clinics—do they strengthen defenses or foster dependency?

Days under care of an outpatient clinic generally accounted for about one-fifth or more of the total time of both UMC and RSH patients. Exceptions were chronic brain syndrome patients from both hospitals and neurotic or personality disorder patients from RSH who spent only one-tenth of their time in outpatient care (Table 4).

About one-third of the released patients had received no further psychiatric care of any kind (Table 3). Days without care accounted for 71 percent of the total time of the UMC patients compared with 41 percent for the RSH patients (Table 4). This discrepancy results from the larger proportion of time under inpatient care for the RSH group.

Discussion and Summary

In response to the first question posed in the introduction, "How are these facilities now used?" our data suggest that the Rochester State Hospital and the University Medical Center (or psychiatric unit of a general hospital), in part, serve different population segments and that they play roles in serving the community which are different and complementary. Patients admitted to the state hospital for the first time tend to be older and more urban; two-thirds have chronic brain syndrome, whereas one-half of the university hospital patients receive a diagnosis of neurosis or personality disorder. Affective psychoses are more frequent among the university hospital first admissions. Patients with schizophrenic reactions comprise almost one-third of the university hospital first admissions but only one-fifth of the state hospital first admissions. The state hospital has many more readmissions, most of whom are schizophrenic patients contributing to the much larger proportion of this group in the state hospital resident population.

TABLE 4. PERCENTAGE DISTRIBUTION OF TIME UNDER INPATIENT AND OUTPATIENT PSYCHIATRIC CARE OF FIRST ADMISSION COHORTS DURING 2-YEAR FOLLOW-UP, BY TYPE OF PSYCHIATRIC CARE, INPATIENT SERVICES OF UNIVERSITY MEDICAL CENTER AND ROCHESTER STATE HOSPITAL, MONROE COUNTY RESIDENTS, 1960-1962

Time under care	University Medical Center					Rochester State Hospital				
	All diagnoses	Schizophrenic reaction	Affective psychosis	Chronic brain syndrome	Other diagnoses[1]	All diagnoses	Schizophrenic reaction	Affective psychosis	Chronic brain syndrome	Other diagnoses[1]
	(N=453)[2]	(N=132)[2]	(N=86)[2]	(N=24)[2]	(N=211)[2]	(N=176)[2]	(N=55)[2]	(N=10)[2]	(N=80)[2]	(N=31)[2]
Proportion of total time spent:										
Under inpatient care	9.4	13.8	9.2	19.0	5.7	44.8	28.7	9.8	71.6	14.9
Under outpatient care	19.9	24.0	19.9	10.4	18.2	13.7	18.0	31.5	9.2	11.8
Not under care	70.7	62.2	70.9	70.6	76.1	41.5	53.3	58.7	19.2	73.3
Total cohort	100.0	100.0	100.0	100.0	100.0	100.0	100.0	100.0	100.0	100.0
Proportion of time spent under inpatient care:										
More than 75 percent	2.7	3.8	1.2	14.3	1.4	35.2	12.7	.0	64.6	9.7
51-74 percent	2.0	3.0	3.5	.0	1.0	2.2	3.6	9.1	.0	3.2
26-50 percent	2.9	3.8	3.5	4.8	1.9	8.9	10.9	.0	12.2	.0
25 percent or less	92.3	89.4	91.8	80.9	95.7	53.6	72.8	90.9	23.2	87.1

[1] Includes personality disorder, neurotic reaction, situational reaction, and psychophysiological disorder.

[2] Number excludes patients who died, moved from county, or were lost to follow-up during the 2-year period, and includes those who were continuously hospitalized.

These data offer new information about factors involved in the use of these two hospitals by the community. It is apparent, however, that there are many patients who could go to either hospital. Obviously, factors other than age, diagnosis, and number of prior admissions help determine to which hospital those patients will be admitted. One such factor is the lack of legal authority for the University Medical Center to admit involuntary patients, whom the state hospital can admit. There undoubtedly are other factors. They need to be sought and their impact measured.

In answer to the second question, "What is the subsequent psychiatric experience of patients hospitalized at either of these facilities?" our cohort data also suggest certain specificity in the use of the two hospitals. The difference in the proportions of diagnostic disorders treated makes it necessary to view the longitudinal experience of each diagnostic group separately in any comparison of the facilities.

Although the university hospital schizophrenic patients are released much earlier than those from the state hospital (median time for UMC patients was 1 month in contrast to almost 3 months for RSH patients), by the end of 2 years more than 85 percent of both groups had experienced their first significant release from the hospital. The hospital first readmission rate within the 2-year period was higher for the schizophrenic patients from the University Medical Center. But once readmitted, the state hospital patients were more likely to remain in the hospital while the university hospital patients were more likely to be discharged and readmitted a second time.

With successive readmissions there was a general drift of University Medical Center patients to the state hospital. Outpatient care did not appear to protect against readmission, but the data available do not justify firm impressions on this point. The total time in the hospital during the 2-year period for the state hospital schizophrenic patients was twice that for those of the University Medical Center. This is accounted for more by the long stay of the readmissions than possible differences in administrative practice, as reflected by the duration of the initial admission. Although the University Medical Center cares for a considerable portion of the early and acute schizophrenic patients, the state hospital continues to carry the brunt of the chronic, schizophrenic patient load.

The other diagnostic groups are distributed far more unevenly between the two hospitals than the schizophrenic patients. Rates for affective psychosis were higher for the University Medical Center at all ages. The patients with affective psychosis differed from the schizophrenic patients primarily in their lower readmission rate. Partly associated with this lower return rate, a somewhat smaller proportion of time was spent in inpatient care.

In general, the psychiatric follow-up experience of the university hospital patients with a diagnosis of psychoneurotic or personality disorder was not greatly different from that of the patients with a diagnosis of affective psychosis, but did differ significantly from that of the schizophrenic patients. A large proportion of the nonpsychotic readmissions of the university hospital cohort were to the county hospital unit for a brief period of observation or as a waiting period prior to transfer to another hospital. Fewer nonpsychotic patients were in the hospital at the end of the 2-year period.

Eighty-six percent of the patients with a diagnosis of chronic brain syndrome were admitted to the state hospital. As noted with other public mental hospitals,[7,8] the chronic brain syndrome cohort admitted to the state hospital was characterized by a high death rate; more than one-half of those who did not die remained in the hospital. Those released had no significantly higher readmission rates than other patients. Primarily because of their low rate of first release, however, 72 percent of the total cohort time (excluding those who died or were lost to observation) was spent in the hospital; for only 9 percent of the follow-up period patients were under outpatient care and 19 percent of the time they were without care. It appears that the state hospital is being used as a depository for terminally ill persons as well as for custodial care of aged, demented persons.

Thus, the profiles of the first admission cohorts and, to some degree, the movement of patients between the facilities during a 2-year followup period demonstrate the different and complementary roles which a state hospital and a university (or general) hospital play in serving the mental health needs of a community. Certainly, such differences must be considered in the planning of psychiatric services.

In the schizophrenic and brain syndrome groups, and to a much lesser degree in the other diagnostic categories, a group of patients became chronically disabled from the time of the first psychiatric hospital admission. It has been noted by Brill and Patton[9] that the proportion of schizophrenic patients becoming chronically hospitalized in the New York State hospital system has diminished in the past several years. However, as they have mentioned, and as we have seen in our studies, the chronicity has not been completely eliminated. As a subgroup of the schizophrenic patients, the "chronic" group is distinguished by a pattern of inpatient care that is frequently distinct from the other patients; they are continuously or repeatedly hospitalized throughout the 2-year period and enter the state hospital either for their first admission or at some later point. A preliminary inspection of hospital records suggests that a feature distinguishing this group from the "nonchronic" patients is a history of parental loss because of death or desertion before the age of 5. This point is being investigated further.

The accumulation of chronically impaired patients plays an important role in determining the character of the state hospital resident population. A knowledge of the admission, release, and readmission pattern enables us to estimate the future magnitude and distribution of the state hospital caseload. The brief duration of the current study, however, permits only a gross prediction of future trends. The high admission rate to the state hospital for patients aged 65 and over with chronic brain syndrome and the comparatively much lower first admission rate for patients with schizophrenia indicates a trend that may change the diagnostic distribution of the state hospital resident population. At the end of the 2-year follow-up period, 43 of the 200 elderly demented patients and 20 of the 205 schizophrenic patients admitted to both hospitals were under inpatient care at the state hospital. Conceivably, our state hospital will, in the future, have a larger proportion of patients aged 65 years and over admitted with a diagnosis of chronic brain syndrome than schizophrenia or any other diagnosis. This would represent a reversal of the present distribution. Although there is currently a large number of persons aged 65 and over in the state hospital, the majority of these are chronic schizophrenic patients who have aged in the hospital.

The descriptive data available in a case register can tell us little about the effect of hospitalization on the course of a patient's disorder without further investigation. Such data can, however, provide leads for further study. The inclusion of the 1961 admissions and a longer period of follow-up will provide more stable figures and better predictability. As such data become available, we hope they can provide a more solid foundation for the planning of future psychiatric care.

REFERENCES

1. Forstenzer, H. M. Problems in Relating Community Programs to State Hospitals. Amer. J. Publ. Hlth. 51: 1152-1157, 1961.
2. Dorken, H. Behind the Scenes in Community Mental Health. Amer. J. Psychiat. 119: 328-335, 1962.

3. Schulberg, H. C. Psychiatric Units in General Hospitals: Boon or Bane? Amer. J. Psychiat. 120:30-36, 1963.
4. Baldwin, J. A. A Critique of the Use of Patient-Movement Studies in the Planning of Mental Health Services. Scot. Med. J. 8: 227-233, 1963.
5. Gardner, E. A., Miles, H. C., Iker, H. P., and Romano, J. A Cumulative Register of Psychiatric Services in a Community. Amer. J. Publ. Hlth. 53: 1269-1277, 1963. Reprinted as chapter 19 of this book.
6. Kramer, M., Pollack, E. S., and Redick, R. W. Studies of the Incidence and Prevalence of Hospitalized Mental Disorders in the United States: Current Status and Future Goals. Comparative Epidemiology of Mental Disorders. New York: Grune & Stratton, 1961.
7. Roth, M. Mental Health Problems of Aging and the Aged. Bull. WHO, 21: 527-561, 1959.
8. Pollack, E. S., Person, P. H., Kramer, M., and Goldstein, H. Patterns of Retention, Release, and Death of First Admissions to State Mental Hospitals. PHS Publication No. 672 (Public Health Monograph No. 58). Washington: U.S. Government Printing Office, 1959.
9. Brill, H., and Patton, R. E. Clinical-Statistical Analysis of Population Changes in New York State Mental Hospitals Since Introduction of Psychotropic Drugs. Amer. J. Psychiat. 119: 20-35, 1962.

Work upon which this report is based was supported by contract No. C-19021 from the New York State Department of Mental Hygiene, and grant No. MH-00381-07 from the National Institute of Mental Health, Bethesda, Md. The material was presented at a meeting of the American Public Health Association in Kansas City, Mo., in November 1963.

27

Size, Staffing, and Psychiatric Hospital Effectiveness

LEONARD P. ULLMANN and LEE GUREL

THERE is general agreement among those who treat mental illness that psychiatric hospitals should be (a) small, and (b) highly staffed.[1] Two previous sources of data provide numerical support for the contention that smaller size and higher staff-patient ratio are related to higher rates of favorable outcome.

The first previous set of data was computed by one of us (LU) from material presented by Bockoven[2] on "Moral Treatment in American Psychiatry." For data concerning operation of Worcester State Hospital over 12 consecutive decades, rank-order correlations were 0.76 ($P < 0.01$) between per cent of admissions released and physicians per patient and —0.89 ($P < 0.001$) between per cent of admissions released and size of patient population. Jenkins,[3] using selected psychotic admissions at 12 hospitals, obtained a 0.64 correlation ($P < 0.05$) between early release and per diem expense (reflecting overall staffing) and a —0.77 correlation ($P < 0.01$) between early release and size of patient population. In short, in these two studies, both staffing and size were significantly associated with patient release. In both studies it was found that hospital size was somewhat more highly correlated with the release criterion than was staffing, but the small number of 12 cases and the presence of a significant correlation between hospital size and staffing ratio precluded determination of the correlation between favorable outcome and one characteristic (size *or* staffing) with the other held constant.

The purpose of the present paper was to ascertain the association between mental hospital size and staffing and several criterion measures of effectiveness. By virtue of using a larger number of hospitals than had been the case in previous research, it was possible to clarify the relationships among the variables.

Procedure

Data Obtained From Hospitals. The following material was obtained from 30 VA psychiatric hospitals: (a) A list of the names, unit numbers, and diagnoses for all admissions for two fiscal years (July 1, 1959-June 30, 1961) and (b) a photocopy of VA Form 10-2593, Record of Hospitalization, for all schizophrenic males admitted during the first of these two years.

Use of the VA's unit (identifying) number procedure permitted a check on possible readmission to the same hospital during the entire second fiscal year. When additional material (because of transfer or readmission) was needed to determine the outcome of a case, the hospital registrars were contacted.

The VA's Record of Hospitalization form is imprinted at time of admission with 34 items of information. Of these the current research used name, identifying unit number, data of admission, date of birth, sex, marital status, and whom to notify in case of emergency. As treatment proceeds, established clinical diagnoses are entered on the form, as are all absences from the hospital. In cases where the patient receives more than one diagnosis, further specification is made of which diagnosis was responsible for the major part of the hospital stay. The form also contains material as to the final disposition of the case: discharge, transfer, or death.

The VA's Record of Hospitalization form was used to identify during a full year all males, under 60 years of age at admission, for whom a schizophrenic reaction was cited as responsible for the major part of their hospital stay. Men whose diagnoses were changed from schizophrenic reaction were dropped from the study.

Early Release Criterion. The material from the VA Record of Hospitalization was used to determine whether each patient achieved an early or late first significant release (FSR). An early FSR was defined as leaving the hospital within 274 calendar days of admission and remaining in the community at least 90 consecutive days. A late FSR was defined as a failure to establish an early FSR. Those few patients for whom an unequivocal early or late FSR could not be established, usually due to death or transfer prior to 275 calendar days of admission, were dropped from the study. In accordance with eliminating from the study all equivocal cases, a minimum length of hospitalization, seven days, was required for inclusion in the sample and the few administrative or "paper" admissions were discarded. Finally it should be explicit that the unit number system permitted checks on readmissions and transfers and made it certain that each man was counted once only.

Selection of Hospitals. The data for this study covered 30 hospitals. All VA psychiatric hospitals were used except those which (a) had a major (greater than 13% of the patient population) nonpsychiatric mission; (b) had undergone major structural (size) changes during the study period; or (c) had fewer than a total of 100 patients establishing unequivocal FSR designations.

Sample of Patients. For the 30 hospitals in this sample there were 7,212 male schizophrenics under age 60 who unequivocally established an early or late FSR. In terms of type of schizophrenic reaction, 37.4% were paranoid, 7.4% catatonic, 3.9% hebephrenic, 1.9% simple, 3.2% schizoaffective, 1.2% residual, and the remainder, 45.0% undifferentiated. Table 1 presents detailed information on the age and marital status characteristics of the patient sample.

Predictor Variables. Because differences in hospital release rates might be ascribed to differences in the favorability of prognosis of patients entering the various hospitals, the effects of marital status and ages were investigated. In the present study, three categories of marital status were used. In the first category, comprising 29.6% of the 7,212 patients, were the men who were married and who listed their

TABLE 1. – THE ASSOCIATION BETWEEN EARLY FSR AND CATEGORIZATION BY MARITAL STATUS AND AGE FOR 7,212 SCHIZOPHRENIC ADMISSIONS

		Married, Notify Wife		
Age	Early FSR	Late FSR	Sum	%Early FSR
17-30	266	67	333	79.9
31-45	1,163	397	1,560	74.6
46-59	155	89	244	63.5
Sum	1,584	553	2,137	x^2, 2df, = 20.16; $P<0.001$
		Married, Notify Someone Other Than Wife		
17-30	147	63	210	70.0
31-45	710	400	1,110	64.0
46-59	100	108	214	49.5
Sum	963	571	1,534	x^2, df, = 21.57; $P<0.001$.
		Never Married		
17-30	684	577	1,261	54.2
31-45	898	1,050	1,948	46.1
46-59	132	200	332	39.8
Sum	1,714	1,827	3,541	x^2, 2df, = 30.96; $P<0.001$

wives as the people to notify in case of emergency. Of this group, 74.1% established an early FSR. The second category was composed of men who had married at some time in their lives but who did not list a wife as the person to notify in case of emergency. This group, which included primarily the divorced and widowed, comprised 21.3% of the patient sample, and 62.8% of these cases established an early FSR. The third category was composed of the men who had never married. This category accounted for 49.1% of the sample, and within it 48.4% established an early FSR. The χ^2 with 2 degrees of freedom was 377.98 indicating a highly significant association between marital status and likelihood of an early FSR. Age was investigated to determine whether it would significantly *add* to the prediction obtained from marital status alone. The sample was divided into three age groups: from 17 to 30, from 31 to 45, and from 46 to 59 years of age.[4] As presented in Table 1, each of the three marital statuses was subdivided into the three age levels. Within all three marital categories, younger age was associated with more favorable prognosis to an extent well past the 0.001 level of significance.

Criteria of Hospital Effectiveness. Four criteria of hospital effectiveness were used. The first of these used the FSR data and involved three separate figures. The FSR criterion scores for each of the 30 hospitals were based on an average of 240 cases (range from 113 to 538 cases). One FSR criterion score was simply *the percentage of cases at each hospital achieving an early FSR*. This figure, called FSR-Raw, varied for the 30 hospitals from 41.4% achieving an early FSR to 74.7%, with an average of 57.9%. In the other two FSR scores a correction was made to take into account sample variations in terms of the predictor variables. For FSR corrected for marital status, the number of cases at each hospital in each marital status was multiplied by the percentage in that marital status *expected* to establish an early FSR. This expected percentage of early FSR was subtracted from the percent of early FSR cases actually *obtained*. After a constant had been added to eliminate negative numbers, each hospital's score reflected the degree to which it had done better or worse than the base rate expectancy derived from the patients in the total sample. This measure, called FSR-M varied for the 30 hospitals from 17% below the expected percentage of early FSR to 16% higher than the expected number of early FSR, with the average hospital having an equality of expected and obtained early FSR. A similar procedure took into account age as well as marital status: the frequency of patients in each of the nine age-marital status categories was multiplied by the appropriate expectancy of early FSR, and this expected percentage was compared with the empirically obtained early FSR percentage. This measure called FSR-M+A ranged from hospitals obtaining 16% below the expected percentage of early FSR to hospitals obtaining 16% higher early FSR than expected, with the average hospital having equal numbers of expected and obtained early FSRs.

Another criterion measure of effectiveness was a measure of *intake per unit size* (intake/size). This measure was the total number of schizophrenics in this study from each hospital who established an early or late FSR divided by the size of the patient population at that hospital. This criterion may be thought of as a measure of turnover: the number of newly admitted schizophrenic patients per bed. It has the advantages of (a) being restricted to a single diagnostic group, schizophrenic reaction; (b) being protected against any patient being counted more than once; and (c) unless a late FSR designation had already been established, eliminating error due to death or transfer to another hospital. That is, this criterion, intake/size, was free of the most common criticisms of turnover figures. For the 30 hospitals, the range was from 8.0% to 38.2% with an average of 17.8%.

A different criterion measure came from the VA Field Station Summaries and was a more typical measure of *turnover*. In these routinely compiled reports, the number of cases terminated in a given period are divided by the size of the patient population. Whereas the previous criterion, intake/size, dealt with admissions and was restricted to schizophrenic reactions, the present turnover criterion measure dealt with termination (discharge, death, and transfer) for all diagnostic categories. Turnover is reported quarterly. The four quarters of each of the two years of this study were separately summed. The correlation between turnover in the successive years was 0.953 for the sample of 30 hospitals, indicating a high degree of stability over time. For criterion purposes, turnover in the two successive years was averaged. The range of this % *turn-over* figure was from 8.80% per annum to 37.85% per annum with an average of 17.12%.

A final criterion measure was percentage of patients with relatively *long hospital residence*. This figure came from the VA Field Station Summaries where once a year information is collected on a 20% sample of all patients in VA hospitals. The measure chosen for this study was the percentage of patients in hospitals who had been in residence two or more years (% 2 + yr). The percent whose residence had been two or more years at each hospital was correlated for successive years. This correlation was 0.904, indicating stability over time. To arrive at the criterion measure used in the present research, the figures for the two successive years were averaged. For the 30 hospitals in the sample, the range of percentage of patients with two or more years residence was from 50.0% to 82.0% with an average of 71.58%.

Hospital Size and Staffing. The purpose of this research was to determine the association between size, staffing, and hospital effectiveness. *Hospital size* was determined from the VA Field Station Summaries report of Average Daily Patient Load (ADPL), during the two fiscal years of this study. The correlation betwen ADPL for one year with ADPL during the succeeding year was 0.999. That is, size was a highly stable characteristic during the period of study. The size figures (ADPL) for the two years were averaged and became the measure of size used in the present study. The range of size (ADPL) for the 30 hospitals was from 604 to 2,390 patients, with an average of 1,453.

To obtain an overall figure regarding *staffing,* data in the VA Field Station Summaries were again used. Here, the number of Full Time Equivalents (FTE), a method for correcting for number of part-time workers, is reported each month. Figures were obtained for three months: June, 1959, June, 1960, and June, 1961, marking the beginning, middle, and end of the study period. Each hospital's number of Full Time Equivalents was divided by the size of the hospital. The intercorrelations of these three figures were 0.929, 0.964, and 0.958 indicating a high degree of stability over time. The average of the three figures (FTE/ADPL) became the measure of staffing used in the present study. At the 30 hospitals the number of employees per patient ranged from 0.594 to 1.145 with an average of 0.705.

Hospital Psychiatric Involvement. A final hospital characteristic which was taken into account was the degree of psychiatric involvement. In the present study, because the focus was on the treatment of psychiatric patients, specifically schizophrenics, hospitals with a high nonpsychiatric mission, i.e., tuberculosis, general medicine, neurology/geriatrics, were eliminated. The measure used was the number of psychiatric cases divided by the total average daily patient load. This figure was derived for each of the 30 hospitals from three successive reports, i.e., June, 1959, June, 1960, and June, 1961, the beginning, middle, and end of the study period. The intercorrelations between the figures were 0.978, 0.945, and 0.967. In short, this characteristic, even when an attentuated sample had been selected, was stable over time. The three figures were averaged to provide the figure used in the present research. The range was from 87% of the inpatient population designated as psychiatric to 100% with an average of 96.5%.

Results

Table 2 presents the basic findings of this study. The first four columns of Table 2 deal with measures of favorable outcome, the next two columns deal with size as measured by average daily patient load, ADPL, and staffing as measured by number of full-time employees per patient, FTE/ADPL, and the final two columns deal with per cent psychiatric involvement and the correlation between staffing ratio (FTE/size) and the other variables in the matrix with per cent psychiatric involvement held constant by means of partial correlation.

Intercorrelations Among FSR Scores. Of the measures of hospital effectiveness, three dealt with FSR: FSR without correction for differences in samples at various hospitals, FSR corrected for marital status (i.e., FSR-M), and FSR corrected for both marital status and age (i.e., FSR-M+A). The intercorrelations among these three measures indicated that they were virtually identical (i.e., 0.99). Two points were involved. The first was that it seemed unlikely that additional corrections for potential differences among samples would lead to major changes in the correlations between FSR criteria and measures of size or staffing.

The second point was that only one of the FSR criterion measures would be useful and nonredundant. Therefore, in Table 2, only the FSR measure corrected for marital status and age, FSR-M+A, was reported.

Effect of Varying Percent Psychiatric. To avoid confounding results dealing with psychiatric patients when the hospital had a major nonpsychiatric mission, hospitals had been selected which had a high percentage of psychiatric patients composing the average daily patient load. Even with such attentuation, the variations in percentage of psychiatric patients (% psychiatric) were highly stable over time. From column 7 of Table 2, it may be noted that the % psychiatric variable was significantly associated only with the staffing per patient measure. As % psychiatric patients increased, the staffing ratio decreased. The final column of Table 2 presents partial correlations to indicate what the correlations between staffing ratio and the other measures would have been if there had been no variation in percentage of psychiatric patients composing the average daily patient load. As may be noted, the effect was to increase the correlations between staffing per patient and measures of effectiveness, but in no case did a previously insignificant correlation become statistically significant. While no further analysis of the % psychiatric variable was within the scope of the present article, in further research dealing

TABLE 2. – INTERCORRELATION OF FOUR MEASURES OF HOSPITAL EFFECTIVENESS, SIZE, AND STAFFING FOR 30 PSYCHIATRIC HOSPITALS

	1	2	3	4	5	6	7	8*
1. FSR M+A		0.55	0.65	−0.49	−0.37	0.15	0.06	0.20
2. Intake /size			0.80	−0.84	−0.46	0.66	0.04	0.77
3. % turnover				−0.88	−0.39	0.48	0.07	0.57
4. % 2 yr stay					0.51	−0.73	0.12	−0.74
5. Size						−0.44	−0.06	−0.53
6. FTE/size							−0.46	
7. % psychiatric								

* Column number 8 deals with FTE/size to variables 1-6 with variable number 7, % Psychiatric, held constant by partial correlation.

with specific aspects of staffing, or in studies in which hospitals have not been attenutated on this variable at time of sample selection, the investigation of % psychiatric will be necessary.

Correlation Between Size and Staffing. As reported in Table 2, the correlation between size and staffing was statistically significant, −0.44. As hospitals became smaller in the present sample, they tended to have more staff per patient. Because this was so, there was empirical evidence for the need to use partial correlation to hold one characteristic, size or staffing, constant while determining the relationship of the other to measures of effectiveness.

Intercorrelation Among Measures of Turnover. There were three measures of turnover. The first was the % turnover figure obtained directly from the VA Field Station Summaries. The second measure was the percent of patients in the hospital whose stay was two or more years (% 2 + yr stay). The third measure was the number of cases establishing an FSR (early or late) at each hospital divided by the size of that hospital (intake/size). Where % turnover was a measure at exit, % 2 + yr stay was a measure of ongoing population, and intake/size was a measure at admission. From Table 2 it may be noted that there was empirical evidence that these three criteria were measuring essentially the same construct. The correlation between intake/size and % turnover was 0.80. The correlation between intake/size and % 2 + yr stay was −0.84 (i.e., high intake/size associated with low % 2 + yr stay), and the correlation between % turnover and % 2 + yr stay was −0.88.

Relationship Between FSR-M+A and Three Turnover Measures. It is logical that measures of effectiveness, in general, be significantly associated. In particular, it may be hypothesized that the more early releases there are, the greater will be the space available for intake of new patients, the lower will be the percentage of inpatients with long stay, and the higher will be turnover as measured by terminated cases. From Table 2 it may be noted that this was in fact the case. All the correlations among criteria were in the predicted direction and significant beyond the 0.01 level. However, while the three measures of the turnover construct were significantly associated with the early release measure, it was possible to determine that these scores were measuring something different from and in addition to early release. Specifically, when FSR-M + A was held constant by means of partial correlation, the correlation between % turnover and % 2 + yr stay decreased minimally from —0.88 to —0.84; the correlation between intake/size and % 2 + yr stay decreased from —0.84 to —0.78; and the correlation between % turnover and intake/size decreased from 0.80 to 0.70. This last correlation, the lowest of the triad, yielded a critical ratio of 4.42, and therefore these three measures of turnover were very significantly intercorrelated even when FSR-M + A was held constant.

Relationship Between Favorable Outcome and Size and Staffing. With 30 cases, a correlation of 0.32 or greater is needed to reject the null hypothesis at the 0.05 level with one-tail test ($z = 1.65$). From Table 2, it may be noted that the correlation between size (ADPL) and FSR-M + A was —0.37, which was in the predicted direction and statistically significant. That is, to a statistically significant extent, small hospital size was associated with high percentage of early releases. The correlation between staffing ratio (FTE/ADPL) and FSR-M + A was in the predicted (positive) direction but was not statistically significant. Both size and staffing were significantly correlated in the predicted direction with all three criterion measures of turnover.

Effect of Size or Staffing With Other Characteristic Held Constant. A major reason for the present undertaking was to increase the number of hospitals so that partial correlation might be used to test the effect of one characteristic, either size *or* staffing, with the other held constant. Table 3 presents this material.

The data reported in Table 3 indicate that even when staffing was held constant, small size was significantly associated with high early release rate (FSR M + A). There was also a trend, bordering on significance, for small size to be associated with the three measures of turnover after staffing had been held constant. On the other hand,

TABLE 3. – PARTIAL CORRELATIONS FOR 30 PSYCHIATRIC HOSPITALS
RELATING FOUR MEASURES OF HOSPITAL EFFECTIVENESS TO SIZE
OR STAFFING

	A: Size, Holding Staffing Constant	B: Staffing, Holding Size Constant
FSR-M+A	−0.34*	−0.02
Intake/size	−0.24	0.57†
% turnover	−0.23	0.37*
% 2+yr stay	0.30	−0.65†

*0.05 level, one tail.
†0.001 level.

while staffing was randomly associated with early release (FSR M + A) when size was held constant, high staffing was significantly associated with all three measures of turnover even after size had been held constant by means of partial correlation. *The results indicate the demonstrable value of both size and staffing, and, perhaps more importantly, do so in such a manner as to specify the particular beneficial effect each has on different measures of hospital effectiveness.*

Additional Computations. Three further analyses were completed to deal with questions raised by the preceding information. The first question dealt with the possibility that small hospitals achieved their superior early release rates by discharging men in less satisfactory symptomatic condition than large hospitals. While the criterion of remaining in the community 90 consecutive days would argue against such a proposal, an additional source of information was available. The hospitals were divided into the 12 with a relatively small number of patients (up to 1,201) and the 18 with a relatively large number of patients (1,316 or more). The cutting point was determined on both an absolute numerical basis and by the fact that a difference of over 100 resident patients separated the largest small hospital and the smallest large hospital. When this was done, it was found that smaller hospitals not only had a significantly higher early release rate, but also that of these early releases a smaller percentage, 14.98%, of patients at the small hospitals started their early FSRs on a status without medical approval than patients at larger hospitals for whom this percentage was 21.21%. The difference between the two figures was significant well past the 0.001 level, the χ^7 with 1 degree of freedom being 25.30.

A second additional analysis was also directed to potential questions concerning the results. It is possible to argue that the findings with a schizophrenic sample, particularly with the intake/size criterion measure, resulted from more highly staffed hospitals providing more careful examinations of patients and therefore diagnosing schizophrenic reaction more frequently. While the intercorrelation of the three turnover measures, at intake, exit, and resident inpatients with long stay, would argue against this, the following was done: the number of primary schizophrenic and the number of primary psychoneurotic diagnoses on admission were tabulated at each hospital for the year between July 1, 1959, and June 30, 1960. The range of number of schizophrenic diagnoses divided by number of schizophrenic and neurotic diagnoses was startling: from 59% to 93% with an average of 76%. However, as the number of schizophrenic diagnoses increased, so did the number of neurotic diagnoses, the correlation coefficient being 0.74, which was significant well beyond the 0.001 level. More importantly, the percentage of schizophrenic diagnoses was not systematically related with any other hospital characteristic. The correlation between the percentage of schizophrenic diagnoses and intake/size was −0.14 which was not only random but also in the direction opposite to the one "predicted." Similarly, the correlation between percentage of schizophrenic diagnoses and staffing, FTE/ADPL, was random, 0.11. When percentage of schizophrenic diagnoses was held constant by means of partial correlation, the correlation between intake/size and FTE/ADPL *increased* slightly rather than decreased.

A final analysis was aimed at the questions of (a) how much smaller hospital size added to the prediction obtained from knowledge of age and marital status and (b) whether smaller hospital size was of particular value with particular patients. Table 4 presents this analysis. For all nine age and marital status categories, smaller hospitals had a higher early FSR rate than larger hospitals. Smaller hospital size was particularly important with the patient group with the poorest likelihood of early release, the men who had never married. Smaller size of hospital seemed to make little difference in the case of men who had been married but who did not list their wives as the person to notify in case of emergency. The difference between small and large hospitals in the rate of early FSR of older single men was, perhaps, the most impressive single finding of this study because these are the men most likely to become continuously hospitalized and forgotten.

TABLE 4. – EARLY RELEASE RATES (FSR) FOR SCHIZOPHRENIC
ADMISSIONS AT LARGE AND SMALL HOSPITALS STRATIFIED BY AGE
AND MARITAL STATUS

	Small Hospitals		Large Hospitals		Difference	
Age	No. Cases	%Early FSR	No. Cases	%Early FSR	%Early FSR	x^2
			Married, Notify Wife			
17-30	122	85.25	211	76.78	8.47	2.94
31-45	569	79.96	991	71.44	8.52	13.84
46-59	91	67.03	153	61.44	5.59	0.55
			Married, Notify Other Than Wife			
17-30	54	75.93	156	67.95	7.98	0.87
31-45	398	66.83	712	62.36	4.47	2.03
46-59	67	50.75	147	48.98	1.77	0.09
			Never Married			
17-30	452	59.07	809	51.55	7.52	6.31
31-45	675	53.48	1,273	42.18	11.30	22.21
46-59	108	55.56	224	32.14	23.42	15.71

Comment and Summary

The present data are limited to Veterans Administration hospitals during a specific period of time.[5] VA hospitals are typically smaller and more highly staffed than state mental hospitals. However, within these limitations, using a sample of every male schizophrenic under 60 years of age who established an unequivocal early or late first significant release, 30 hospitals were studied in terms of size and staffing. Marital status and age of patients were found to be significant predictor variables, but correction for these variables did not influence the status of the hospitals. Additional data obtained from the VA's administrative statistics were used to round out the picture. Finally, differential diagnostic practices and rate of early release with or without staff permission were investigated.

Both small size and high staffing were significantly associated with hospital effectiveness. However, small size was found to be of greater importance in establishing a high rate of early release, while high staffing was found to be of greater importance in obtaining turnover in terms of number of admissions, number of terminated cases, and percentages of patients with long-continued hospitalization. The data dealing with size support the trend to build smaller hospitals, or if this is not feasible, to utilize unit system plans. The data dealing with the effect of staffing on turnover criteria as distinct from early release may be taken as an indication of the value of increased staffing on continued treatment, chronic, or back wards, rather than the current possibly disproportionate emphasis on staffing of acute or admission wards. This thought, put forward tentatively, derives not only from the staffing to turnover correlations, but also from the finding that when size of hospital was held constant, there was a random relationship between staffing per patient and early release. In short, both small size and high staffing contribute to the effectiveness of mental hospitals, but these two characteristics may influence different aspects of effectiveness and have different areas of impact.

NOTES AND REFERENCES

1. Joint Commission on Mental Illness and Health. Action for Mental Health. New York: Basic Books, 1961.
2. Bockoven, J. S. Moral Treatment in American Psychiatry. J. Nerv. Ment. Dis. 124: 167-194, 292-321, 1956.
3. Jenkins, R. L. Preliminary Report on Psychiatric Evaluation Project, Cooperative Study. Psychiat. Res. App. Ment. Ill. 6: 361-366, 1961.
4. To determine whether a finer discrimination would be worthwhile, each age category was further subdivided. There were not enough extremely young or extremely old patients to warrant further computation, while there was no significant predictive difference between the 31-37 and the 38-45-year old age groups.
5. During the period under investigation, there was evidence for overall programmatic improvement. The average per cent of patients resident with two or more years of stay for Oct. 31, 1960, was 72.67% while the average for the survey of Oct. 31, 1961 was 70.40. The difference between correlated means yielded a t-ratio of 2.58 in the direction of improvement and could have occurred by chance less than once in 100 times. In a similar fashion, the average turnover during the first fiscal year of the study was 16.32% while the average turnover across the 30 hospitals during the second fiscal year of the study was 17.95%. The difference between these correlated means yielded a t-ratio of 3.82 in the direction of improvement and could have occurred by chance less than once in 1,000 times. These measures of improvement took place within a population which, for administrative reasons of eligibility for admission to VA hospitals, was, even more than the general population, an aging one.
   Another way of making this point, with data obtained from VA Field Station Summaries, but which were not within the immediate scope of this paper, was that comparing the first fiscal year during which this study was made with the second fiscal year of the study, the ratio of applications for hositalizations to

average daily patient load across 30 hospitals increased from 85.50% to 90.17%. This increase was statistically significant, $t = 2.52$. During the same period, the waiting list decreased from an average for the 30 hospitals of 22.20% of the average daily patient load in June, 1959 to 18.63% of average daily patient load in June, 1961. The difference between correlated means yielded a t-ratio of 2.87. In short, *during the period of study, while the number of applications increased significantly, the size of the waiting list decreased significantly.*

This material is relevant to a point which should not be overlooked: the data reported were obtained within a dynamic rather than a static system.

Veterans Hospital registrars coöperated in this study, which was completed as an individual hospital project within the Veterans Administration Psychiatric Evaluation Project.

28

The Cost of Mental Health Care Under Changing Treatment Methods

KENNETH M. McCAFFREE

METHODS of treating the mentally ill have changed radically in recent years. Prior to World War II most mentally ill persons were isolated and confined under minimally adequate living conditions to protect the rest of society from them and the patients from themselves. In the past two decades, however, there has come increased understanding and use of psychotherapy. The application of drugs has been an extremely impressive development. Drugs alone, when properly administered, have permitted many persons to lead normal lives and, in other circumstances, have made others amenable to further treatment. Group therapy, family therapy, and social milieu therapy have provided treatments which have improved the patient's competence to perform in primary social roles. It is literally true that in comparison with an earlier period it is now possible to restore to useful and productive lives many, if not most, persons who previously would have been held in custody.[1]

Although the health prognosis of the mentally ill has been markedly improved, it is not immediately nor clearly evident that relative economic costs have been affected. On the one hand, the average length of hospital confinement for the mentally ill has dropped substantially and the number of persons who can be effectively treated in outpatient facilities has increased. But, on the other hand, the costs of treatment have risen greatly. The new treatment methods have increased the use of psychiatrists, psychologists, and other skilled therapists. Both more personnel and more highly trained professionals have been required by the more intensive treatment of the new technology. Thus, since both the period of disability from a mental illness is shorter and at the same time the costs of care per unit of service have gone up, the net effect upon relative economic costs is uncertain and requires more careful and detailed evaluation. Does it, in fact, make economic sense to undertake a modern intensive therapy program or should a "comfortable" custodial care program be followed?

In this paper I have made a comparison of the relative economic efficiency in an institutional (hospital) setting between the traditional program of custodial care and the new intensive therapies. After a brief statement of the methods and basic assumptions underlying the analysis of costs and treatment results, I present the experience of the state mental hospital system in Washington State which has replaced the custodial care program with a more intensive therapy during the past several years. The final section is devoted to a consideration of the public policy issues raised by the results and analysis of the comparative economic efficiency of the alternative treatment technologies.

Assumptions and Methods of Analysis

The results and costs of treatment and the costs of the illness must be reduced to a common denominator in order to estimate the efficiency of alternative methods of care. This has been accomplished by using the average cost per patient as the measure of economic efficiency.[2] Average patient cost is the arithmetic product of the length of hospital stay and costs per capita per time unit, as day or month. Length of stay is the proxy measure of the mental health care "product."[3] It can be affected by the method of production (treatment). Since hospital stay is a function of time, costs, which can also be affected by the technology of care, are appropriately put in time units. The average cost per patient can thus be computed for alternative treatment methods and compared.[4]

The Experience of the Washington State Hospital System

Between the bienniums of 1954-1956 and 1962-1964 traditional custodial care has been essentially replaced by intensive treatment methods in the major mental hospitals of the state of Washington.[5] I have first estimated the effects of the change in treatment methods upon the average length of hospitalization. Changes in the economic costs are considered second.

Length of Hospitalization

The average length of stay of a first admission cohort in the Washington State hospitals has declined by at least 18 months, and perhaps as much as 26 months, since the mid-1950's. The proportion of all admissions released from the hospitals within 12 months has risen from about 70 per cent in 1950-1958 to over 85 per cent in 1962-1964.[6] The length of stay of those who remain in the hospital for more than one year of treatment has stayed close to 12 years.[7] Thus the estimated average length of stay under the custodial program was probably about 42 to 44 months. With intensive treatment available in the state mental hospitals similar computations gave an average period of hospitalization of 23 months in 1962 and just over 18 months for the year ending June 30, 1964.[8]

This apparent reduction in the average length of hospitalization with the introduction of intensive therapy may be offset somewhat by several sets of circumstances. In the first place, the readmission rate is up slightly from what it was in the period prior to 1957. Readmissions in 1963 were approximately 42 per cent of total admissions which is three to five percentage points higher than in 1955 and 1956. Exactly what effect this change had, if any, on hospital stay is difficult to determine. All of the increase in the readmissions rate took place in 1955 and 1956. Since 1957 readmissions as a percentage of total admissions have remained relatively stable and, during this period, most of the decline in the average length of hospital stay has taken place.[9] Probably there has been a very negligible effect, if any at all, upon average length of hospitalization under the intensive treatment program relative to custodial care by the readmissions since 1954-1956.

Further facts suggest that the type and severity of illness may have changed sufficiently between the admission cohorts of the fifties and those of the 1962-1964 period to affect the average length of stay. For example, the major changes were, first, that the proportion of patients diagnosed with psychoneurotic reactions rose from 6.9 per cent in 1956 to 14.9 percent in 1963. At the same time those admitted to the hospitals in the diagnostic category of chronic brain syndrome fell from 27 percent to 15.2 percent.[10] Since the average period of hospitalization for psychoneurotics is usually less than for those with chronic brain diseases, these shifts in proportions of patients in such categories would have the effect of shortening the average length of stay even though there had been no change in the treatment methods at all. Unfortunately data are not available to permit any kind of exact estimate of the magnitude of the effect of these changes, and the others of a minor character.[11]

The severity of the illnesses of those admitted in 1962 and later may have been less than for the persons committed in the mid-fifties. Voluntary admissions rose from only 15 percent of admissions and readmissions in 1956 to over 40 percent in 1962-1963.[12] State hospital officials believe that the increase in voluntary admissions means that earlier treatment of mental disease is being given. Illnesses may well be less advanced in these circumstances than would be the case otherwise, since it is unnecessary to obtain court orders to admit patients to the hospitals and treatment can begin more quickly. Of course, the period of hospitalization would be shorter for persons with less severe illnesses than for those more seriously ill, whether treated by the new therapies or held for recovery under a custodial program.[13]

The exact reduction in average length of stay over the past several years, which is attributable to the introduction and use of intensive treatment methods at the state mental hospitals, is obviously not precisely determinable. I have concluded, however, that the new treatment program led to a fall in average length of hospital confinement by about 20 months for the following reasons. The actual decline in the average period of hospitalization probably lies between 19 and 26 months. This range represents the minimum and maximum differences between the estimated average length of stay from 42 to 44 months in the mid-fifties and from 18 to 23 months for 1962-1964 reported above. Part of the over-all fall in the length of hospitalization probably resulted from other factors. The increased proportion of patients with diseases which usually lead to short hospital stay or the possible decline in the severity of illness of patients admitted to the hospitals account for some of the decline in average length of hospitalization. It is doubtful if these factors would have affected the estimated reduction in average length of stay by more than 10 percent. Thus taking the midpoint of the range of 19 to 26 months as the most representative of the actual decline in the average period of hospitalization, the decline of 20 months in average length of hospital stay attributable to the new therapies is reached. For subsequent computational purposes, I have concluded that 42 months would reasonably represent the length of hospital stay under the custodial program and, after adjustment for other factors, that 22 months is a best estimate for the average period of hospitalization in 1962-1964 under the intensive treatment program.

Economic Costs

The costs of mental illness and its treatment fall into four major categories: (1) subsistence costs as for board and room, housekeeping expenses, charges for depreciation on facilities, and so forth; (2) treatment costs as the expenditures for doctors and nurses, drugs and medical supplies, and a portion of maintenance overhead on equipment and facilities directly related to treatment; (3) costs which result from losses in productivity (real income) because resources are not employed or because they are withdrawn from one use to be employed in the care of mentally ill persons; and (4) costs of transfer payments, i.e., any economic cost which may result from taking income from one unit in society and giving it to another.

The first three categories have been conveniently rearranged into direct and indirect costs. The former constitute the actual expenditures on subsistence and treatment; the latter are costs primarily determined by the "economic loss in dollars (or work years) that society incurs because a part of society is suffering from mental illness," i.e., what would have been added or contributed to the economy if they had not been ill.[14]

Direct Costs

The operating budgets of the state hospitals provide the data for most of the subsistence and treatment costs. These expenditures are summarized in the published per capita daily costs of the state institutions. In the middle of the 1950's the per capita daily cost was approximately $3,[15] and had increased to an average of $7.93 for the 1962-1964 fiscal years.[16] The increase reflects both the rise in the number of staff employed per patient and also the rise in prices of medical services and supplies. Since the comparison of costs of the alternative treatment programs at different times is the desired objective, these daily costs must be adjusted for changing prices. The medical care component of the Consumer Price Index rose 30 per cent between 1955 and 1963.[17] Thus, if the same items bought in 1963 were obtained at 1955 prices, per capita daily costs would have been only $5.55 rather than nearly $8.[18]

The average cost per patient for subsistence and treatment costs, as developed from estimates here, indicates no preference between the two types of hospital care and treatment. At a custodial program cost of $2.97 per day per person, the per patient costs over an average hospital stay of 42 months would be $3,825. Alternatively, with more spent per day on personnel and drugs for an intensive therapy program, the per patient cost for 22 months at $5.55 per day would total $3,714. The difference between the two estimates is quite small and not significant when possible errors of computing the average length of stay under either the custodial care program of the mid-fifties or the intensive treatment methods of more recent years are taken into account.

Direct costs in addition to state budgeted operating expenses result from capital carrying costs, depreciation, and obsolescence allowances on the investment in hospital and treatment facilities.[19] These costs depend upon the capital value of facilities, the expected length of life of those facilities, and the net rate of interest. Since neither state budget agencies nor the Department of Institutions maintains a capital budget from which initial costs and subsequent depreciation charges on present plant, land, and equipment can be taken, the best alternative for computing estimated value of invested capital is replacement cost. The new construction cost per bed for a complete hospital as those already in use would have been about $15,000 in 1955.[20] Thus, if a 1 1/2 percent depreciation allowance is provided,[21] and the net market rate of interest is estimated at 4 percent,[22] the annual per bed total for capital carrying costs and depreciation allowance would be $825.

The conversion of per bed costs into per patient costs must take into account both length of stay and the hospital occupancy rate under the different systems of care and treatment. Obviously, the shorter stay and therefore the greater turnover of patients under the intensive treatment program leads to a lower occupancy rate than for the hospitals under the traditional custodial care arrangements. During the 1962-1964 period, on the average about 90 percent of the beds were filled.[23] In the mid-fifties the resident hospital population exceeded the rated hospital capacity for some time.[24] If the hospital is considered filled to capacity under a custodial program, the per bed capital carrying and depreciation costs estimated above can be translated directly into per patient costs. On the basis of a 42-month average hospital stay, the implicit and direct costs would be $2,887 under the custody program of care. On the other hand, if only 90 percent of the beds are kept filled when the new therapies are used, the per bed cost must be increased by one-ninth when converted to a per patient basis. The patients occupying the 90 percent of the beds must also "pay" for the fixed cost of maintaining all 100 percent. Thus, the annual per patient cost is $917, or for a 22-month average period of hospitalization under the intensive therapy program, the capital carrying costs and depreciation allowances would be $1,682.

Indirect Costs

A reduction in the average length of hospital stay will have significant economic effects other than on the costs of subsistence and treatment. There are indirect economic costs as well. First, the mentally ill person is incapacitated for the period of his confinement, as a minimum, and accordingly is unproductive during this period. A return to useful employment eliminates the loss of income and augments national product. Second, resources may be taken from present uses and employed to perform what formerly were noneconomic (nonmarket) functions. In the event a mother is hospitalized, who performs the home and child-rearing (nonmarket) tasks for the family? Not infrequently, private family resources are used to hire housekeepers, who were previously otherwise employed, to manage the home.

The loss of income from an illness is a function both of the length of confinement and the rate of earnings. Table 1 presents data for estimating the effects upon earnings of hospital tenures of varying length. Mean incomes, by age group and sex, were computed for 1956 for Washington, and a weighted average annual income determined for the age-sex distributions that appeared in the first admission cohorts to the three tax-supported mental hospitals in 1956 and in 1962. The weighted average per capita income, using only income of those persons between 15 and 65 years of age, was $1,973 for 1956 and $2,262 for 1962. If the average length of stay under the custodial program was 42 months, the loss of income per patient for those persons was $6,906. If, on the other hand, the age-sex distribution among the 1962 admissions prevailed and these persons were confined in hospitals for an average of only 22 months, the loss of income per patient, on the basis of 1956 average incomes, would have been $4,146.[25]

Private resources may also be allocated from alternative productive uses to the care of the dependents and families of mental hospital patients. Resources may be shifted from market to nonmarket uses. For example, funds which could otherwise be used in the home or family are frequently required for child care, or are unearned because the "well" parent is unable, in the absence of one spouse, to earn his usual full-time pay.

Any estimate on the cost of family care can only be a guess. Obviously some, if not many, of those admitted to the state hospitals are themselves only family dependents. The family resources may therefore be little affected by the hospital stay of a family member.[26] It would seem reasonable, however, to argue that at least as large a proportion of families with a mentally ill member would provide for their own emergency needs and to as great an extent economically as are given public assistance. Approximately 10 percent of the first admissions to one state hospital received full or part support from public assistance in 1962.[27] Another randomly selected sample of 50 patients from the case history records at one hospital disclosed that 18 percent of this sample had dependents on public welfare rolls.[28] If these samples are representative and the proportion of patients dependent on welfare is considered to be about 15 percent, the diversion of private (family) resources from productive market uses to the care of children or

TABLE 1 – ESTIMATED AVERAGE ANNUAL INCOMES FOR
WASHINGTON STATE RESIDENTS WITH SAME AGE AND SEX DISTRIBUTION
AS FIRST ADMISSIONS TO THE THREE TAX-SUPPORTED STATE MENTAL
HOSPITALS IN WASHINGTON STATE, 1956 AND 1962

Age in Years and Sex	1956 Mean Income*	1956 New Admissions		1962 New Admissions		1962 Mean Income*
		Per cent in Age Group†	Average Income Weight (1956 Incomes)	Per cent in Age Group†	Average Income Weight (1956 Incomes)	
Male						
Under 14	$ 000	0.0‡	$ 0.00	2.5	$ 0.00	$ 000
14-19	654§	5.9	38.59	4.9‖	32.05	709§
20-24	2,813	4.4	123.73	3.7‖	104.05	3,051
25-34	5,376	8.0	430.08	8.4	451.58	5,831
35-44	6,568	5.8	380.94	8.1	532.00	7,124
45-54	6,141	5.2	374.60	6.7	411.45	6,661
55-64	5,095	5.2	264.94	5.8	295.50	5,526
65 and over	§	19.5	0.00	12.2	0.00	§
Female						
Under 14	000	0.0‡	0.00	1.1	0.00	000
14-19	416§	2.9	12.07	4.1‖	17.05	451§
20-24	1,154	2.3	26.54	3.3‖	38.09	1,252
25-34	967	7.0	67.69	9.6	92.83	1,049
35-44	1,265	7.6	96.14	9.2	116.38	1,372
45-54	1,543	5.6	86.41	6.8	104.92	1,674
55-64	1,429	5.0	71.45	4.6	65.73	1,550
65 and over	§	15.2	0.00	8.9	0.00	§
Total		99.6 ¶	$1,973.18	100.1¶	$2,261.63	

*Mean incomes per age and sex group were computed from data in Bureau of Census, U. S. Department of Commerce, 1960 Census of Population: Detailed Characteristics, Vol. 49. Washington, D. C.: Government Printing Office, 1962, pp. 398ff., and adjusted to 1956 and 1962 by the same proportion as average per capita income increased in the State of Washington between 1956 and 1959 and 1962. (See U. S. Department of Commerce, Survey of Current Business, April, 1963, p. 9). Incomes were further adjusted to 1959 dollars. The 1962 mean income is not used in table, but is included for information only.

†Washington State Department of Institutions, First Biennial Report. Olympia: State Printing Plant, 1956, p. 61. The 1962 age sex distribution was provided the author by the Washington State Department of Institutions from unpublished data.

‡A few persons under 14 were in the hospitals in 1956 but the exact numbers were not available.

§ Mean incomes for age class 14-19 years is only for ages 15-19 years. Persons over 65 years of age did have income. It is assumed, however, that none who were hospitalized returned to active employment.

‖ Age breakdowns were available only for ages 14-24 for 1962. The subclasses of 14-19 years and 20-24 years were computed on the same basis as was the case in 1956. The 20-24 year class may have been underestimated. See Section of Research and Program Analysis. Washington State Department of Institutions, Research Rev. No. XV (Oct.), 1964, p. 40.

¶Totals do not equal 100 because of rounding.

family members would amount to an average of $410 for those under the longer custodial program and about $215 for families whose members were being cared for by intensive treatment.[29]

Transfer Payments

Any costs related to a reduction in transfer payments will be small. The redistribution of income via public assistance to the mentally ill is an infinitesimal fraction of state income.[30] Similarly any reduction in taxes of current taxpayers through the ability of rehabilitated persons to pay a portion of their income to the state would be quite small in relation to the magnitude of state taxes and to the size of state income.[31]

Summary of Findings

The economic costs of mental illness and its treatment by traditional custodial care or by the intensive therapy methods are summarized in Table 2. The first and overwhelming fact is the substantial economic advantage for the intensive therapy program over custodial care. The grand total state and private costs per patient are 30 percent less under intensive care than under a custodial program. Furthermore, the private costs, which bear a direct relation to the average length of stay under the alternative treatment methods, are only 60 per cent as much when results of modern therapy are compared to those of traditional custodial care. Only when direct public expenditures on maintenance and treatment of patients are considered is there no clear economic advantage for intensive therapy. The conclusion is clear, however, that the economic efficiency of new treatment methods of psychotherapy and intensive care in the Washington State mental hospitals is greater than that under the care and treatment of the mentally ill by the programs of the mid-1950's.[32]

Economic Implications and Public Policy

Several implications for social policy follow from the comparison of economic efficiency among alternative treatment methods. First, and most obvious, is a mandate to encourage and to promote the use of intensive therapies in the care of the mentally ill. The economic advantage is unmistakably clear and supports the intensive treatment whether public or private costs or the combination of the two are considered. Furthermore, an expansion of the purchase of psychiatric service and further appreciable growth in the mental health industry surely can be expected. The decline in relative costs of care by the use

TABLE 2 – COMPARATIVE COSTS OF MENTAL ILLNESS AND
ALTERNATIVE TREATMENT METHODS IN THREE WASHINGTON STATE
MENTAL HOSPITALS, 1954-1964

Average per Patient	Custodial Care 1954-1956 Actual Experience	Intensive Therapy 1962-1964 Experience in Terms of 1954-1956 Prices
1. Length of hospitalization for admission cohort (in months)	42	22
2. Daily maintenance and treatment costs	$ 2.97	$ 5.55
3. Direct budgeted costs of maintenance and treatment*	3,825.00	3,714.00
4. Implicit state capital carrying and depreciation costs	2,887.00	1,682.00
5. Total State (Public) Costs	$ 6,712.00	$5,396.00
6. Loss of income (private)	$ 6,906.00	$4,146.00
7. Emergency family expenditures	410.00	215.00
8. Total Private Costs	$ 7,316.00	$4,361.00
9. Grand Total State and Private Costs	$14,028.00	$9,757.00
10. Transfer payments: Public welfare and assistance	$ 410.00	$ 215.00
Loss in tax revenue from loss in personal income	690.00	361.00
Total Transfer Payments	$ 1,100.00	$ 576.00

*Approximately 15 percent of the maintenance and treatment costs are paid directly by patients and thus are, in effect, private costs. The remainder comes from public funds.

of the new treatment therapies will clearly stimulate the demand for mental health services.[33] This is already evident in the increased rate of new admissions per 1,000 population at the state mental hospitals, in the increased number of private psychiatric beds available in general hospitals, and in the general expansion of the private practice of psychiatry.[34]

The remarkable progress in reducing the period of hospital confinement by intensive care and the substantial decrease in the private costs of mental illness and treatment open the way for a reduction of public support through taxes and an increase in private payment for mental health care. The basis for tax support of a mental health program has been weakened. Public payment of the excessive costs of long periods of hospitalization, which rapidly exhaust the private resources of even the well-to-do, is of course, defensible on welfare grounds. The costs to society to do otherwise would likely be substantially more. Caring for the mentally ill would appear less costly than providing for, and suffering the consequences from, a number of poverty-stricken and disintegrated families which result from unsuccessful attempts at caring for long-term patients with private resources only. But if half the patients now admitted to mental hospitals are treated by intensive therapies and improved, and released in eight or nine weeks, the burden of the illness is clearly much less overwhelming than a confinement of 40 or 50 weeks, or years.[35] Patients are in a much better position to contribute to treatment costs. Patient-households gain personal income which otherwise would have been lost through the longer confinement under a custodial program. Additional private assets are therefore available to offset the higher daily costs of maintenance and treatment which are connected with the more intensive therapies. Furthermore, it should not be overlooked that average real per capita income in the nation is steadily rising. A portion of this increase can readily be, and in the market under free enterprise usually is, diverted to buying more and better services. Finally, the probabilities of reduced costs of treatment for many persons have opened the door to the application of insurance to mental illness and the payment for psychiatric services, including limited hospitalization.[36] Catastrophic costs can be avoided largely by insurance coverage at costs which increasing numbers of persons can afford without jeopardizing the financial stability and security of the family.[37]

A further implication of the relative economic advantage of the more intensive care over a custodial program, in part a corollary of any increase in the private payment for psychiatric services, is the stimulation and growth of the private practice of psychiatry and the development of additional nongovernment inpatient facilities in local communities. The lower cost of care, of course, makes it possible for more persons to finance treatment. In addition, the shorter average length of hospital stay, especially for the one-fourth who now are confined for only 20 or 30 days, makes possible the handling of many patients in psychiatric wards of general hospitals. Both of these factors support the growth of psychiatric insurance which is heavily relied on by the general and nonpsychiatric facility for private payment of the costs of hospital care. Also, psychiatrists in local communities can expand their practices. Patients can be placed in nearby general hospital psychiatric wards and continuing care made available by the same doctor.

The role and character of the state mental hospitals are being and will be affected by the further development and use of the intensive therapies. The economic advantages of the latter over the traditional custodial program provide justification for the immediate extension of the intensive treatment program even under state control and financing. Such an expansion in state systems, however, will be limited not only by the willingness of legislatures to provide funds for growth, but also by the need to avoid building new facilities to accommodate increasing populations under a custody program and, in the long run, by the extent to which private practice of psychiatry and local community outpatient and inpatient mental health facilities can meet the needs of the mentally ill at prices most families can bear.

Many nonmedical public officials have been loath to press for substantially increased moneys for psychiatric care. State legislators have generally refused to appropriate additional funds for expanded personnel requirements of the more intensive treatments in most state hospital systems. These attitudes reflect a fear of rapidly rising annual appropriations to meet a rapidly rising demand for mental health services. As shown in Table 2, direct budgeted expenditures per individual are about the same whether one type of care or another is used. But with shorter hospital stays, the lower over-all cost per person of intensive care will bring forth more persons seeking treatment, and total annual appropriations and tax burdens will rise accordingly. This creates some short run reluctance to shift from one type of treatment to another.

Furthermore, even though total state or public costs per patient are nearly 20 per cent less for intensive therapy than for custodial care, the difference arises from the implicit capital carrying costs and depreciation allowances. This difference, however, is not very meaningful in the short run. The costs of facilities are a sunk cost and become significant in determining alternative courses of action only if additional mental hospital facilities must be provided.

The growth in population and an increased awareness on the part of citizens of the improved technologies for treating mental illness will soon place extra pressure on state bodies to provide additional facilities for mental health needs. When legislatures must make the choice between expanded facilities for custodial care and the acquisition of more personnel to effectuate an intensive therapy program, the latter will undoubtedly be chosen. If further discoveries in psychotherapy and drugs reduce even more the prognosis for hospitalization, community inpatient facilities may even replace the state hospital for short-term care. Current thinking in the mental health field concludes that treatment in the community is much preferred to care provided at a large state psychiatric hospital. Exact economies of staffing and operation, however, have not yet been fully determined.

There will be state mental hospitals for some time, but exactly what function they will perform will depend on several factors. Some institution will be required for the confinement and care both of the seriously and violently disturbed individuals and of others who are chronically incapacitated.[38] In both cases public provision and support are the best alternatives available and the state mental hospital is a logical institution to provide such services, just as they have been doing in the past.

Over the long run the extent to which state hospital systems will provide intensive treatment for the acutely ill depends to a great degree upon the rapidity and success with which private practitioners with private or nongovernmental inpatient facilities can meet the growing demand for psychiatric care in local communities. As suggested above, successful adaptation of insurance principles to the incidence and treatment of mental illness will also reduce the need for public support and accordingly will curtail the significance of state mental hospitals on the mental health scene.

In the meantime, as the demands for psychiatric services continue to expand, the state mental hospitals will be called upon to provide a large share of inpatient care for the mentally ill. The intensive therapy and rehabilitory care, which can generally be made available with present hospital and other physical plant, is clearly the preferable program. It is advantageous economically to provide the intensive care, on the grounds of total state costs, total private costs, or on the basis of both combined. Research and training activities, from which significant benefits may be derived, are more compatible with intensive care than a custodial program. Finally, for some time during the period of rapidly changing technology and treatment methods in mental health care, in which the direction of mental health treatment programs will be more fully determined, the intensive treatment program provides a greater flexibility for further developments. Less is invested in facilities. Personnel and administrative structure can be altered and the state hospital system more readily adapted both to further changes in technologies and to subsequent developments in the private sector of mental health care.

NOTES AND REFERENCES

1. See the statement by Dr. Robert H. Felix, director of the National Institute of Mental Health, Public Health Service, in the Hearings before the Subcommittee of the Committee on Appropriations, House of Representatives, Eighty-Seventh Congress, First Session, March 23, 1961, p. 589. See also, Engel, L. New Trends in the Care and Treatment of the Mentally Ill. New York: National Association for Mental Health, 1959, pp. 3-11.

2. Economic efficiency is the relation of the value of output to the value of inputs. Thus, if results are equivalent, whichever method can produce them at the lowest cost will be regarded as the most efficient.

    Average cost is the practical measure even though marginal cost is, on principle, the most appropriate. The cost which is needed is the addition to total costs occasioned by caring for one more patient under each of the alternative treatment programs. Marginal cost is most difficult to estimate, whereas average cost is relatively easy to obtain and easily computed. Probably there is little difference between the two, given the high proportion of variable costs in the total costs of mental illness and its treatment. In fact, all that is required is for the ratios of average costs under the two programs of care to approximate the ratios of marginal costs. There is not a priori reason to suppose the ratios are not approximately equal. For further discussion on this matter see, Fein, R. Economics of Mental Illness. New York: Basic Books, 1958, pp. 9ff., and the discussion below on economic costs.

3. There are grounds for broad philosophical differences over the nature of "product" or "goals" in the health care and mental health industry. I do not intend to argue them here. Let it suffice for now that the most generally accepted product unit, although still quite an imperfect one, is the effect of care upon the length of the period of disability (length of hospital stay, for example, in the present study) from a particular illness or disease. For an interesting discussion of the many issues involved, see Jahoda, M. Current Concepts of Positive Mental Health. New York: Basic Books, 1958.

4. The comparison can only be "ideal" when the "material" worked on under the different treatment methods is identical. This implies if different methods of care are used on different patient populations and the economic efficiency of the alternative methods compared, that the characteristics of the patient populations, which are relevant to psychiatric treatment, should be the same or closely comparable. Any comparison will undoubtedly be faulty to some extent until psychiatrists and the medical profession can clearly identify and label the diseases of the mentally ill and can measure the degree of severity of the illness.

5. The essential difference between custodial care and intensive treatment methods is the ratios of professional staff to patients. Exactly what ratios make the treatment intensive is not precisely determinable because of the various combinations of professional personnel with varying degrees of training which can be used and because of the multiplicity of hospital conditions under which these personnel are employed. Furthermore, there are many levels of care

among which there are grounds for disagreements on which are "intensive" treatment and which are not. However, for the purposes of this analysis, I have relied upon the American Psychiatric Association minimum staffing standards and upon standards of hospital accreditation.

In all categories of professional personnel, staffing ratios failed by an appreciable amount to meet minimum professional standards in the mid-1950's. One of the three state hospitals was given probationary accreditation in 1956 but this was subsequently withdrawn in 1957. By 1962-1964 the hospitals were fully accredited and had increased staffing ratios to meet the APA standards. For example, the hospitals employed only one-third enough psychiatrists and clinical psychologists in 1956 but effectively meet the standards in 1963. At present the number of psychiatric nurses in relation to patients is below the APA minimum but for other auxiliary personnel the staff-patient ratio is substantially above the standards. Nursing personnel of all categories in the mid-1950's fell far below the APA requirements.

In a "Report of the Washington State Mental Hospitals," the Department of Institutions concludes that "the state hospitals no longer serve primarily a custodial function.... They are now active treatment centers geared to handle psychiatric emergencies for the communities which they serve.... In all areas the number of professional employees has been increased to provide intensive treatment...." (Section of Research and Program Analysis, Department of Institutions, State of Washington. Research Rev. No. XV (Oct.), 1964, pp. 3, 62.) For a detailed factual discussion of APA standards and the actual statistics of staffing, see, ibid., pp. 49-52, 62, and McCaffree, K. M. Some Economic Aspects of Mental Health Care. Univ. of Washington Business Rev. 18, 7: 15-16, 1959.

6. Department of Institutions, Section of Research and Statistics. Research Bull. 1: 2 (Feb.), 1955; Research Rev. VI: 7, 1962; Ibid. XV, 1964.

7. Op. cit. Research Bull. Vol. 3, 1957, Table 1; Research Rev. VI: 9, 1962; XV: 17, 1964. The exact years for which computations were made and the results obtained were 1956—12.07 years; 1961—11.91 years; and 1963—11.81 years. It, therefore, is possible that the average number of years of those who are not released by the end of a year of hospitalization is declining gradually. In each case these data have been estimated from the average length of stay of the resident population of the hospitals. Exact data on admission cohorts are not available for recent years, and the decline may be much greater than indicated.

8. A special tabulation on length of hospitalization of those admitted in 1957, which was provided by the Washington State Department of Institutions, gives an average length of stay of 43 months. The 1962 estimate in the text is computed from the same special tabulation.

Preliminary data for fiscal 1964 for the Washington State hospitals indicate that the average length of stay may have dropped to almost 18 months. Median length of stay, for example, declined from 4.7 months in 1957 to less than 2.7 months in 1964. See op. cit., Research Rev. XV: 15, 1964.

9. Ibid., p. 20. See also Section of Research and Program Analysis, Washington State Department of Institutions. Characteristics, Diagnosis, and Length of Hospitalization of Patients Admitted to Washington State Mental Hospitals, 1955-1961. Research Bull., 1961, p. 9.

A special tabulation of the number of persons returning to the state hospitals who were released to a noninstitutional environment in each year, 1956 through 1959, showed no difference in the proportions returning to the hospitals after six months, one year, two years, or three years. Ibid., p. 9.

The preferred statistics for estimating readmission rates are the proportions of each first admission cohort which return to hospitalization at each of several intervals over a period of, say, three years. Such data, however, were unavailable.

10. Ibid. Research Rev. XV: 36, 1964.

11. If the average length of hospital stay for patients within the diagnostic category of psychoneurotic reactions is only half that of the patients included in the category of chronic brain syndrome, the shift in proportions could have reduced average length of stay of the 1954-1956 admission cohorts by about two months, given the average length of stay from 42 to 44 months estimated above. Other changes in diagnostic categories would appear to have even less effect on the average length of stay when estimated by similarly rough computations.

12. Ibid., p. 31.

13. The treatment of less severe illnesses may be a function of the intensive therapy directly. At the margin, some persons would remain partially incapacitated and stay in the community if intensive treatment and short hospital stays were not available. Thus, even if hospital stay is shorter under intensive care by reason of treating less severe illnesses, the alternative may well be some "permanent" disability for the ill person who otherwise avoids hospitalization altogether, and consequently does not show up in the statistics of the average period of hospitalization under a custodial program in the state hospitals.

14. Fein, op. cit., pp. 10-11.

15. Department of Institutions. First Biennial Report, 1954-1956. Olympia: State Printing Shop, 1956, p. 267. Costs were somewhat less at the beginning of the biennium and ended at approximately $3.20 daily per capita in June, 1956.

16. Average was computed from data supplied the author by the Washington State Department of Institutions. Per capita daily cost for each of three fiscal years was 1962—$7.08; 1963—$7.88; 1964—$8.82. See also op. cit. Research Rev. XV: 45-46, 1964.

17. Consumer Price Index data were taken from various issues of the Monthly Labor Review between 1955 and 1964.

18. There is some possibility that a small portion of the increase in prices was offset by increases in the quality of products purchased by the state hospitals. Drugs would be an example; however, the total spent on these items is so small in relation to total costs that the effect on the above computation would be negligible. On the other hand, the rise in salaries and wages may represent a disequilibrium price in the medical care market because the rapid rise in the demand for medical and mental health care services during this period was not accommodated by an elastic supply of personnel. In the long run, costs under the intensive treatment program would therefore not rise as much as indicated above. It is interesting to note that the development of intensive treatment programs in the mental health field, in adding substantially to the demand for personnel, has contributed further to the general rise in salaries and wages of mental health professionals and the creation of "shortages" of health care personnel.

19. The capital carrying costs and the depreciation or obsolescence allowance are implicit costs and not explicitly a part of the budgets of the state hospitals.

They are nevertheless "real" economic costs. The capital carrying cost of an investment is the return which could have been obtained by having made that investment in the best alternative use. In this case the taxes paid to the state for construction and investment in mental hospitals could have been invested alternatively in other enterprises. The net return which that investment would have yielded in the best alternative enterprise is the cost of investing the tax funds in mental hospitals. The return foregone is a function of the size of the investment and the net market rate of interest on invested funds.

Depreciation or obsolescence allowances constitute that part of the gross return from invested capital which is necessary to maintain the same quantity (value) of capital over time. In the case of a building (as an example of a capital investment) some part of the gross rent for that building must be set aside each year in order to maintain the building and/or must be saved each year so that when the building is fully used up (collapses or condemned) sufficient amounts of the gross rent have been accumulated that the building can be replaced.

20. Op. cit. First Biennial Report, p. 23.

21. The length of time over which depreciation or replacement reserves should be accumulated will be different for different types of property. Land values may change little; some temporary buildings and equipment, as boilers and the like, may have exhausted their usefulness within ten years. Permanent structures, on the other hand, probably will last for efficient service for 35, 50, or possibly 75 years. Most hospital facilities will fall in the middle class, such that between 1 and 2 per cent annual depreciation allowances (40 to 80 years capital life) would seem appropriate.

22. The insurance earnings rate, which represents a conservative level of earnings from a diverse and large volume of investments, was 3.63 per cent in 1956. See Life Insurance Fact Book, 1957. New York: Institute of Life Insurance, 1957, p. 55.

23. The rate capacity of all three Washington State hospitals during this period was 5,836. The average resident daily population was 5,604, 4,984, and 4,534 in 1962, 1963, and 1964, respectively. See op. cit. Research Rev. XV: 47, 1964.

Only about 15 to 20 per cent of the patients in the hospitals at any one time were actually under an intensive therapy program. The remainder represents those persons whose illnesses are chronic or for whom a longer confinement period appears necessary. The intensive treatment wards operate similarly to most general hospitals so far as admission and discharge are concerned, and therefore do run much lower occupancy rates than for the hospital as a whole.

24. Washington State Department of Institutions. Research Rev. IV: 1-3, 1962. See also op. cit. First Biennial Report, pp. 32, 40, 49.

25. One of the differences between the 1962 cohort and the 1954-1956 groups was the smaller proportion of persons over 65 and an increased proportion of those in the middle high income years. Had the age-sex distribution remained the same in 1962 as in 1956, the income loss from 22 months average length of stay would have been only $3,617 instead of the estimated $4,146 in the text. In other words, the income loss would have been over $500 more for the 1956 groups relative to the 1962 cohort were it not for the additional high earners who sought treatment in 1962.

26. About 15 per cent of the 1954-1956 expenditure of the state hospitals was

covered by collections from patients or their families. See Department of Institutions. Research Bull. Vol. 3, no. 9, 1957, Table 2. This amount was still about 15 per cent in 1964. See op. cit. Research Rev. XV: 46, 1964.

27. Data taken from an analysis of first admission cohort at Western State Mental Hospital, Ft. Steilicom, for 1962.

28. McGough, P. S. Some Economic Aspects of Mental Illness in Washington State. Unpublished M.A. thesis, Department of Economics, Univ. of Washington, p. 29.

29. Average monthly public assistance payment for all Washington State cases (families) for the period July, 1955 to June, 1956 was approximately $65. Washington State Department of Public Assistance. Public Assistance in the State of Washington. Vol. 18, Nos. 1-12 (July), 1955 through 1956. Olympia: State Printing Shop, 1956.

Thus, if families of 15 of each 100 mental hospital patients received relief or public assistance for an average of 42 months the total payments would equal $40,950, or about $410 per patient family. Or alternatively, if the length of stay was only 22 months, the total for 100 patients would be $21,450, or an average of $215 per patient family.

30. See note 29.

31. To the extent that citizens pay a portion of their incomes to the state in the form of taxes, and on the basis that approximately $1 in each $10 of income in Washington in 1956 was collected in taxes, the state (taxpayers as a whole) could, on the average, expect to receive one-tenth of the private income obtained by reemployment of the rehabilitated mentally ill. From the income estimates made above about $300 in taxes were "lost" because of longer stay for patients under hospital care in the custodial program than was the case under the more intensive therapies.

32. There are also, in addition to the measured economic gains indicated, substantially reduced psychic costs from the faster treatment and shorter periods of disability both to the patient and to his family. The desire to quantify results and to show explicit economic benefits should not obscure the less measurable, but nevertheless increased well-being of persons returned to good health.

33. The demand for medical care generally is income-elastic, and probably some expansion of the demand for treatment of the mentally ill can be attributed to rising per capita real income.

34. For example, total admissions in the Washington State mental hospitals rose from 104.6 per 100,000 population in 1955 to 137.6 per 100,000 in 1964. See op. cit. Research Rev. XV: 4, 1964.

35. Median length of stay for new admissions in the Washington State mental hospitals in 1963 was 2.7 months. Ibid., p. 15. General hospitals report average periods of hospitalization for psychiatric cases at between 10 and 21 days.

36. See Masco, F. H. Is Psychiatric Care Insurable? Unpublished M.A. thesis, Department of Economics, University of Washington, 1964.

37. The basis for urging private payment and the reduction of public support is the fact that it is primarily the patient (and/or his family) who benefits from the health care. Economically, little difference exists between mental health care and physical health care. The latter, except for the indigent and the poor, is paid for by the individuals receiving the hospital or medical services. The public charge among the mentally ill, however, includes not only the indigent and the poor, but the criminally insane, from whom society requires protec-

tion, and the incurably chronically ill, for whom the costs of care are an un-
bearable burden for the individual household. The rest of the population
could well pay for mental health care in the same manner as for medical
services.

It is frequently argued that the price of psychiatric and mental health services
is relatively high and precludes or substantially reduces its purchase by many
people. This is true. But a high relative price is not specific grounds alone for
public purchase and distribution of an economic good or service. A relatively
high price for psychiatric care is no different than for a great multitude of
other services and economic goods. Many people cannot afford college educa-
tions, cannot finance extended law suits, cannot take trips to visit grandmother
and friends, or buy long vacations, and so forth. Most goods and services are
scarce and thus exact a price. The greater the scarcity the higher the price,
and more difficult it is for many people to obtain certain economic goods or
as much of them as some of us think those persons should have.

38. There is also the possibility that individuals suffering from certain kinds of
disturbances may generate pathology in others. This situation would be
analagous to public control of contagious diseases, and as argued by Weisbrod,
a situation which requires public (governmental) support. See Weisbrod, E.
Economics of Public Health, Philadelphia: University of Pennsylvania Press,
1961, pp. 1-24.

The study was supported in part by a grant from the National Institute of Mental
Health. I am indebted to Kenneth R. Smith for assistance in compiling some of the
data and for making some of the statistical computations.

29

Rehabilitation of Former Mental Patients: An Evaluation of a Coordinated Community Aftercare Program

TRAVIS J. NORTHCUTT JR., THEODORE LANDSMAN,
JOHN S. NEILL, and JOANNA F. GORMAN

DUE to the progress made in the treatment of the mentally ill in recent years, an increasing percentage of the patients hospitalized are soon able to return to their communities. Unfortunately, however, complete rehabilitation after discharge is not readily nor frequently attained. A substantial proportion of patients leaving the hospital eventually have to be readmitted, and many of the ex-patients who remain in the community are unable to perform the roles that are normally expected of them. In an attempt to facilitate the posthospital adjustment of former patients, communities around the nation have utilized various approaches.

In a metropolitan Florida county, representatives of various social and health agencies and professional organizations developed a plan by which their services could be coordinated to aid former hospitalized mental patients and their families. They believed that through such a plan a broader service program could be made available to these returned persons and their families, and duplication of effort could be avoided.

After working with the problem for some time on an informal basis, the group decided that the goals could be achieved more readily through a formal organization with a full-time staff. In January, 1958, at a general meeting of representatives from interested agencies and professional groups, an organizational plan was presented and adopted. The name selected for the organization was the Mental Health Resource Council. At this time membership was extended to 24 agencies and organizations and plans were made to secure the financial support needed to employ a staff and operate the program.

In the following months the number of participating agencies and organizations increased from 24 to 33, and financial support for the operation of the council was secured through a demonstration grant from the National Institute of Mental Health (NIHOM239). The council then employed a full-time psychiatric social worker and a secretary. The psychiatric social worker, who had previously worked in the social service department of a state mental hospital, served as coordinator and assistant project director. Medical direction for the project was provided by the assistant director of the county health department on a part-time basis. The offices of the council were located in the county health department.

In brief, the program was operated in the following manner. The general membership formulated the policies of the council and direction was provided by a 12-member Executive Committee. The nucleus of the program was the Professional Services Committee, which was composed of a psychiatrist, psychologist, nurse, rehabilitation counselor, and social worker. The membership was drawn from practicing representatives of these professions in the community, all of whom served without remuneration. The members served for a two-month period on a rotating basis. The Professional Services Committee met semimonthly to staff the cases of patients on trial visit and to make recommendations regarding the services which they should receive. Prior to each meeting the project coordinator collected pertinent information regarding each case to be considered. Following the meetings she made the referrals which were recommended by the committee. Almost without exception these referrals were accepted by the agencies and professional persons to whom they were made. This cooperation which was a distinctive feature of the program from the early stages of its development, in addition to the unusually large amount of time contributed by the members of the Professional Services Committee, are indicative of the high level of coordination attained.

Plan for Evaluation

From the inception of the program, plans were made for evaluating the effectiveness of this approach to the rehabilitation of former mental patients. In brief, the council wanted to test the hypothesis that: A program designed to coordinate services to patients returning to the community following hospitalization for mental illness is more effective in facilitating their posthospital adjustment than is a community program in which there is no designated coordinating service for this purpose. To make such an assessment, the evaluation plan included a comparison of the posthospital adjustment of patients returning to the county with the coordinated aftercare program with that of patients returning to a control county.

The control county was selected for its high degree of similarity in population characteristics and economic structure, as well as mental health resources. There were, of course, some differences between the counties with regard to these variables. In the county with the coordinated aftercare program there was one county-wide health department, while in the control county there were two separate health departments, one serving the central city and the other serving the smaller municipalities and rural areas. The health departments in both counties were similar, however, in that they received routine notices from the state mental hospitals regarding returning patients and provided aftercare services when indicated. For purposes of this study the major difference between the two counties was that the control county had no individual or agency designated to coordinate services to patients returning from state hospitals. It was this difference which allowed the testing of the above hypothesis.

The Mental Health Resource Council was in operation for two years before the study of posthospital adjustment of returning patients was undertaken. This allowed time for the details of the operation to be worked out and stabilized. Following this two-year period, all patients returning to both the experimental and the control counties from state hospitals during the succeeding year were seen by trained interviewers who followed a structured schedule to obtain comparable data.[1] The interviews were conducted 12 months after the patients left the hospital.

During this one-year period, information was gathered regarding 269 patients; 147 in the county with the coordinated program and 122 in the control county. In most instances the interviews were conducted with the patients themselves; in those cases where the patient was in the hospital or was too disturbed to be interviewed, the necessary information was obtained from a family member, relative, or close friend. In all, only 18 patients furloughed to the two counties were lost to the study; ten from the county with the coordinated program and eight from the control county. The reasons for failure to complete these interviews were as follows: (a) patient moved out of county (eight cases), (b) interviewer was unable to locate patient or family (seven), and (c) refusal to be interviewed (three).

Limitations in Interpretation of Data

The study was designed to collect information regarding the patients in the two counties in the following areas: social characteristics, diagnoses and psychiatric histories, employment, economic adjustment, social participation, hospital and other medical care, community services received, restoration of civil rights, and homemaking role. Despite the fact that excellent coverage of the planned sample was achieved, a number of factors prevented the collection of all of the information desired. First, the time limitation of the interviews prevented a full exploration of the areas being studied. Next, due to the fact that some of the patients had returned to the hospital and others were too disturbed to be interviewed, it was not always possible to obtain a first-hand report regarding the desired information. Finally, the length of time that some of the patients had been hospitalized made the recall of prehospital information difficult. For these reasons, data are presented in the findings only in those areas where sufficient information was available.

While the use of a control county in the study added to the rigor of the design and provided an opportunity to test the hypothesis, it was anticipated that a perfect control could not be obtained. As shown in the findings which follow, the patient population of the control county was found to be comparable to that of the county with the coordinated aftercare program with regard to most of the characteristics which were believed to be relevant. It must be recognized, however, that the significant differences which were found to exist regarding several characteristics place some limitations upon the conclusions which may be drawn from the study.

Since comparable data are not available regarding patients' post-hospital adjustment before the coordinated program was started, definite conclusions cannot be drawn regarding the impact that the program has had upon patients' rehabilitation in that county. While there is evidence that the follow-up programs in the two counties were quite similar before the start of the coordinated program, the question remains unanswered as to whether the council was more successful in facilitating the rehabilitation of patients through a coordinated program than the traditonal approach had been in that county.

No attempt should be made to draw global conclusions regarding the efficacy of coordinated or noncoordinated programs from the findings of this study. It is quite possible that entirely different results might be obtained through different methods of coordinating services or through other noncoordinated approaches.

Findings

To facilitate the reading of this report, the major findings are presented in the text in summary tables.[2] In order to avoid the temptation to interpret any superiority in numbers or percentages as indicative of actual differences between the two counties, the Chi Square (X^2) test was used to determine the significance of observed differences. In the summary tables which follow, the level of significance is shown only for those differences which were found to be significant at the 0.05 level or higher. An abbreviation (N.S.) is used to designate those variables in which no significant differences were found between the patients from the two counties.

Comparison of Patient Populations

A comparison of the social characteristics, prehospital employment status and income, diagnoses and psychiatric histories, revealed few significant differences between the patients from the two counties. As shown in Table 1, significant differences were found for five of the 25 characteristics studied. The significantly different characteristics were: (1) race, (2) marital status, (3) diagnosis, (4) prehospital social participation score, and (5) prehospital acceptance-rejection score.[3] While the extent to which these variables influence all the aspects of the patients' rehabilitation is not known, subsequent analysis revealed that readmission to a mental hospital within the study year was not associated with any of these characteristics.[4]

In general, it seems reasonable to assume that the patient populations are sufficiently similar to permit the necessary comparisons.

Comparison of Services to Patients

As shown in Table 2, several significant differences were found regarding follow-up services to the patients in the two counties. During the year 91.7 percent of the patients in the control county received services from community agencies as compared to 71.9 percent of the patients in the county with the coordinated program. In most cases patients in the control county had been out of the hospital a shorter period of time before services were initiated; 81.3 percent of the patients in the control county as compared to 36.3 percent in the county with the coordinated program had their first contact with a community service within one month after leaving the hospital. It was also found that a significantly higher percentage of the agency-patient contacts were initiated by community agencies in the control county. No significant differences were found regarding (1) patient reaction to community services, (2) number of visits to physicians and outpatient clinics, (3) use of medication recommended by hospital, and (4) source of medication.

TABLE 1–COMPARISON OF PATIENT POPULATIONS IN COUNTY
WITH COORDINATED PROGRAM AND CONTROL COUNTY *

Characteristics	Significance	Direction of Observed Differences
I. Social Characteristics		
1. Age	N.S.†	
2. Sex	N.S.	
3. Race	Sig. 0.01	Higher percentage of patients in the control county were Negroes.
4. Education	N.S.	
5. Social class	N.S.	
6. Marital status	Sig. 0.05	Higher percentage of patients in the county with coordinated program were married.
7. Number of children	N.S.	
8. Number of dependents	N.S.	
9. Number of living relatives	N.S.	
10. Stage of family life cycle	N.S.	
11. Prehospital social participation score		
12. Prehospital acceptance-rejection score	Sig. 0.05	Patients in the county with coordinated program were more active in community organizations.
	Sig. 0.05	Patients in the county with coordinated program were more accepted in community organizations.

TABLE 1–COMPARISON OF PATIENT POPULATIONS IN COUNTY
WITH COORDINATED PROGRAM AND CONTROL COUNTY *

Characteristics	Significance	Direction of Observed Differences
II. Prehospital Employment and Income		
1. Monthly income	N.S.	
2. Source of income	N.S.	
3. Occupation	N.S.	
4. Employment status	N.S.	
5. Monthly earnings	N.S.	
6. Role in self support	N.S.	
7. Role in family support	N.S.	
8. Number of jobs during year prior to hospitalization	N.S.	
9. Job satisfaction	N.S.	
III. Diagnosis and Psychiatric History		
1. Diagnosis during last admission	Sig. 0.05	Higher percentage of patients in the county with co-ordinated program were diagnosed as involutional (no significant difference when diagnoses are grouped into broader categories of (1) schizophrenia, (2) other functional, (3) organic).
2. Total number of hospitalizations	N.S.	
3. Total time in hospital	N.S.	
4. Length of time since first hospitalization	N.S.	

*The Chi Square (X^2) test was used to determine the significance of observed differences.
†Not significantly different.

TABLE 2 – COMPARISON OF COMMUNITY SERVICES AND MEDICAL
CARE RECEIVED BY PATIENTS IN COUNTY WITH COORDINATED PROGRAM
AND CONTROL COUNTY*

Services	Significance	Direction of Observed Differences
1. Percent receiving community services	Sig. 0.05	Larger percentage of patients in the control county received community services.
2. Length of time patient out of hospital before initiation of community services	Sig. 0.01	Patients in control county received services earlier.
3. Initiator of contact between patient and community services	Sig. 0.01	Higher percentage of contacts in control county were initiated by community agencies.
4. Patient reaction to community services	N.S.†	
5. Number of visits to physician	N.S.	
6. Number of visits to outpatient clinics	N.S.	
7. Use of medication (tranquilizers) recommended by hospital	N.S.	
8. Source of medication during trial visit	N.S.	

*The Chi Square (X^2) test was used to determine the significance of observed differences.
†Not significantly different.

Subsequent analysis of the data revealed that differences found between the counties regarding receipt of services were not associated with the differences in the racial composition of the two groups.

Comparison of Patients' Rehabilitation

In general, the findings regarding rehabilitation of patients did not support the hypothesis that: A program designed to coordinate services to patients returning to the community following hospitalization for mental illness is more effective in facilitating their posthospital adjustment than is a community program in which there is no designated coordinating service for this purpose. As shown in Table 3, no significant differences were found between the patients from the two counties with regard to 16 of 19 areas of posthospital adjustment studied. While patients from the county with the coordinated aftercare program scored somewhat higher in several areas of social adjustment, this evidence must remain in doubt in as much as they had scored higher in these areas during the prehospitalization period. Patients in the control county were found to achieve a higher work performance level. However, since comparable measures could not be obtained for the two groups regarding the prehospitalization period, the importance which should be attached to this finding also remains somewhat in doubt. While 46.9 per cent of the patients from the county with the coordinated program compared to 38.5 per cent of the patients in the control county were readmitted to the hospital during the study year, this difference was not found to be significant at the 0.05 level.

Summary and Conclusions

In an attempt to evaluate the effectiveness of a coordinated community aftercare program, follow-up interviews were conducted with all patients returning to the county from state hospitals over a period of one year. Similarly, patients returning to a control county were interviewed to determine the relative contributions of a noncoordinated approach in which individual agencies contact former patients as they deem necessary. In all, data were collected regarding 269 patients, 147 in the county with the coordinated aftercare program and 122 in the control county. A comparison of the characteristics of the patient populations of the two counties indicated that they were comparable except for five of the 25 characteristics. (Subsequent analysis of the data revealed that none of the characteristics of the patient populations which were found to be significantly different were associated with readmission to the hospital during the study year.)

TABLE 3 – COMPARISON OF POSTHOSPITAL ADJUSTMENT OF PATIENTS
RETURNING TO COUNTY WITH COORDINATED PROGRAM AND CONTROL COUNTY*

Area of Adjustment	Significance	Direction of Observed Differences
I. Readmission and Hospital Status		
1. Readmission to mental hospital during year of trial visit	N.S.†	
2. Amount of time out of hospital during year of trial visit	N.S.	
3. Hospital status at time of interview	N.S.	
II. Civil Rights		
1. Restoration of Civil Rights	N.S.	
2. Attempts at Civil Rights restoration	N.S.	
III. Employment and Income		
1. Employment of eligible persons	N.S.	
2. Return to job held prior to hospitalization	N.S.	
3. Number of jobs held during year of trial visit	N.S.	
4. Monthly earnings of persons employed	N.S.	
5. Work performance level	Sig. 0.05	Higher performance attained by patients in control county.
6. Role in self support	N.S.	
7. Role in family support	N.S.	

TABLE 3 – COMPARISON OF POSTHOSPITAL ADJUSTMENT OF PATIENTS
RETURNING TO COUNTY WITH COORDINATED PROGRAM AND CONTROL COUNTY*

Area of Adjustment	Significance	Direction of Observed Differences
IV. Social Adjustment		
1. Social participation score	N.S.	
2. Acceptance-rejection score	Sig. 0.05	Higher percentage of patients in county with coordinated program were accepted by the community organizations. (It should be noted that this was also true in the prehospital period.)
3. Number of persons considered to be friends	Sig. 0.01	Higher percentage of patients in county with coordinated program reported that they had friends.
4. Get together with friends	N.S.	
5. Friends in neighborhood	N.S.	
6. Change in relationship with friends	N.S.	
V. Homemaking Responsibility		
1. Homemaking responsibility assumed by adult females	N.S.	

*The Chi Square (X^2) test was used to determine the significance of observed differences.
†Not significantly different.

While the study does not provide a basis for extensive generalizations concerning the relative efficacy of coordinated and noncoordinated aftercare programs, the findings strongly challenge the assumption that coordination of existing community services provides an adequate solution to the problems associated with posthospital adjustment of former mental patients. The data regarding posthospital adjustment of the patients in the two counties studied failed to support the hypothesis that: A program designed to coordinate services to patients returning to the community following hospitalization for mental illness is more effective in facilitating their posthospital adjustment than is a community program in which there is no designated coordinating service for this purpose.

Further, it was not demonstrated that the county with the coordinated aftercare program was more effective in providing services to patients. It was found (1) that significantly more patients in the control county received services from community agencies and (2) services were initiated sooner after the patients returned from the hospital.

Discussion and Implications

In view of the considerable significance placed upon coordination in the Community Mental Health Services Act which Congress recently passed and the current emphasis that is being placed upon coordination in the planning of state and local mental health programs, the findings of this study are of more than incidental concern. While on the basis of simple logic the coordinated approach may appear to facilitate the provision of services to returning mental patients and to enhance their chances of making a satisfactory posthospital adjustment, the findings of the present study indicate that this is not always accomplished. Due to the financial costs and the amount of professional time required to operate a coordinated aftercare program, it would seem that further research should be conducted to determine the contribution that this approach makes in comparison with other approaches. Also suggested here is the need for evaluation of the effectiveness of the various individual services provided returning mental patients. It would appear that little or no additional benefit would be derived from coordinating numerous services which themselves are ineffective.

Finally, communities which utilize a coordinated approach for providing services to returning patients should make certain that the focus of the program is centered upon the patients and their needs. Where such precautions are not taken, coordination itself can become the primary goal and as the observer of one such program remarked, "You can't rehabilitate patients by holding conferences and shuffling papers."

NOTES AND REFERENCES

1. The writers wish to express their appreciation to Howard Freeman, Ozzie Simmons, John James, and Associates for their permission to utilize portions of questionnaires which had been developed for use in somewhat similar studies of posthospital adjustment. See Freeman, H. and Simmons, O. The Mental Patient Comes Home. New York: Wiley, 1963; James, J. et. al. The Oregon Study of Rehabilitation of Mental Hospital Patients. Vols. I and II. Salem, Ore., 1960.

2. Detailed findings and data collection instruments may be obtained by writing the Bureau of Mental Health, Florida State Board of Health, Jacksonville, Fla.

3. Both the social participation and the acceptance-rejection scores are measures of the individual's participation in formal community organizations. The social participation score reflects both the extensity and intensity of the individual's participation in community groups. It is derived through a weighted score of his organizational memberships, attendance, financial contributions, committee memberships, and offices held. The acceptance-rejection score reflects the individual's acceptance or rejection within community organizations. It is derived through a weighted score of his organizational memberships, committee memberships, and offices held. In the present study these measures were obtained through the use of the Social Participation Scale designed by F. Stuart Chapin. See Chapin, F. S. Experimental Designs in Sociological Research. (rev. ed.) New York: Harper, 1952.

4. The data are currently being analyzed in an epidemiological study of rehabilitation; through this analysis the extent to which these variables influence other aspects of rehabilitation will be determined.

This paper was presented before the Mental Health Section of the American Public Health Association at its annual meeting in Kansas City, Mo., November 1963.

The evaluation study was made possible by a grant from the Florida Council on Mental Health Training and Research.

Section V

Implementing Research Findings

30

Scientific Communication: Five Themes from Social Science Research

HERBERT MENZEL

THE recent upsurge of interest in the behavioral aspects of scientific and technical communication and information flow has two distinct sources, a theoretical one in the development of communication research, and a practical one in the concerns of policy makers in scientific organizations and information services.

For some time past, the attention of sociologists and social psychologists studying communication processes, once focused on so-called mass phenomena and mass publics, has turned to the interplay of communication processes with more and more definitely delineated and mapped aspects of social structure. One aspect of this shift in interest has been the increasing attention paid by behavioral scientists to the systems supplying information of a specialized sort, and to the publics which are consumers of this specialized information. The scientific and applied professions have been most prominent among the publics so studied.

At the same time those concerned with the planning of science information policy have become increasingly interested in so-called "user studies" as possible sources of guidance. For a decade or two, as the mushrooming of the scientific enterprise has led to a multifold increase in the supply of scientific information as well as in the demand for such information on the part of scientists and technologists, the adequacy of the science information system whose task it is to link this supply and this demand has become a matter of increasing concern. A multitude of astonishing new services has been introduced into the system, alleviating some of the concerns, but also generating new questions of optimal allocation of resources and even giving rise to some additional strains in the information system itself. Concerns have led to attempts at planning and these have, after some lag, more recently led to demands in some quarters that the information needs of science be ascertained as a basis for wise planning. While some have asked that the scientist users of scientific information be studied in order to ascertain these needs, others have countered that these needs can better be estimated by those who are experts in information handling. Both proponents and critics of the so-called "user study" approach have often confused it with opinion polling—that is, with quizzing scientists on what should be done.[1-3]

Actually, studies of the information gathering behavior and experiences of scientists have been going on, in one form or another, for at least 20 years (reviewed in Paisley).[4] Behavioral scientists have taken some part in this work for about 10 years. Many of the studies have been quite primitive in the techniques of data gathering, simplistic in the conceptualization of variables and research goals, poor in comparability, and questionable in generalizability. But although many of the shortcomings remain, sounder and more sophisticated approaches have increasingly been used, with an especially gratifying concentration in the last 3 years or so.[5] Outstanding among these most recent accomplishments is the Project on Scientific Information Exchange in Psychology of the American Psychological Association,[6,7] which has refined and innovated research techniques and has used them in a battery of studies giving comprehensive coverage to the communication situation in a discipline. It has drawn together the results in a process model which has suggested several policy changes and has aided in the choice between them. Recent highlights from this work are reported in other articles in the November, 1966 issue of the *American Psychologist*.

Enough of this work has now accumulated to make it possible to discern certain themes which emerge with increasing insistence as the sophistication of the studies advances. A discussion of five of these interrelated themes will constitute the bulk of this paper. The selection of these particular themes was, no doubt, influenced by the author's sociological bias, but it is believed that they warrant special attention in the interest of both practical and theoretical advances in the field of science communication research.

Acts of Scientific Communication Constitute a System

The first of these themes is that of the desirability of taking a systemic view of the scientific communication in any discipline. It is necessary to look upon any one arrangement, institution, facility, or policy for scientific and professional communication as a component of the total system of scientific communication for a profession, a system which includes *all* the provisions, *all* the publications, *all* the facilities, *all* the occasions and arrangements, and *all* the customs in the discipline that determine how scientific messages are transmitted.[8]

The systemic view, however, means more than comprehensiveness with regard to the channels and mechanisms encompassed. Thus, for example, it also seems useful to conceive of the flow of scientific information as a set of interaction processes in a social system. The information-receiving actions of any one individual often involve several of his roles (as researcher, teacher, consultant, editorial referee, etc.) and approaches to several different channels, including individuals standing in diverse relationships to him and serving now as sources, now as relays, of information. The scientists who generate and use the information in a given discipline can therefore be usefully looked upon as interconnected publics.

Furthermore, it is necessary to be comprehensive with regard to the varied functions served by the science information system. And finally, it is necessary to be comprehensive in the delineation of transactions of scientific information, for these frequently involve much more than a single encounter between a scientist and some one communication channel.

The systemic view is urged upon us by a number of considerations. One cannot obtain a true picture of what the functions of the science communication system are, how often the need for each function arises, and how well each is performed, unless one considers all the channels through which scientific information travels. Conversely, one cannot obtain a true picture of the significance of any particular channel or arrangement unless one considers all the information functions that it may perform. Changes and innovations introduced in any one component of the system will have their consequences on the utilization and efficacy of other components. (This is made very clear in APA,[9] pp. 127-140.) Numerous transactions of scientific information within a public of scientists may have to be considered before aggregate regularities and patterns are revealed behind what appears to be accidental and idiosyncratic in the individual case.[10] And finally, even the effective transmission of a single message to an individual scientist may involve a multitude of contacts with diverse channels extending over a period of time—a topic to which we now turn.

Several Channels May Act Synergistically to Bring About the Effective Transmission of a Message

Any given transaction between a scientist as a receiver of information and the channel that brings him that information usually has a history behind it and a future ahead of it that may be very relevant to the evaluation of the success of that transaction and to the prognosis of whether this kind of transaction will happen again with similar results.

Often one channel of communication calls attention to a message to be found in another; sometimes a third channel is required to locate the precise document in which the message is contained; frequently one or more persons serve as relays between the source of a message and its ultimate consumer; and contacts at each intervening step may be initiated now by the receiver, now by the bringer of the message. The events which thus interplay are often distributed over a period of time. The possible relevance of a message to a man's work may not become apparent at the time it is first received, but only when that same message is repeated, sometimes more than once, or when it is put together with other information yet to be received, or when changes occur and needs come up in the course of the scientist's own future work.

In fact, not only an individual scientist, but an entire scientific community may for years turn its back on some already published and significant piece of work, until it is "brought home" by repetition, appearance in new media, rediscovery in new contexts, or other supplementary messages. Information must often be publicized repeatedly or through diverse channels before it will enter the stream of communications which will lead it to its ultimate user; and from the point of view of the consumer of information, it is frequently necessary to be exposed to the information repeatedly before it will make an impact.[11] Much of this crucial multiple exposure is brought about in informal ways, largely through contacts between individual scientists. This phenomenon will be discussed in the next section.

Informal and Unplanned Communication Plays a Crucial Role in the Science Information System

There is by now a fair amount of documentation[12-19] for the great role played by informal, unplanned, person-to-person communication in the experiences of scientific investigators, often in ways that affect their work quite vitally. This comes as no surprise to communications researchers familiar with the "multistep flow of communications" that prevails in so-called mass communications. (For a recent summary, see Lazarsfeld and Menzel[20]). However, the situation in the sciences differs from "mass communication" in fundamental ways: The mass communication audience is typically apathetic, while the scientific audience is highly motivated; the familiar multistep flow serves to diffuse messages already contained in the mass media, while informal transmission of messages among scientists often antecedes their appearance in print; in mass communication, interpersonal links play their role primarily in persuasion, while in the sciences they seem to be crucial even in mere cognitive transmission. (For an example of persuasive communication in an applied profession, see Coleman, Katz, and Menzel[21]). For these reasons, the importance of interpersonal communication in the sciences cannot simply be explained by the same factors as in mass communication, but will have to be accounted for through the specific characteristics of the scientific public. (For one attempt to do this, see Menzel[22]).

While informal communication in the sciences is largely unplanned, and sometimes appears accidental, there is actually a good bit of regularity to it. Certain individuals, for example, tend to be the most frequent carriers of information from one place to another, the recipients of correspondence, the hosts of visiting scientists, the visitors to other institutions—largely due to the positions or obligations that researchers assume in addition to their primary activity as researchers. It is the people who serve as editors of journals, who serve on grant-application review committees, who go to summer laboratories, and so on, that play the role of "the scientific troubadour," as it has been called.

There is also some regularity in the kinds of occasions, places, and times at which these information exchanges take place: at summer laboratories, in the corridors of scientific meetings, during and after colloquia and conferences. There is some regularity as to the patterns of initiative on the part of the conveyor and of the recipient of information through which unplanned communication comes about: seeking one kind of information and obtaining another; informing a colleague of current work and being rewarded with a relevant item of information; information brought up spontaneously by a colleague with whom one is together for another purpose; being sought out deliberately by a colleague who has information to convey; and so on.[23]

And finally, there is some regularity as to the content of the information that seems preferentially to flow through these kinds of channels rather than through the more regular and systematized mechanisms of the printed word and the attendant bibliographic control devices. For example, there is a certain level of know-how information about the use and setting up of scientific apparatus that seems to go by preference through the word-of-mouth channels, perhaps because this kind of information is regarded as unworthy of being handled in detail in the printed word, and does not find a ready place under the subject terms of indexing procedures. Information that helps interpret results and information that helps a person become acquainted with a new field also seem to make their way differentially, often through the personal channels. [24-26]

The regularities inherent in the apparently accidental and unplanned ways of communicating hold out the hope of planned improvements in the system. On the one hand, as more is learned of the kinds of information that seem to go through these kinds of communication-switching devices, needs for better and more effective sources on the part of the formal devices become clear. On the other hand, as it is realized that some kinds of information will continue to be carried primarily through interpersonal interchanges, formal devices for making these informal interchanges more effective may be developed—planned mechanisms to make the so-called lucky accidents happen more often. These mechanisms may range from directories and newsletters that tell scientists who is doing what to the scheduling of working hours and the location of new institutes in such a way as to facilitate visits.

Scientists Constitute Publics

The populations which are served by the science information systems—scientific researchers, practitioners in various disciplines and professions—can be usefully looked upon as publics, and described under the same categories that one uses when describing the more familiar publics of the mass media. These publics can, for example, be described in terms of size, in terms of turnover, and in terms of the interaction that exists within them. They can also be described in terms of their interests in a range of topics, in terms of the fidelity with which they attend to given channels and in terms of the norms that they have created with regard to exposure to various channels.

Yet, while the scientific publics share certain characteristics with the mass publics, in certain other respects they are very different from the public of the newspaper, of the TV program, or the neighborhood public library. Number one, the scientists have a very high motivation to obtain the information that is channeled in their direction through the system that is designed to serve them. They go out of their way to reach out for this information. Second, they want this information to help in very specific activities—activities that form very essential parts of their professional roles and therefore of their lives. Third, because of both of these facts, they have very well-developed and very well-structured behavior patterns with regard to professional communication. In more concrete language, these professions have, in the course of their development, worked out a rich set of customs, habits, traditions, mechanisms, tricks, and devices as to how one goes about obtaining information, what one does by way of screening and listening for information, and what one need not listen or attend to. Planners of information policies must take into account this body of behavior patterns, of traditions, customs, and learned behavior. The members of these specialized publics have developed communication institutions and learned ways of interacting with them and with one another to a much higher degree than is true, for example, for the public of a newspaper. Furthermore, scientists themselves look upon the communications services and systems as instruments, and take an interest in their improvement as technologies.

Of course, the several scientific publics also differ from one another in many of these aspects.[27] All of these aspects have implications for the wise planning of information services for these publics.

Science Information Systems Serve Multiple Functions

The last theme to be taken up here is that it is rather important to draw qualitative distinctions between the several kinds of things that the science information systems are called upon to perform, especially in this current age of streamlining, of great technological strides, of great advances in logical systems. The reason is that these advances bring with them some risk that they may make some of these functions be served more efficiently and satisfactorily, while neglecting or even hampering others. Most of the great innovations have been instituted under the guiding themes of speed, efficiency, and comprehensiveness. The overriding aim has been to bring information to scientists promptly, to bring all the information that is relevant to the scientist's specific query, and to do so with a minimum of waste motion. The prototype of that activity is the exhaustive search. But this is only one of several types of services that are required of the science information system. To give but one example of another type, with characteristics almost the opposite of those of the exhaustive search, there is the requirement to call the scientist's attention to relevant developments in fields which he has not recognized as pertinent to his own work.

Can policies designed to satisfy some of these requirements really work to the detriment of others? If search and retrieval services and selected distribution arrangements were working optimally, they would bring to each scientist exactly that which he has asked for and nothing else. But, by that very fact they would eliminate browsing, and would thereby put an end to the occasions when a scientist's attention is called to information which he had not appreciated as relevant to his own interests. This is just one example of perhaps the crudest kind of optimizing one science information function to the detriment of others.

But what actually are all the various kinds of functions that these information systems must perform; how many of them is it worth distinguishing? Distinctions along a number of axes have been suggested. The most basic criterion of classification is probably that of the scope and permanence with which the information needed by a particular scientist can be described in advance.[28] Along this dimension one can distinguish the exhaustive search; the reference function (to give the scientist the single best answer to a specific question); the current awareness function (to keep the person abreast of developments in his predetermined area of attention); a function which consists of stimulating researchers from time to time to seek information outside of their predesigned areas of attention; and a function which consists of enabling a scientist to follow through on this stimulation by "brushing up" or familiarizing himself with a well-defined field of inquiry which he had not previously included in his attention area. The two last-mentioned functions, it should be noted, transcend the informational requirements that each scientist can define for himself.

Conclusion

The themes enumerated above have implications for science information policy, but the translation of these implications into concrete steps requires that the themes be specified through a considerable amount of empirical research. As indicated in the opening paragraphs, much research on the use of information and information sources by scientists has been carried out, but until very recently the great variety and subtlety of potentially useful research questions and approaches was not realized. Discussions of "methodology" in this field all too often are confined to a consideration of data-gathering techniques. Insufficient attention has been paid to the more fundamental questions of the conceptualization of units of observation, the choice of variables to be considered, the causal models to be employed, and the analytic designs to be used.[29]

REFERENCES

1. Menzel, H. Comment. Coll. Res. Lib. 20: 419-420, 1959 (a).
2. Menzel, H. The Information Needs of Current Scientific Research. Lib. Quart. 34: 4-19, 1964.
3. Shaw, R. Review of "Flow of Information among Scientists." Coll. Res. Lib. 20: 163-164, 1959.
4. Paisley, W. J. The Flow of (Behavioral) Science Information—a Review of the Research Literature. Stanford: Stanford Univ., Institute for Communication Research, 1965. (Mimeo.)
5. Menzel, H. Information Needs and Uses in Science and Technology. In Cuadra, C. (Ed.) Annual Review of Information Science and Technology. Vol. 1. New York: Wiley, 1966 (c).
6. American Psychological Association. Reports of the American Psychological Association's Project on Scientific Information Exchange in Psychology. Vol. 1. Washington: APA, 1963.
7. American Psychological Association. Reports of the American Psychological Association's Project on Scientific Information Exchange in Psychology. Vol. 2. Washington: APA, 1965.
8. For an excellent and thorough laying out of the information system and its components in biomedical research, see Orr, R. H., Abdian, G., Bourne, C. P., Coyl, E. B., Leeds, A. A., and Pings, V. M. The Biomedical Information Complex Viewed as a System. Federation Proceedings, 23: 1133-1145, 1964.
9. APA, 1965, op. cit.
10. Menzel, H. Planned and Unplanned Scientific Communication. In Proceedings of the International Conference on Scientific Information. Washington: National Academy of Sciences, 1959 (b), pp. 199-243.
11. Menzel, H. The Flow of Information Among Scientists—Problems, Opportunities, and Research Questions. New York: Columbia University, Bureau of Applied Social Research, 1958, pp. 14-17, 32-49, 92-124. (Mimeo.) (Available as Technical Report 144390 PB from the Clearinghouse, Department of Commerce, Springfield, Va.)
12. Ackoff, R. L., and Halbert, M. M. An Operations Research Study of the Scientific Activity of Chemists. Cleveland: Case Institute of Technology, Operations Research Group, 1958. (Mimeo.)
13. APA, 1965, op. cit.
14. Herner, S. Information-Gathering Habits of Workers in Pure and Applied Science. Ind. Eng. Chem. 46: 228-236, 1954.
15. Menzel, 1959 (b), op. cit.
16. Orr, R. H., Coyl, E. B., and Leeds, A. A. Trends in Oral Communication among Biomedical Scientists. Federation Proceedings, 23: 1146-1154, 1964.
17. Pelz, R. C. Social Factors Related to Performance in a Research Organization. Admin. Sci. Quart. 1: 310-325, 1956.
18. Price, D. J. de S. Little Science, Big Science. New York: Columbia University Press, 1963.
19. Rosenbloom, R. S., McLaughlin, C. P., and Wolek, F. W. Technology Transfer and the Flow of Technical Information in a Large Industrial Corporation. Boston: Harvard Univ., Graduate School of Business Administration, 1965. 2 Vols. (Mimeo.)

20. Lazarsfeld, P. F., and Menzel, H. Mass Media and Personal Influence. In Schramm, W. (Ed.) The Science of Human Communication. New York: Basic Books, 1963, pp. 94-115.
21. Coleman, J., Katz, E., and Menzel, H. Medical Innovation—a Diffusion Study. Indianapolis: Bobbs-Merrill, 1966.
22. Menzel, H. Informal Communication in Science: Its Advantages and its Formal Analogues. In Bergen, D. (Ed.) The Foundations of Access to Knowledge. Syracuse: Syracuse Univ. Press, in press. (b).
23. Menzel, 1959 (b), op. cit.
24. APA, 1965, op. cit.
25. Menzel, 1959 (b), op. cit.
26. Rosenbloom, McLaughlin, and Wolek, op. cit.
27. Menzel, H. Sociological Perspectives on the Information-Gathering Practices of the Scientific Investigator and the Medical Practitioner. In McCord, D. (Ed.) Bibliotheca Medica: Physician for Tomorrow, Dedication of the Countway Library of Medicine. Boston: Harvard Medical School, 1966 (d).
28. For a fuller treatment, see Menzel, 1964, op. cit.
29. Some remarks on the conceptualization of units and on certain related methodological questions will be found in Menzel (30) on the variety of analytic designs embodied in recent studies in Menzel (31) and on the feasibility of inferring science information needs from the past uses made of information services in Menzel (32).
30. Menzel, H. Review of Studies in the Flow of Information among Scientists. New York: Columbia University, Bureau of Applied Social Research, 1960. 2 Vols. (Mimeo.) (Available as Technical Report 156 941 PB from the Clearinghouse, Department of Commerce, Springfield, Va.)
31. Menzel, 1966 (c), op. cit.
32. Menzel, H. Can Science Information Needs Be Ascertained Empirically? In Thayer, L. (Ed.) Communication: Concepts and Perspectives (Proceedings of the Second International Symposium on Communication Theory and Research). Washington: Spartan Books, 1966 (a).

Communications as a Basic Tool in Promoting Utilization of Research Findings

HAROLD P. HALPERT

WEBSTER'S New International Dictionary defines the word *communication* as "the act or action of imparting or transmitting." For those who are concerned with the utilization of research in mental health programs, this is only a partial definition. It needs to be expanded to include the purpose of communication. The people with whom we wish to communicate need to be specified and their anticipated action identified. Specifically, the communications are concerned with getting people who plan and conduct service programs to put into practice those principles and methods which incorporate the new knowledge gleaned from research and experimentation. A test of the efficacy of communication is its ability to translate research into altered behavior of key individuals.

Merely imparting or transmitting the results of research is usually insufficient. For example, as a guide for future planning, one mental hospital undertook to study the effect of the furnishings in dayrooms on patients' socialization patterns. One dayroom was furnished with Swedish Modern furniture and the other with Early American. Observation over a considerable period of time showed that the patients constantly favored the room with Swedish Modern furniture; they found it more congenial and comfortable. However, when the hospital needed new furniture, the staff responsible for requisitioning new supplies paid no attention to the results of this study. They ordered what they had always ordered, Early American furniture.

Here was research that was not utilized. Unfortunately, this is not an uncommon kind of occurrence. If the efficiency of research utilization was measured in terms of a rate developed by dividing the number of units applying the results of a particular piece of research by the total number of units capable of applying such results, it is probable that a very low score would ensue. Why it it that communications do not communicate in the full sense of the word? What goes wrong in such cases? What are the resistance and barriers to effective communication? How can these barriers be overcome and make communications effective in terms of research utilization?

Barriers to Useful Communication

One of the principal barriers to effective communication is the lack of transmission of findings. Operators of mental health programs who develop new methods and techniques frequently do not write them up—doers often are not writers. Allied to this problem is the lack of support for publication of research results. Who will pay the practitioner's salary while he writes his report? Where will he find space for his article in journals already filled up for a year or more in advance? Who will help defray page costs?

Increasing attention is being given to this problem. At a conference of editors of biological journals and national leaders meeting to study problems of scientific communication and information, Dr. David E. Price, then Deputy Surgeon General of the Public Health Service, declared, "It is clearly not enough to say that journals are simply reporting mechanisms. They are part of the research process itself." The conference took to task the attitude common among clinicians and practitioners that "any fool can write." Dr. Burton Adkinson of the National Science Foundation stated: "Information is an integral part of research and development. It should not be considered free for the asking. Publication charges should be accepted as an integral part of research and development costs." The conference had no ready answers to the problems of scientific communication. Various suggestions were made, such as facsimile newspapers and central and regional banks of information, but there was no clear definition of how to achieve effective communications. The underlying problem for any system of communications, mechanized or otherwise, is that it must be geared to meet specific and complex human needs.

People who operate programs frequently do not have time to read the literature extensively enough to pick up new findings—doers are not readers. Practitioners often find it easier to learn by looking, listening, and talking than by reading. Besides, the tremendous amount of scientific publication makes it extremely difficult to keep up with the literature. Even professional meetings have become "3-ring circuses" with much more material being presented than any one person can assimilate. In addition, a large percentage of research reports have little significance in terms of direct utilization. A good deal of winnowing of the literature needs to be done. Even where research reports contain material that can be utilized in operating programs, persons in service agencies often find it hard to see the practical implications. Researchers generally address themselves to an audience of other researchers or to the administrators and trustees of the foundations which have supported their research. In many instances, researchers are insufficiently motivated or unprepared to attempt to interpret their findings in terms useful for program implementation.

Methods to Overcome Barriers

Abstracts of reports and teaching manuals. A number of different methods are being used to help overcome this particular barrier to communication. One method is to analyze new knowledge in terms of the needs of operating agencies and to abstract and pinpoint the usable material so that busy doers will not become engulfed in a mass of new knowledge. Another method is the preparation of review papers containing comprehensive surveys of different mental health fields, i.e., aging, delinquency, and alcoholism, with guidelines for application of new techniques. It has been proposed that a group of research reviewers and lecturers be employed to prepare substantive reports on new research knowledge in various mental health areas, and that they give lectures on their specialities. There is increasing need for teaching aids, training and instruction manuals, and similar packages of helpful information with built in methods of evaluation.

Interdisciplinary conferences. To help develop such packages, some professional organizations are experimenting with special or regular meetings concentrated around specific themes in order to pull together accumulated knowledge in important areas. Research utilization conferences are proving to be extremely useful communication tools. There is also much need for conferences that will encourage greater communication among researchers themselves, particularly in mental health areas where research is being conducted concurrently in the biological, psychological, and social science disciplines. Adequate and readable reports of all such meetings and conferences need to be prepared and given wide distribution.

Written documents alone, however, are often insufficient to stimulate a change in practice. The reaction to such reports frequently is: "This may be all right for these people, but it won't work for us—our situation is different." Practitioners who read these reports frequently say, and often with some justification, that they make "specialty shop" recommendations that cannot be adapted to program operation on "bargain basement" budgets.

Evaluative visits to operating programs. Personal exposure to new programs may provide the necessary motivation for adoption of new practices—"Seeing is believing." One method of bringing this about is to provide funds so that people in operating programs can visit other programs to see what is new. Seeing it for themselves can help them make the necessary bridge to their own programs in terms that have meaning for them. This practical kind of demonstration can be of considerable value, particularly if visitors get a chance to talk to, and get to know the principal experimenters and prime movers in the new types of programs. If the demonstration is to lead to utilization, it must clearly indicate where the program is, how it got there, and where it is going. Frequently, new and very worthwhile programs are not as widely adopted as they might be because the lack of evaluative measures in the report or presentation makes it difficult for outsiders to see what the whole thing really proves. In their study on *Changing Attitudes Through Social Contact,* Festinger and Kelley[1] found that contacts are not effective in producing change if information alone is transmitted; value judgments and evaluative statements are essential to effective communication.

Shirt-sleeve consultants. The same study indicated that the effectiveness of communication depended upon a relationship between the person communicating and the person receiving the communication. Interest in a common task provides good soil for opinion and attitude changes. Some agencies have found it useful to engage consultants who do more than consult at the verbal level. These consultants actually become part of the operating program. They work along with the regular employees and show them how they can put new practices into effect. This kind of shirt sleeve consultation has proved to be successful in getting kitchens, laundries, and various other departments in mental hospitals to adopt new methods.

Practitioners Block Change

Of course, the extent to which such strategies can be employed to encourage research utilization is limited. It is much more difficult to get mature practitioners to admit that they ought to change. People who have been trained in a professional discipline tend to become professionalized, and to think in terms of their particular discipline rather than the area of need. This may explain part of the reason why many of the changes that come about as a result of research are inconsistent with the research findings. Findings often are reinterpreted to fit into preconceived patterns of behavior.

Though all practitioners are for progress, they frequently tend to see researchers as strangers and as members of alien professions. This, essentially, is the core communication problem that needs to be solved if we are to have effective research utilization. How can we reach people across the barrier of widely different system identifications?

Studying Research Utilization

Much attention was given to the subject of communication in the report submitted to the White House in April 1962 by the Behavioral Sciences Subpanel of the President's Science Advisory Committee. In summarizing the development and present state of knowledge in this field, the report emphasized two directions in which profitable research on communication has been conducted:

> The one assumes that contacts between individuals are governed largely by geographic distance ... the other takes account of the tendency of social networks to turn back on themselves, by giving numerical expression to the degree to which the friends of my friends are my friends ... [2]

The most recent studies of communication appear to indicate that there are limits to the spread of information dictated by geographic distance and social interrelationships. These limits serve as fire lanes which prevent the spread of new ideas and new practices from one system to another, and make it necessary to develop a planned set of linkages to help bridge the gaps.

Lippitt, at the Research Center for Group Dynamics, has enumerated three types of linkage that might be of conceptual value in dealing with problems of research utilization. The first of these is the establishment of intermediary roles. This type of linkage implies the development and use of consultants and other individuals who serve as communication links between researchers and practitioners. The second kind of linkage consists of planned interactions. This includes conferences, institutes, workshops, and other groupings which bring researchers and practitioners together. The third type of linkage involves administrative arrangements, such as appointing individuals to perform joint research-service functions. It also encompasses research training for clinicians, clinical experience for researchers, and similar methods of enforced dual functions. All three of these types of linkages, and particularly the first two, i.e., use of intermediaries and planned interactions, have been employed with less than optimum results in terms of research utilization.

Values and self-images within a system. Lippitt points out that the
effectiveness of linkage functions depends upon factors within the
systems that need to be linked together. The hierarchy of goals within
a system determines the extent to which it will utilize new knowledge
from outside the system. Scientific evaluation of practice, for example,
has a much lower status in the scale of organizational purposes in a
service agency than it does in a research agency. Values and self
images within a system are particularly crucial in determining whether
new ideas can penetrate. If anything, the practitioner who derives his
satisfaction from meeting people's needs is motivated against changing from practices which apparently have been successful. He is unwilling to change to a theoretically better procedure unless he can be
thoroughly convinced that it is better. This bar to communication,
this fire lane between systems, can be a very valuable safety device, it
can prevent premature assimilation of new practices.

Each system maintains its own integrity by the establishment of
boundaries which set it off from other systems. Researchers are researchers, practitioners are practitioners, and there is a difference between the two. The degree to which these boundaries are permeable
to influence from outside rests upon an awareness of their interdependence. The extent to which clinicians recognize their dependence
on new research knowledge will determine their willingness to accept
and to attempt to put that knowledge to use. The degree to which
researchers are interested in seeing their findings put to use will determine the efforts they make to relate their research to program needs.

Courses of Action

Two major courses of action are open to those who set about to insure greater research utilization. Completed research can be reviewed
and analyzed in terms of its applicability to service programs. Consumer needs can be analyzed before research is undertaken and an
attempt made to interest researchers in filling needs.

Classify research for consumer. Whichever course of action is taken,
the ultimate consumer must be determined. It is possible to pinpoint
consumers of specific kinds of research knowledge. Not all new information in the field of mental health is equally applicable for all program people working in the field. Planners of programs are consumers
for new knowledge resulting from epidemiological studies and research
on appropriate preventive measures. Professional workers who plan
and conduct clinical services are the logical consumers of research
knowledge on etiology, treatment, and rehabilitation. It is possible

to go down the line and classify research knowledge in terms of the practitioners who have the most need for, and can make use of, each type of knowledge.

Key practitioners as advocates of new ideas. Differentiation of target audiences can also help open the way to more effective communication with the various groups and organizations to which the different target practitioners belong. This will permit working through the in groups whose values they accept. Since members of any group or system are apt to be influenced more by active leaders within their own group or system than by outsiders, research utilization depends upon finding the kingpins in selected practitioner agencies and professional organizations and getting them to advocate the new practices. It is not easy, however, for the mature and respected practitioner to make a radical change with dignity. The most privileged members of any social system tend to resist change the most. One must find a key to help open the door to interpenetration of new ideas. One must find a privileged person, a respected practitioner, who is willing and wants to change, and can serve as a port of entry to a system of practitioners. Sometimes this key may not exist and it will take time to develop one. Where there is such a key, the whole research utilization process can be materially shortened. Sometimes prominent and respected public officials and political leaders, working through special commissions or conferences can help set new trends in motion.

Low paid staffs resist new practices. Rank and file practitioners also play an important role in determining whether new research findings will be put to use in changed services. Although it is true that the less privileged persons in any system usually do desire change, they are in a relatively poor position to bring it about. If their desire for change has been constantly thwarted, they may reach a point where they not only lose such a desire, but actively resist any effort to change. They fear that any change will be a change for the worse because no change they favored had ever been put into effect. The lower paid staff of some of the larger mental hospitals, for example, have tended to be less than enthusiastic about such new practices as the open ward and the therapeutic milieu.

Need of research in application methods. In addition to measuring the applicability of research and pinpointing the ultimate consumer of different types of new knowledge, it is essential to analyze the steps intermediate between research and its application. In many instances, basic research needs to be followed up with developmental research in order to find ways of putting the new knowledge to use.

After the developmental research has been conducted, inservice and professional training programs are required to teach people how to apply the knowledge. Inservice training programs are particularly important in motivating people to apply research findings. This training is intimately related to the values and rewards of service personnel and the practical structure of the system in which services are provided. Often, resistance to change can be overcome by personal involvement in the new types of programs. If practitioners, following the lead of a respected member of their profession or the administrator of their program, try out a new procedure, behavior change can serve as the prelude to attitude change. In itself, the adoption of the new technique can be a learning process.

Recommendations

Whatever methods of communication are employed, there are certain factors that must be kept constantly in mind in order to overcome the usual resistances to change.

1. Frames of reference within which individuals perform their professional tasks, and within which they think about and deal with social and health problems must be understood. For this reason, it is essential to work through leading practitioners and professional associations.

2. It is essential to take into consideration the motivation of the target audience, and the motivations they are likely to attribute to the people who ask them to change their ways of thinking and behaving. Appropriate ways of creating a desire for change in target audiences must be found and developed.

3. The validity and desirability of new practices must be related to the past experience of the target audience. New procedures need to be tied in with old ways of doing things as much as possible. One cannot "win friends and influence people" by telling them that everything they have been doing to date has been wrong. Rather, one must show people how new procedures can help them do the job they have been trying to do in a better way.

4. The things to which people are personally committed by direct participation are the things to which they usually owe greatest allegiance. The more ways in which practitioners can become directly involved in trying out new procedures, the more effective research utilization will be. It sometimes is possible to get practitioners to try out new procedures and techniques before they are fully convinced that these are the best possible procedures. If the new practices do prove to be useful, then attitude change will follow behavior change.

5. There is wide variation in individual response to communications of any kind. The changes in attitude and behavior that result from any form of communication vary in duration. Some people will accept change and then revert to former practices. Others will reject new ideas at first, but then later accept and apply them. Whatever method of communication is utilized, whatever the audience or target group, the message must be repeated over and over again to encourage utilization of new research knowledge.

REFERENCES

1. Festinger, L., and Kelley, H. H. Changing Attitudes through Social Contact. Ann Arbor: Research Center for Group Dynamics, Univ. of Michigan, 1951.
2. Life Sciences Panel, President's Science Advisory Committee. Strengthening the Behavioral Sciences. Washington: Government Printing Office, 1962.

This material was presented at a Conference on Research Utilization in Aging, in Bethesda, Md., May, 1963.

32

Symbolic and Substantive Evaluative Research

JOSEPH W. EATON

MUCH value is attached to research in a technologically oriented society. Research is frequently equated with development and progress.[1] Verbal espousal of research as a "good idea" is noncontroversial. But research costs money that could be used for more immediate operational purposes, and findings have to be interpreted. If the data are about organizational problems, their interpretations may be administratively disturbing, especially if suggestions for change are implied. As a consequence, ambivalent attitudes arise toward evaluative research, particularly in large organizations.

Symbolic Versus Substantive Evaluative Research

Research has two very different functions for organizations: a *symbolic* function and a *substantive* one. Science thrives on substantive research: the asking of questions, the gathering of data to explore them, the application of theory to explain the findings, and the communication of findings to others. Symbolic research, in contrast, characterizes studies of socially controversial topics. It involves ritualistic avowal of the value of research by staff members in organizational committees and in policy statements. Such a favorable verbal climate for research can be maintained as long as findings are not seen as threatening to positions of power or as questioning professional traditions or organizational policies. Symbolic research is an unintended consequence of the uncertainty element between two conflicting attitudes—the belief in the value of exploring the unknown, and the fear of disturbing positions of power or raising questions about existing agency operations.

In social work, as in nursing, psychiatry, and similar professions, an increasing number of evaluative studies are being published, but many of the findings of the more gifted practitioners are never written up, or they are filed away as being "inconclusive." Acceptance of the scientific credo favoring the publication of research is often overbalanced by organizational concern for disturbing the *status quo*. A symbolic approach is especially likely in studies that examine the validity of key policies normally taken for granted.

The discrepancy among professionally trained persons between their research interest and readiness to communicate research findings was explored in two large organizations by means of questionnaire surveys. The bulk of the data came from a sample of 282 Veterans Administration social workers.[2] An organization with a well-developed general policy favorable to research,[3] the Veterans Administration has also set high standards for the selection of social work personnel in keeping with its goal of maintaining a progressive organization.[4]

Supplementary data came from a survey of 94 per cent of the personnel of the California Department of Corrections. The department's interest in research is expressed in its large Research Division and in more than a decade of top echelon encouragement by staff persons for the examination of fundamental questions about key agency policies.

Three attitude clusters of employees were investigated:

1. *Research interest:* readiness to give research high priority among alternate organizational functions and to recommend allocation of resources for this purpose.

2. *Interpretation readiness:* predisposition to infer meaning from specific research data.

3. *Communication readiness:* predisposition to publicize research findings verbally and in written form.

Research Interest

The Veterans Administration social workers gave research a high priority in the use of unbudgeted funds, spare time, and training opportunities. More than one-third (35 per cent) ranked research first out of five alternate organizational activities that would warrant expansion (Table 1). Twenty-two per cent of the direct-service social workers and 32 per cent of their supervisors and administrators checked "do research" as their first or second choice in response to a question asking what they would want to do personally if they had more time (Table 2). Fifteen per cent would devote their time to study research and 4 per cent would engage in studies of miscellaneous subjects toward a Ph.D., in response to the following question: "What would you want to study or observe most if you were given a six months leave of absence with pay to study anything, anywhere you were interested?"

TABLE 1. FIRST AND LAST CHOICES OF VETERANS
ADMINISTRATION SOCIAL WORKERS TO SPEND A
$10,000 ANNUALLY RENEWABLE GIFT* (IN PER CENT).

Use of gift	First choice (N=275)	Fifth choice (N=227)†
Raise the starting social work salaries to recruit more qualified case workers	41	2
Support work on a research project regarded as important by the agency	35	7
Hire a psychiatric consultant	13	26
Improve the buildings, food, and facilities for inmates	8	43
Raise the starting salaries for custodial officers	3	22
Total	100	100

*Responses to the question: "If your agency received a ten thousand dollar annually renewable gift, what would be your priority for its use (number from one as highest to five as lowest)? Please rank all items."

†Some respondents did not rank all five items as instructed

Research was regarded highly by a significant minority of the Veterans Administration social work respondents. More than one-third were willing to give this function a top *organizational* priority. Not quite so many, 15 to 32 per cent, saw research as an activity in which they would *personally* participate.

California Department of Corrections personnel were somewhat less inclined to give research a high organizational priority. Twenty-five per cent of 337 persons with advanced education and 22 per cent of all 3,659 employees gave first choice to "hire research personnel" in response to a question about alternate uses of extra funds placed at the Department's disposal (Table 3).

Were the expressions of research interests related to what the respondents would recommend doing with evaluative research findings? To examine this question, the respondents were asked a number of questions designed to measure the readiness to *interpret* and the readiness to *communicate*, two prerequisites for performing a research role.

Readiness to Interpret

For the research scientist, it matters little whether a hypothesis is proved or disproved. Research is his primary function. For practi-

TABLE 2. HIGH PRIORITY PREFERENCES OF VETERANS
ADMINISTRATION SOCIAL WORKERS FOR
UNASSIGNED FUNCTIONS* (IN PER CENT).

Professional activity	1st and 2nd choices		
	Social caseworkers (N=210)	Supervisors & administrators (N=78)	Total (N=288)†
Do research (N=72)	22	32	25
Read books and journal articles relevant to my practice (N=70)	26	21	24
Engage in about the same kind of practice that I am doing (N=53)	17	23	18
Take on a few (more) cases for very intensive treatment (N=65)	26	14	23
Organize a special nonintensive service program for clients (N=28)	9	10	10
Total (N=288)	100	100	100

*Responses to the question: "Please assume that your agency received funds to permit each of its professional employees to reduce their present work load, giving you the freedom to devote *one day a week* to a professional activity of your choice. Which of the following would you choose? And in what order of priority?"

†Some of the 282 respondents give more than one response.

tioners, it is at best an ancillary function. Practitioners also have reason to react quite personally to evaluative research data. Findings may raise questions, not only about technique, but also about their own competency as users of the technique. Contrast, for instance, the role of physicians evaluating a new drug. They are examining a chemical, something in which they have no emotional involvement. In social work, as in psychotherapy, the treatment instrument, the professional worker, is also the main instrument of action. Discouraging findings tend to be interpreted as reflecting more than uncertainty about an impersonal technique. They could be a reflection on the competence of the person applying it. Only practitioners with a secure self-image will find it easy to become involved in evaluative re-

TABLE 3. PREFERENCES OF EMPLOYEES OF THE
CALIFORNIA DEPARTMENT OF CORRECTIONS FOR
SPENDING A GIFT OF $100,000* (IN PER CENT).

Recommendation	Professionals with advanced schooling (N=337)	All employees (N=3,659)
Hire more professional treatment staff (psychiatrists, psychologists and social workers)	34	31
Hire more research personnel	25	22
Pay merit bonuses to staff who do their work well	2	8
Establish a travel fund for needy dependents of prisoners who could not otherwise visit them	7	7
Build additional recreational facilities for inmates	2	7
Other (specify)	28	22
No answer	2	3
Total	100	100

*Responses to the question: "Assume you are an administrative assistant to the Director and you are asked to recommend how to spend a gift to the Department of $100,000, to be spent in any manner. What would be your recommendation? Check *only* one."

search about so personalized an aspect of treatment as their effectiveness as instruments of treatment.

It was not surprising, therefore, that the readiness to interpret was highest for findings which most respondents viewed as "encouraging" (Table 4). Preference for checking the "meaning unclear without more information" item was highest for findings judged by many as "discouraging." Forty-six per cent of all Veterans Administration social workers made *only* encouraging responses or avoided committing themselves. An additional 18 per cent never hazarded an interpretation. The readiness of the majority to interpret can be epitomized in the motto: *If you can't be positive, be tentative.* But a minority, about one in three, was ready to identify both the encouraging and discouraging implications of evaluative research data.

Accentuation of the "positive" can also be inferred from the responses of Department of Corrections employees to two similarly

TABLE 4. FINDINGS WHICH VETERANS ADMINISTRATION
SOCIAL WORKERS WERE ASKED TO INTERPRET.

Would you please read the following statements? Each is part of a plausible but imaginary outcome of a hospital program in an organization like yours. After each statement, please indicate what you think it means. Please check only *one* response to each statement, the one which comes closest to representing your opinion.

In January, 1955, the VA assigned a social worker to an intensive casework "Demonstration Ward" of patients. The following facts were discovered during a review of all case records and of work done in 1956-57. *

01. The average patient referred to the social worker was seen three times during the month. Weekly consultation meetings of varying length were held by the social worker with the ward nurse.

Encouraging evaluative evidence	67%
Discouraging evaluative evidence	3%
Meaning unclear without more information	30%

02. A record kept of 250 telephone calls from relatives about patients at the VA station showed the following evidence about anxieties:

	Patients without contact with the social worker	Patients with contact with the social worker
Per cent of relatives expressing anxiety about quality of the patient's care	75%	25%

Encouraging evaluative evidence	33%
Discouraging evaluative evidence	6%
Meaning unclear without more information	60%

03. Over one-third of the patients receiving intensive social casework were reported by ward nurses as "becoming more of a problem than they used to be" within the first six months of the beginning of participation in this therapeutic program. Among 100 patients on whom such information was collected, 10 went AWOL (absent without leave), 25 refused more than three times to go to their work detail, 8 had to be transferred to a closed ward.

Encouraging evaluative evidence	17%
Discouraging evaluative evidence	23%
Meaning unclear without more information	59%

04. Patients reported by the nurse to have a "very satisfactory " adjustment to life on the ward and a "good relationship" with her accounted for the majority (7 out of 10) of patients reported by the social worker as refusing casework help.

Encouraging evaluative evidence	15%
Discouraging evaluative evidence	20%
Meaning unclear without more information	64%

*Percentages are based on the opinions expressed by 282 respondents. No more than 1 percent failed to answer any one question.

phrased questions, one summarizing an encouraging finding about the effects of a treatment technique, the other having discouraging implications for practitioners. While the findings used in the Veterans Administration questionnaire were not based on any actual research report, those used in the Department of Corrections questionnaire summarized a trend that emerged from a number of departmental studies. It is probable that this fact was known to many employees, particularly the mental health personnel, who were providing therapeutic services. However, the 159 mental health specialists (social workers, sociologists, psychologists, psychiatrists, and correctional counselors with various academic backgrounds) did not differ much in their attitudes from 1,473 correctional officers. As Table 5 shows, both recommended "further study" for the discouraging finding more often than for the encouraging finding. All departmental staff members were more willing to publicize positive rather than negative data.

The readiness to interpret in both the Veterans Administration and the Department of Corrections was not related to research interest, as indicated by the respondents' priorities for the importance of research as an organizational function. The two attitudes seemed to be independent of each other. Employees who wanted to use a gift to do research or to hire more research personnel were as reluctant to accept discouraging implications of data as respondents giving a low priority to research.

Personal discussion with respondents elicited three attitudinal sets to explain their reluctance to interpret research findings. One might be termed a scientific rationale: Each of the findings mentioned in the questionnaire was sketchy. But if scientific prudence was a major factor here, why were so many Veterans Administration respondents reluctant to discuss these findings with fellow professionals who could be of help in interpreting them? As will be shown later, the respondents displayed little general readiness to communicate.

Other practitioners expressed reluctance to assume an unfamilar role—that of data interpretation—without consulting a research specialist. Practitioners have experience in dealing with individual cases, but many are hesitant to make generalizations in writing from their individual experiences to a category of cases. They do not see generalization as one of their job functions. Often they had the stereotyped notion that advancement of knowledge can come only through "experts."

There is also a tendency to believe that interpretative statements about practice involve organizational policy, and on policy matters organizational personnel are understandably cautious. They can

TABLE 5. READINESS OF PROFESSIONALS TO INTERPRET
ENCOURAGING VERSUS DISCOURAGING EVALUATIVE RESEARCH FINDINGS,*
DEPARTMENT OF CORRECTIONS, CALIFORNIA, 1959 (IN PER CENT).

Recommendation	Correctional officers (N=1,473)		Mental health personnel (N=159)	
	Encour-aging	Discour-aging	Encour-aging	Discour-aging
Recommend no release of findings at this time	6	10	1	3
Recommend that methodology and sampling techniques be re-examined and that the study be continued to get more information	24	44	31	50
Recommend findings with careful interpretation be released as confidential memo to staff only	10	10	7	7
Recommend that findings with careful interpretation be released as a technical report to a professional journal such as *Journal of Criminal Law and Criminology*	33	20	29	16
Recommend that findings with careful interpretation by agency research specialists be issued to newspapers	20	10	29	20
Recommend that the facts be released to newspapers for interpretation by their own feature writers	6	5	3	2
Unknown	1	1	–	2
Total	100	100	100	100

Encouraging finding: "Suppose a study showed that inmates in group counseling have *less trouble* in prison (violate fewer rules) than those who refused to participate. Assume you are a member of a Department-wide research advisory committee. What would be your recommendations with regard to publicizing the findings? Check one *only.*"

Discouraging finding: "Suppose a study showed that people in group counseling do *no better* on parole than those who refuse to participate. Assume you are a member of a Department-wide research advisory committee. What would be your recommendation with regard to publicizing this finding? Please check one *only.*"

count on departmental support only when they restrict their communication to the proper channels, beginning with their immediate
supervisor.

Readiness to Communicate

The advancement of knowledge comes from the sharing of discoveries. Information of general interest comes to the attention of every
professional, but professionals vary in their attitudes regarding its
communication. The evidence is strong that unfamiliarity with the
role of clinical research was common among Veterans Administration
social workers. To explore the balance of forces favoring or inhibiting
communication of research results, each of the 282 respondents was
asked to answer ten questions about every one of four hypothetical
research findings: "What would you do with the foregoing fact about
casework on the 'demonstration ward?' Assume that it applies to your
hospital and you are the first to learn about it. If in doubt about an
answer, please select the one that corresponds most closely to what
you would do." Five verbal and five written communication channels
were then mentioned. The respondents were asked to indicate whether
they would agree, be doubtful, or disagree with communicating the
facts through each of the channels. The results are given in Tables 6
and 7.

Verbal channels were preferred over written channels as a communication device for research results. In almost half the responses
(49 per cent) the Veterans Administration social workers were willing
to share the information verbally, but only 16 per cent were willing to
do this in writing. Supervisors and administrators expressed themselves
more often in favor of communicating research findings verbally, but
they and the more directly service-related social workers were equally
reluctant to have research data written up. Silence and ambivalence
predominated. Reluctance to communicate research findings was also
expressed by professionally trained persons in the California Department of Corrections. More recommended publishing a favorable evaluative research finding than a discouraging one. This was about equally
true of 41 master's-level social workers, 25 sociologists, and 35 psychologists, all of whom had at least a master's degree. Specialists in public
administration, education, and business administration seemed somewhat more public-relations minded. Table 8 indicates that they were
even less inclined to release discouraging data.

In both organizations, the readiness to communicate was unrelated
to expressed research interest. Respondents who gave research a high

TABLE 6. PREFERENCE OF VETERANS ADMINISTRATION SOCIAL
WORKERS REGARDING VERBAL CHANNELS FOR COMMUNICATION
OF EVALUATIVE RESEARCH FINDINGS.

Preference	Per cent agreeing to communicate		
	Social caseworkers (N=201)	Supervisors & administrators (N=81)	Total (N=282)
Report facts orally to your immediate supervisor	85	89	86
Keep this fact to yourself until someone asks about it	73	84	76
Report the facts orally to a special staff meeting of social workers, staff physicians and nurses	46	52	48
Tell fellow workers I can trust	20	21	20
Informally tell hospital administrator	8	33	15
	(N=1,005)	(N=405)	(N=1,410)
Summary of responses to all 5 questions	46	56	49

or a low priority as a personal or agency activity were equal in their degree of disinclination to publish research information. The two attitudes appeared to be independent variables.

Verbal Communication

The usage of verbal communication channels generally conformed with organizational expectations. The social workers (86 per cent) were quite willing to report research data verbally to their immediate supervisor, but less than half thought it wise to report the facts verbally at a special staff meeting of social workers, physicians, and nurses. Interprofessional teamwork is espoused strongly to improve the quality of service to patients, but when research data about social work practice were involved, more social workers expressed self-censorship attitudes than a readiness to discuss these findings with colleagues from related disciplines, although the findings involved thought-provoking data about interprofessional relationships.

Very few respondents were willing to discuss their research findings with the hospital administrator. Only 8 per cent of the direct-service social workers and one-third of their supervisors and administrators

TABLE 7. PREFERENCE OF VETERANS ADMINISTRATION SOCIAL
WORKERS REGARDING WRITTEN CHANNELS FOR COMMUNICATION
OF EVALUATIVE RESEARCH FINDINGS.

Preference	Per cent agreeing to communicate		
	Social caseworkers (N=201)	Supervisors & administrators (N=81)	Total (N=282)
Report the facts in writing to your immediate supervisor	30	42	34
Suggest this fact be included in the next monthly administrative report	27	35	29
Suggest the facts with detailed interpretations be incorporated in an article about your agency for publication in a professional journal	18	10	16
Submit the facts to patient newspaper	1	0	1
Suggest that the public relations officer furnish this information to the press. This fact could be newsworthy	0	0	0
	(N=1,005)	(N=405)	(N=1,410)
Summary of responses to all 5 questions	15	17	16

were willing to tell the hospital administrator informally about the research findings. One plausible explanation for their reluctance might be that very few of the respondents knew the administrator well enough to discuss any hospital problem informally. But even two-thirds of the supervisors and administrators who interacted frequently with the chief administrator were doubtful or disagreed with the idea that he be told informally about research findings that had come to their attention.

Supervisors and administrators were more ready than social workers to recommend the communication of evaluative research findings through verbal channels. But they were more reluctant than their practice-oriented colleagues to put their ideas in writing. This finding would not have been predicted since supervisors are very dependent on the willingness of lower-echelon professional personnel to write records about their work with clients. Only 17 per cent of the super-

TABLE 8. READINESS OF UNIVERSITY–TRAINED PROFESSIONALS TO
COMMUNICATE ENCOURAGING AND DISCOURAGING EVALUATIVE RESEARCH
FINDINGS,* DEPARTMENT OF CORRECTIONS, CALIFORNIA, 1959.

	No public release		Journal or newspaper publication	
Professions (N=337)	Encouraging finding	Discouraging finding	Encouraging finding	Discouraging finding
Master of Arts or more	%	%	%	%
Social work (N=41)	45	61	54	36
Sociology (N=25)	44	64	56	36
Psychology (N=34)	47	59	53	39
Public adm. (N=9)	44	78	55	22
Psychiatry (N=21)	38	67	62	33
Bachelor of Science				
Education (N=126)	40	70	60	29
Correctional adm. (N=38)	48	66	50	32
Business adm. (N=43)	37	70	63	30

*Encouraging and discouraging finding defined as in Table 5.

visors expressed a definitely favorable attitude toward communication through written channels. Their strong inclination toward self-censorship was not consistent with their dependence on written data from others in order to perform their jobs.

Written Communication

Verbal communication of research findings is restricted to persons who meet each other and can interact directly; wider dissemination of scientific knowledge is obtained when research findings are published. Social worker respondents showed great reluctance to use written channels, in spite of the fact that they were accustomed to writing detailed clinical reports. As many as two-thirds of them agreed with the idea of reporting research findings in writing to their immediate supervisor, but only 29 per cent were willing to have the information disseminated through the entire organization in the next monthly administrative report. Not quite 16 per cent were willing to have "the facts with detailed interpretation incorporated in an article about your agency for publication in a professional journal." The vast majority of respondents, including 90 per cent of the supervisors and administrators, were doubtful or disagreed with the use of scholarly journals to report the research data.[5]

Supervisors and administrators were somewhat more favorably inclined than direct-service practitioners toward the use of intra-organization written channels, such as getting the facts reported in writing to their immediate supervisor or having them included in the next monthly administrative report. Nonadministrative social workers were more willing than their superiors to communicate research findings to the general public and to fellow professionals and scientists.

Readiness to Self-Censor

Professionally trained persons in two large treatment-oriented organizations with high standards of service to clients exhibited a marked degree of readiness to censor evaluative research findings. In the Department of Corrections academically trained members of professions exhibited self-censorship attitudes even when the research findings had favorable implications. In the Veterans Administration only one of twenty social workers expressed a readiness to use all of five verbal channels of communication. Six per cent would use none. Not a single one of the 282 respondents was willing to use more than three of the five *written* communication channels. And almost half (49 per cent) were not willing to communicate research findings through any of the written channels suggested. (See Table 9.)

The reluctance to communicate evaluative research findings was observed in organizations other than the Veterans Administration and the Department of Corrections. Essentially the same schedule used in the Veterans Administration study was administered to small samples of social workers in two mental hospitals, a university hospital, and a prison. The findings were essentially the same.[6]

Practitioners in the social service professions are not alone in their reluctance to communicate evaluative research data. Military, governmental, and hospital administrators tend to mark as "secret" research data about important operational variables. Theodore Caplow and Reece J. McGee report that some universities, which have as their primary function the dissemination of knowledge, show strong tendencies toward censorship of information about their own administration. This generalization is derived from a study of hiring, firing, and other personnel practices in ten leading universities:

> The presidents of five state universities responded promptly and favorably to the request to cooperate, but five private universities

TABLE 9. READINESS OF VETERANS ADMINISTRATION SOCIAL
WORKERS TO COMMUNICATE RESEARCH FINDINGS (IN PERCENT).

Communication readiness	Verbal channels*	Written channels*
Always (five times)	5	–
Four times	14	–
Three times	29	4
Twice	31	19
Once	15	28
Never	6	49
Total (*N*=282)	100	100

*Verbal and written channels as defined in Tables 6 and 7.

that were approached proved somewhat less responsive. One of
them rated "among the greatest of the world" never answered
the letter requesting their cooperation. In a subsequent personal
interview, the President refused to countenance any research not
conducted by persons who were not alumni. Another university
president refused to participate for technical reasons. The three
remaining private institutions required rather elaborate explanations and eventually gave consent and cooperated fully. But at
one of them the researchers were requested to avoid any discussion of salaries. At a state university the Dean of the Arts College
objected at one period to the inclusion of "controversial" cases in
the sample, but subsequently he withdrew this objection.[7]

Discussion

Communication of research findings is necessary for the advancement of knowledge. Some scientific research is even exempt from the
cold war. Research results are shared between Russian and American
scientists in many nonmilitary areas. The strongly positive value
placed on unhampered communication distinguishes scientific from
business and governmental organizations, where secrecy is often in-
sisted upon. The creed of the scientist favors communication; so do
the mores of professionally trained practitioners. In social work
agencies, for instance, workers are expected to share what they learn
with their supervisors. Collaboration among practitioners from several
professions can only be successful if each shares knowledge which is
relevant to the work of others. Administrators cannot make rational
policies without access to findings obtained by their subordinates.

The normative pressure to communicate is further enhanced by
the positive value attached to dissemination of news in our society.
The "right to know" is avowed by a powerful press, radio, and television industry. "Secrecy" or "censorship" are not popular words;
they have to be defended when employed. Regard for communication is perhaps greatest among scientists. Their reputation is related
to the knowledge they are able to transmit to others. Keeping specialized knowledge secret, patenting it, or maintaining a monopoly regarding its use is more characteristic of business than of science and
the professions. But these social forces favoring communication are
opposed by forces which discourage it. Individuals and groups in all
professions are reluctant to communicate findings that reflect nega-
tively on their work. Access to disappointing medical information is
often withheld from persons outside the profession on the assumption that "they lack the background" for interpreting the data. This
is often done in the name of medical "ethics."

Communication of research is also inhibited by standards of mod-
esty and reluctance among certain practitioners to assume the role of
scholar. "Who am I to make pronouncements?" or "Probably everyone knows this already" are expressions often used to explain the
failure to publish research data. Others question that generalizations
can be made about practice, which they view as an "art," too elusive
for substantive research. Still others may be reluctant to become involved in controversy, which is likely to arise when people publish
research with action implications. Their professional standing might
be tarnished, they feel, by those who could cite contradictory data and
engage them in a scholarly battle of wits.

The communication of research findings is also influenced by bureaucratic considerations. Many workers in large organizations feel
inhibited about expressing themselves about the results of their work
without prior clearance through complex administrative channels.
Such permission is on occasions denied, especially if top-echelon administrators have fears that the findings could lead to organizational
problems.

In this study the reluctance of professionals to make interpretations
of evaluative research data and the even greater disinclination to
communicate their findings contradicts the strongly favorable policy
of both the Veterans Administration and the Department of Corrections toward research. In both organizations the publication of findings is officially encouraged and is a way to hasten promotion. The
question therefore arises: What accounts for the discrepancy between

the readiness to censor research findings and the official policy of these organizations? While our Veterans Administration data are based on the responses of social workers, a comparison of the communication readiness of social workers, sociologists, psychologists, and other professionals in the Department of Corrections shows no significant difference between them. (See Table 8.) Why did all these university-trained professionals more often favor symbolic than substantive research?

Caution and tentativeness are functional for many people working in a bureaucracy. In the type of bureaucracy studied here, the day-to-day operations of a department are evaluated on the basis of such criteria as the number of cases seen, the working relationships between one specialty and other professionals, the infrequent occurrence of remission, the frequency of cures, and testimonials about the value of a practice by clients and their families. Professional services like social case work and group counseling have grown, expanded, and become accepted on the basis of circumstantial evidence; their validity is often uncertain.

The discussion or publication of research findings carries with it the threat that organizational attention will be focused on the section of the institution in which research is done. In a Veterans Administration hospital, in which social work may be the only segment ready to study its own operations, such attention could lead to widespread discussion of the role and functions of the social work department. Practices and policies that have been taken for granted for a long time could be reviewed and perhaps modified. Reasoning such as this led some of our respondents to conclude that it might be best "not to be noticed" rather than to take the risk of attracting too much attention to their department.

Like other loyal members of an organization, they accepted the notion that it is necessary to be selective about what is to be communicated to "outsiders." They question that their work can be assessed by persons who are not specialists. Such reluctance to communicate involves the risk of losing public support, since the success of a program is largely dependent on the understanding and support of "outsiders." Boards of directors, budget makers, and the public must be convinced of the necessity for a social service if it is to continue and, if need be, to expand.

The possibility should also be considered that the reluctance to make interpretations of the data and to communicate them is to some extent an expression of the preference of scientists and practitioners not to jump to premature conclusions. The hypothetical research findings in our questionnaire were sketchy. They raised many more questions than they could possibly answer. Investigators often prefer to deliberate in private, during which time they are free to engage in trial and error methods. Some of the Veterans Administration social work respondents who expressed a high priority for research as an agency and a personal activity but were reluctant to publish the findings might have acted on the basis of this preference. But even more of them were unwilling to communicate these findings verbally to colleagues in other departments of the hospital whose knowledge and experience could contribute to explaining them. It is therefore hard to escape the conclusion that the great majority of these respondents were generally inclined to be tentative about interpretation and censorship-minded about evaluative research data. While acknowledging the desirability of supporting and doing research in theory, they rejected in practice the substance of this function: interpretation of findings and their communication.[8]

Attention needs also to be given to the existence of a minority of respondents in each organization with favorable attitudes about interpretation and communication of findings. This minority is an available reference group for those who conduct research in practice settings. The fact that the studies on which this report is based could be undertaken illustrates that organizational cautiousness in many employees is not an absolute barrier to evaluative research. Ritualistic concern with data collection and a tendency to censor findings that might give rise to administrative problems are characteristic of all bureaucratic institutions. Such tendencies can best be overcome if research workers are aware of their existence and make appropriate allowance for them in planning their research.

Summary

Social programs are always evaluated by the professional worker, his administrative superiors, clients, and the public. But the methods used in evaluation and the degree to which the resulting findings are communicated are affected by the practitioners' attitudes about research as a personal and organizational function. A symbolic rather than a substantive approach to research predominated among the respondents studied in this research. Those expressing a high priority for the use of agency funds or staff time for research were not willing to publish findings. The majority of respondents expressed a reluctance to interpret evaluative data. There was greater readiness to interpret encouraging findings than discouraging ones. The predominant attitude was to be tentative unless one could be positive.

The Veterans Administration social workers were particularly reluctant to favor the communication of research findings to persons whom they regarded as "outsiders," whom they did not trust to understand the complications of their work. The immediate supervisor was most often the person chosen to be informed about research findings. Much less often was there willingness to report to an interdepartmental staff conference and even less to inform hospital administrators. Verbal communication channels were preferred over written ones. More practitioners were willing to report research findings in writing to their immediate supervisor than to see them reach a more general professional audience or the general public. The inclination toward self-censorship was not consistent with the dependence of all professionals in general and supervisors in particular on getting information from others to perform their jobs.

Most of these generalizations are based upon a sample of social workers in one large organization. But supplementary data from other service organizations and professions suggest the existence of a general preference for a symbolic rather than substantive use of research about practice problems. In such evaluative studies the ideology of science, which favors the communication of research results, is often believed to conflict with organizational mores and interests. Only a minority of respondents clearly expressed an attitude favorable to assuming the risk of criticism which exists when information with evaluative implication is widely disseminated. The future of evaluative research may rest on this minority and on organizational encouragement of their readiness to communicate.

NOTES AND REFERENCES

1. Novick, D. What Do We Mean by "Research and Development"? Ill. Bus. Rev. 16: 6-8, 1959. Novick estimates that about ten billion dollars were spent in 1960 on research and development. The high prestige of research as a function is largely derived from the fact that new discoveries are made on occasion which advance the existing level of general knowledge. But only about 1 per cent of the funds go into what he calls "brave new worlds" or basic research. Many of the activities undertaken in the name of research are applied investigations in large organizations to make more use of existing knowledge.
2. Twenty-seven Veterans Administration stations in the western region and nineteen stations in other parts of the United States were included in the study. For more details about the characteristics of the Veterans Administration respondents, see Eaton, J. W. Professional Participation of Social Workers. Social Work, 6 116-118, 1961.

3. Office of the Chief Medical Director, Veterans Administration. Program Guide, Social Work Service (Series G-1, M-2, Part XII; Washington, D.C., Aug. 16, 1957), pp. 37-41. For details about ongoing research see the following publications prepared for the House Committee on Veterans Affairs: 85th Congress, 1st Sess. Vol. I, Print No. 50, April 26, 1957; 85th Congress, 2nd Sess., Print No. 188, May 6, 1958; 86th Congress, Print No. 4, Vol. I, Jan. 30, 1959, and Print No. 50, Vol. II, May 29, 1959; and 86th Congress, 2nd Sess, Print No. 218, June 15, 1960.

4. Only about 5 per cent of the social work employees had less than two years of graduate education. The 282 respondents who participated in our survey had the same sex distribution as all social workers in the Veterans Administration; 60 per cent were female. But persons with professional education were over-represented. Only 2 per cent of our sample had less than two years of graduate education, and 11 per cent had three or more years of postgraduate work, 1 per cent higher than that in the Veterans Administration at large.

5. Almost no one was willing to submit the findings to a patient newspaper or to suggest that the public relations officer furnish the information to the press. Reluctance to use the press to publicize research data is common among research scientists. It is related to fear of being misquoted and the occasional sensationalized reporting of findings.

6. Beal, L., Daygee, J., Gendel, S., Kosower, G., La-Anan, J., Premak, S., and Spiegel, D. The Nature of Communication of Program Outcome. A joint report submitted in partial satisfaction of the requirements for the degree of Master of Social Welfare. Los Angeles: Univ. of California School of Social Welfare, 1958. This pilot study, under the supervision of the writer, plus the administration by him of the instrument to a small sample of the social service staff of another mental hospital, showed results consistent with those of the Veterans Administration.

7. Caplow, T., and McGee, J. The Academic Market Place. New York: Basic Books, 1958, pp. 33-35.

8. Symbolic research is an adaptation to value conflicts which Robert K. Merton calls ritualism. Lofty cultural goals (discovery of knowledge) are scaled down or abandoned, but the means to obtain them are not rejected. Symbolic research involves a lowering of the level of aspiration of professionals for the outcome of research, while retaining espousal of the data-gathering process. See Merton, R. K. Social Theory and Social Structure. Glencoe: Free Press, 1957, pp. 149-152.

Data used in the report were gathered with the help of persons employed in the Veterans Administration and the California Department of Corrections. Research assistance and faculty time for this study were provided by a small grant of the Southern Senate of the University of California, Project OM 89-R of the National Institute of Mental Health, and the University of Pittsburgh.

33

Research, Program Planning, and Evaluation

PAUL M. DENSEN, GEORGE JAMES, and EDWARD COHART

RESEARCH has been an integral part of the activities of the New York City Department of Health since its inception. The department has had a succession of commissioners who were not only able administrators but who recognized the intimate relationship between research and the service functions of the department. They were also aware of the debt that modern public health owes to the early researchers in bacteriology and sanitary science.

Control of infectious diseases requires constant vigilance, but the need for research in chronic diseases has become more pressing. The attack on the chronic diseases proceeds in three stages: study of the fundamental biological mechanism at work producing the disease state, study of the epidemiologic characteristics of the various chronic diseases, and program research and evaluation to translate the gains achieved through laboratory or epidemiologic investigation into programs of benefit to the population.

This three-way research approach is mounted through three units of the department of health. The oldest of these, the Public Health Research Institute, was organized in 1941 as a private nonprofit corporation to perform fundamental health research in New York City. Its activities focus on fundamental biological research in the laboratory. It is concerned, for example, with such basic biological questions as the nature of the antigen-antibody relationship.

The second unit is the Health Research Council of the City of New York. The council's major aim is the mobilization of the resources of the medical community of New York City against the municipality's health problems. It provides grants for studies both in the laboratory and in the community. In 1965 the council supported 172 research investigators, thus increasing the trained research manpower available for the study of city health problems. From the biological point of view, New York's health problems do not differ from those of other communities—except in size—so the work supported by the Health Research Council also contributes to public health in the country as a whole.

With these major research approaches mapped out, the health department felt that it should create an internal focus charged with the responsibility of stimulating activities in the chronic disease area. In a letter to the director of the bureau of the budget, dated March 29, 1956, Commissioner of Health Leona Baumgartner explained her reasons for establishing what was then called the "Office of Scientific Program Planning and Development." The name was later changed to the Office of Program Planning, Research, and Evaluation:

> I am more convinced than ever of the necessity for a section within the department devoted to public health program planning and development. While it is recognized that program planning constitutes an essential element of good administrative practice and should not be divorced from administration, experience has shown that the pressures of day-to-day administration are such, as to limit very severely the time and the thinking devoted to evaluation and development. Often, despite the best intentions of program directors to examine their programs critically, evaluation is deferred indefinitely in the face of more immediate claims upon their time. As a result, programs or parts of programs that have outlived their usefulness and methods that no longer mesh with the mechanisms of a changing society, continue in operation.

Having set forth the reasons for the establishment of an office of program planning, research, and evaluation, it is the purpose of this paper to describe how the office carries out these functions, to illustrate the reciprocal relation of the work of the office and the service programs of the department, and to consider certain requirements which must be met if this relationship is to realize its potential.

The functioning of the Office of Program Planning, Research, and Evaluation (termed the Office of Research subsequently in this paper) is best described through specific activities. These may be grouped under three headings: (a) evaluation, (b) program planning, and (c) research on emerging problems.

Two Examples of Evaluation

Lower East Side Manhattan cardiac program.[1] A 1946 survey by cardiologists suggested that many school children with heart disease were not being identified and that others with neither organic heart disease nor valid histories of rheumatic fever were being followed as "cardiacs." In addition to routine casefinding and follow-up by the school health service, two types of specialized services were provided then to assist school physicians. The health department's division of physically handicapped children provided approval or disapproval by a reviewing cardiologist of all applications for changes in type of class placement and referral for examination by a cardiologist at borough cardiac consultation clinics of children not already under care.

Because these services reached only a small, selected group of children, a pilot program, the Lower East Side rheumatic fever project, was established in the department of preventive medicine of New York University. It was sponsored by the department of health, the board of education, and the New York Heart Association and financially supported by the heart association and the Public Health Service. Its objectives were the following:

1. Find all children with suspected heart disease or rheumatic fever.

2. Attempt to confirm all reported diagnoses.

3. Follow all children with diagnoses in need of clarification as well as those with confirmed heart disease or histories of rheumatic fever to be sure that they received the medical and nonmedical services they needed and that the services were integrated.

4. Serve as a clearinghouse for information on individual children suspected of having rheumatic fever or heart disease and on the community services available to them.

5. Collect information on the incidence and prevalence of rheumatic fever and heart disease among school children in one area of New York City and on the services available to them, and stimulate improvement of existing services and development of new ones when the need arose.

The table from the report of this program illustrates the need for such activity. Brownell and Stix[1] indicate that "These efforts have paid large dividends in terms of the 'delabeling' of children falsely diagnosed as having rheumatic fever or heart disease and thus of fewer children followed needlessly by the school health service. At the same time follow-up of those correctly diagnosed has improved."

In 1963, after the program had been evaluated, conversations were begun by the Office of Research with the administrators of maternal and child health and the division of nursing about extending the program to the entire city. Handling of rheumatic fever cases was found to differ considerably in various parts of the city. Therefore a set of uniform procedures was developed and recommendations made to the commissioner for putting these into effect. A plan for the evaluation of the citywide experience was also developed, and evaluation data are now being collected.

PERCENT OF ADMISSION DIAGNOSES CONFIRMED AND CHANGED
ON REGISTER, LOWER EAST SIDE RHEUMATIC FEVER PROJECT,
JANUARY 1, 1951 – DECEMBER 31, 1958

	Heart disease diagnosis on admission to register				
Last heart disease diagnosis	All diagnoses (N=4,259)	Possible disease (N=525)	Rheumatic fever (N=2,818)	Congenital defect (N=863)	Other or unknown etiology (N=53)
Total	100.0	100.0	100.1	99.9	100.1
Confirmed:					
No disease	14.1	52.4	9.3	6.6	13.2
Possible disease	4.4	23.8	.9	4.1	3.8
Rheumatic fever	50.2	[1]6.4	74.0	.3	28.3
Congenital defect	18.0	[1]5.9	.7	82.7	5.7
Disease of other or unknown etiology.	.8	[1]1.0	.3	.2	34.0
Unconfirmed	12.5	10.5	14.9	6.0	15.1

[1] Cases with insufficient information on first report to make a more definite diagnosis possible.

Satellite clinics. Recently the U.S. Children's Bureau embarked upon a nationwide maternal and infant care project. This program was designed to concentrate efforts for improving the care of mothers and infants in areas in which vital statistics revealed serious problems. In the City of New York the program, designed as clinics functioning as satellites of a hospital, costs nearly $1.5 million a year, and it is imperative that an evaluation of effectiveness be an integral part of the program. The commissioner of health directed the heads of the Office of Research and the maternal and child health program to collaborate on an evaluation of the satellite clinics. Its main feature is that the geographic residence area of women coming to a satellite clinic will be delineated and designated as the "study area." A geographic area without a satellite clinic, where women receive their care through the normally available facilities, will be designated as the "control area." Women in the control area will be matched with those in the study area by a number of characteristics. Three examples of measurements to be made follow:

1. RESIDENCE AREA MEASUREMENTS. These will generally consist of the usual vital statistics pertaining to maternal and child health, such as infant mortality rate, perinatal mortality rate, and proportion of women who first come in for care during the various trimesters of pregnancy.

2. PATIENT MEASUREMENTS. For example, the pattern a woman follows who comes to the satellite clinic in her third pregnancy will be compared with her actions in her second pregnancy, when no satellite clinic was available. The outcome of the woman's third pregnancy will also be compared with the outcome of the third pregnancy of a woman coming to the clinic during her fourth pregnancy. The stage of pregnancy in which she first sought care will be examined, and other measurements will be made. Thus, measurements will be made specific for the particular order of pregnancy and the number of previous infant losses of the mother.

3. PROGRAM MEASUREMENTS. What is the efficiency of the program? At what rate are appointments kept? What referrals are made? How many persons carry them out?

These examples illustrate the need for concern with the process of evaluation and review of continuing activities. They also illustrate the desirability of building evaluation into a program from its inception. Finally, they demonstrate the intimate relationship between evaluative processes and program development.

Program Planning Activities

Selective Service. Early in 1961 the Armed Forces Selective Service System and the Public Health Service began discussions about the men rejected by Selective Service for health reasons. The New York City Department of Health at that time received a phone call asking if the department would be interested in developing a demonstration program for referring these men to community resources to help them with their health defects. The telephoner from the Public Health Service was a former Service trainee who had spent a year with the New York City Department of Health on research, program planning, and evaluation. He had called New York's health department because he knew of its interest in new approaches to community health problems.

In October 1962 the department began a demonstration program. Each man rejected for health reasons by the New York City Selective Service System was referred by public health nurses of the health department referral service to an appropriate community health resource (private physician or agency) for care. By August 1, 1965, 18,270 rejectees had been registered for the program.

The procedures have served as a model for the development of similar programs in other cities and states, and staff members have been consulted in the development of referral services. The findings formed part of the request to Congress for funds to develop a nation-wide program. This referral service is now integrated into the health department under the assistant commissioner, preventable and chronic disease services.

In addition to the immediate objective of taking care of health problems of selective service rejectees, this program is significant for two other reasons. First, the Selective Service System may be viewed as a kind of community health screening program which identifies the individual citizens with health problems. Before the health department's referral service was developed, these men were returned to the community with no provision for health care. Assuming that the earlier health problems are brought under care the better the prognosis, the desirability of referral programs is clear.

The experience of the selective service referral program suggests the possible use of other already available screening procedures as a source of cases for referral services. Some of these would be pre-employment examinations for industry, applications for disability insurance in the programs of the division of vocational rehabilitation, and applications for life insurance. These screening points could be developed into a generalized casefinding mechanism and referral service if systematic procedures were instituted.

Second, the selective service program offers the opportunity for development of two specific research projects, health of the school child and mental health problems. The rejectees for health reasons have been out of school but a short time. A Public Health Service grant to study the relationship between the school health records of these former students and the reasons for their rejection by the Selective Service System has recently been awarded to the department.

The opportunity for mental health research is an outcome of the finding that in New York City 38 percent of the health rejectees were rejected for psychiatric reasons. "Psychiatric reasons" is an Armed Forces classification; the percentage cannot be taken as representing the prevalence of psychiatric conditions among young men subject to the Selective Service System because not all men receive a psychiatric examination.

The number of these young men is sizable—4,544 in the New York City area in the first 2 years of operation of the selective service program. Many are difficult to motivate to take care of their health problems. One approach is to develop a demonstration program offering psychiatric rejectees a variety of services preparatory to referral in addition to the normal services available to all rejectees. Those in the special service program would then be compared with those in the regular program.

Another approach is to follow for 5 years a group of men rejected for psychiatric reasons (but not served by a special department program) to determine how well they adjust to civilian life. This group would be compared with a group entering the health department's special referral program. A grant application is being developed to study this approach.

Thus the initial inquiry from the Public Health Service led to the development of demonstration programs to aid young men rejected from the Armed Forces for health reasons and the assumption of these programs as part of the normal activities of the department. The findings led to a national program for these young men and development of further research on important health problems, growing out of the original project, made possible by the availability of data on a particular population. The research is directly related to the planning of effective school health services and the best means of meeting the mental health needs of young men.

Medical care. Today health departments are called upon to exercise leadership in seeing that adequate medical care programs are provided for people in their jurisdictions. The pressing reasons for such leadership were listed recently.[2]

1. Increasing numbers of persons with chronic diseases. The only adequate method at the present time for control of the diseases is good medical care.

2. Increasing urbanization. It is largely in urban centers that the demand exists for adequate medical care for large populations.

3. The need to find new ways to move the results of research in laboratories and at the bedside into the community to benefit the entire population.

For these reasons the health department has entered into a number of cooperative arrangements with voluntary hospitals in the city, seeking new ways to provide better medical care for citizens. While details of the arrangements differ, each hospital assumes responsibility for the complete medical care of the persons in the population which it serves. The Office of Research aids each project director in developing methods of evaluation. The Office of Research, at the request of project directors, also takes the initiative in bringing groups together periodically to discuss mutual problems and to consider how comparable information can be obtained from the various projects, so that the entire program can be assessed and made more generally useful for those planning programs for the entire city.

Specific chronic diseases. Much research has been done on specific chronic diseases, such as coronary disease and cancer, and additional information is constantly becoming available about the epidemiology of these conditions and the risk factors involved. However, translating research findings into service programs to control these diseases in the population has received relatively little attention. It may be argued that control programs would be premature since the etiology remains clouded, but certain risk factors have been identified. Perhaps a broad casefinding program to identify persons with these risk factors might suggest ways to develop control programs or initiate demonstrations.

The Framingham studies show that persons with raised serum cholesterols, who smoke, and who are overweight have a much greater risk of developing coronary disease than those without these risk factors. Could a health department offer practicing physicians a service to help identify high-risk persons in their practice? Could a control program, perhaps involving dietary advice for those with increased cholesterols, be developed? The Office of Research and the appropriate program directors are exploring ways of developing such programs.

Research on Emerging Problems

Chronic respiratory disease. Death certificate information routinely analyzed by the health department confirms that the chronic respiratory diseases are of growing importance in public health. However, research in these diseases is hampered by a lack of adequate diagnostic criteria. Therefore, to determine the frequency of symptoms in a study of chronic respiratory diseases among 5,000 New York postal workers and 8,000 transit authority employees, it was decided to use a simple test of pulmonary function and a questionnaire adapted from the one formulated by the British Medical Research Council.

In addition to yielding data on frequency of symptoms and abnormal pulmonary function, the study suggested additional lines of investigation, such as the possible prognostic significance of symptoms and pulmonary abnormalities and comparisons of subgroups among the 13,000 study subjects. The subsamples ranged from a group of nonsmokers, free of respiratory symptoms and with normal pulmonary function, through groups with intermediate degrees of impairment and symptoms to a group of heavy smokers with abnormal pulmonary function and high frequency of symptoms. These subgroups are now being followed for 5 years.

Epidemiologic research requires that degree of exposure to risk should be clearly defined. One hypothesis on chronic respiratory disease points to increased air pollution, but present methods of measuring exposure to pollutants are relatively crude. Areawide measurements do not relate one person's symptoms to his particular exposure to contaminants. A solution being investigated by the Office of Research and New York University under a grant from the Health Research Council is the development of a personal air monitor which an individual can wear to measure his exposure to pollutants.

Another difficulty is how to define a pollutant. There will probably be no agreement on this until the concentrations of various pollutants are linked to effects on health. These effects are not necessarily specific but may manifest themselves through such general phenomena as increases in disability and death, as suggested by the Meuse and Donora Valley episodes. Under examination now are two other measurement problems in the study of chronic respiratory disease—classification of smoking habits and methods of describing pulmonary function.

Current activities related to the chronic respiratory diseases thus illustrate several points: (a) use of routine vital statistics to reveal emergence of public health problems, (b) use of epidemiologic techniques to define their nature and size, (c) testing hypotheses in the literature on reasons for an increase, and (d) need for better measuring instruments.

Medical care and health economics. Chronic disease programs are expensive. Partnership between government and private resources will probably be required because health departments cannot provide medical care to large populations. Nevertheless, some agency must be responsible for serving the interests of the whole community; in New York City the health department assumes this function in concert with other city departments which have health components within their activities. The roles and interrelationships of government and voluntary medical care agencies must be determined in such matters as the proportions of the population receiving care from various community agencies and the degree of overlapping and duplication of services. This is the domain of health economics, a continuing activity of the office of research. "Metropolitan Medical Economics," a recent article by N. K. Piore, the office's director of health economics, sets forth some issues and problems.[3] The chart adapted from data in this article illustrates some complexities of the problem. More research is needed along the lines laid down in the report of the National Committee on Vital and Health Statistics.[4] It is part of the long-range plan of the office of research to carry out activities along these lines.

Application of computer technology. Chronic disease studies often

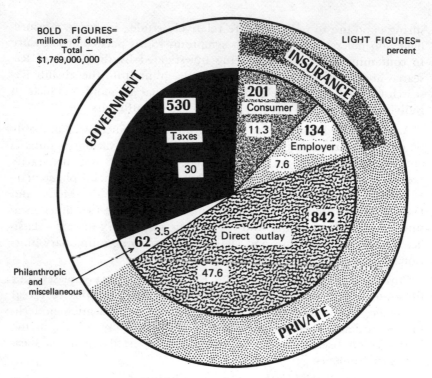

EXPENDITURES FOR MEDICAL CARE OF NEW YORKERS, 1961

require long-term follow-up, and more demands are thrown upon statistical units of health departments to determine whether or not a given individual has died and the cause of death. The mechanics of answering these questions are largely outmoded today. Modern electronic data processing equipment makes it possible to match these requests against death certificate files without resort to slow, costly, and clumsy hand methods. The office of research is now studying the feasibility of matching, by computer, to determine (a) probability of making a match, (b) how probability varies with the number and kinds of items to be matched, and (c) cost of matching on any given number of items. The research directed at solving this technological problem for the department would have wide applicability. A national death clearance program, available to investigators anywhere, might then be possible. Such a death clearance mechanism would, for example, permit clearing out the Social Security files regularly to determine which persons have died.

New sources of health information. Other methods than the use of vital statistics are needed to measure the population's health status. The National Health Survey is another method of measurement, but there is a vacuum at the local level. Therefore, to fill this vacuum, a New York City household survey was begun in 1964, using mechanisms similar to those of the National Health Survey. It has the following purposes:

1. Obtain new measures of the population's health status not available from routine vital statistics or program statistics but needed for program planning and evaluation.

2. Compare differences between National Health Survey findings and data for New York City. Large differences are expected for certain variables.

3. Identify groups needing more intensive study, such as those suffering from a particular disease.

Although the household survey in New York City is just beginning to yield data, its potential is great. Local areas need up-to-date information on numbers and characteristics of their population, particularly as the mobility of the population increases. Continuing sampling should provide more accurate population estimates than the decennial census and other information such as school registration currently used. Such estimates are needed not only for the city as a whole but also for particular neighborhoods, because many urban problems must be approached on a neighborhood basis.

Data useful at the local level resulted from a recent study of health insurance coverage in New York City among various ethnic groups. Although 83.3 percent of the white population have health insurance, only 50.7 percent of the Negro and 42.2 percent of the Puerto Rican populations are so covered. These findings have attracted citywide attention.

A gauge of the economic impact of illness, perhaps measured in days lost from work, would be useful in evaluating such service activities as community rehabilitation programs. Data on the proportion of the population in various neighborhoods confined to the home, by type of disability, should prove important in planning rehabilitation programs. The household survey will eventually provide such data.

Setting up the mechanisms for obtaining basic information on a community problem is often the most difficult, expensive, and time-consuming part of such research. With its continuing household survey project, the office of research has at hand the mechanisms for answering many of the emerging questions in the health field. It is thereby equipped to take on some of the more difficult kinds of research and to shorten the time lag between the appearance of new community problems and their final solution by action.

Future Problems and Needs

The growth of the health department's research, program planning, and evaluation activities is attributable largely to the existence of an internal unit to initiate and develop such functions. Also, the chief of the office has the rank of deputy commissioner, enabling him to explore all of the department's activities. This freedom and policy-level rank is essential in developing research, program planning, and evaluation and in engendering the creativity and effectiveness that move research findings into services of the department.

To incorporate the findings of a project or demonstration into service programs requires a forum before which the research can be discussed and implications considered. In New York the deputy commissioner in charge of research has access to the commissioner and his first deputy, and through them to program directors; also, staff meetings can be used to discuss findings. Some mechanism of this sort for feeding findings into service programs is vital to prevent a dichotomy between research and service programs.

Good research starts with an idea; there must be flexibility to explore this idea, to consider its ramifications, in short to play with it. Without flexibility research loses its chief characteristic of impertinent curiosity. To achieve flexibility some health departments have set up independent, nonprofit corporations to serve as research affiliates. The Medical and Health Research Association of New York City, Inc., serves this function for the department and carries out much of the research done under grant funds.

Both the financing and the organizational structure for conducting research require flexibility. In general, governments do not have the kind of money that industry plows into furthering its general growth and development. Health departments greatly need fluid funds to further their research programs. Federal project money is available, but project applications must be specific and the plan of action clear. Often research ideas are half formed and need to be played with before they become specific enough for a project grant. Also, the ability to recruit outstanding personnel is vital to the development of research activities. A relatively small amount of fluid funds would enable the commissioner of health to recruit and hold good men and further the total program. In short, fluid funds can make the difference between a mediocre and an inspired operation.

The need for research and evaluation by operating health agencies will continue to grow. The degree to which official agencies discharge their responsibilities to the public through imaginative programs depends upon the support of such research. Statesmanship will be required to provide the financial and administrative mechanisms to further research by operating agencies.

REFERENCES

1. Brownell, K. D., and Stix, R. K. A Public Health Program for Children with Heart Disease or Rheumatic Fever. Amer. J. Publ. Hlth. 53: 1587-1593, 1963.
2. Densen, P. M. Research and the Community Functions of a Health Department. New Eng. J. Med. 269: 781-789, 1963.
3. Piore, N. K. Metropolitan Medical Economics. Sci. Amer. 212: 19-27, 1965.
4. U.S. Public Health Service: United States Statistics on Medical Economics. Present Status and Recommendations for Additional Data. Report of the U.S. National Committee on Vital and Health Statistics. PHS Publication No. 1125. Washington: U.S. Government Printing Office, 1964.

34

The Use of a Psychiatric Case Register in the Planning and Evaluation of a Mental Health Program

ELMER A. GARDNER

A PSYCHIATRIC case register constitutes a central file to which are reported all persons with a diagnosed mental illness or all contacts with a group of psychiatric services over a long period of time.[1] Thus, the case register aims at (a) identification of persons with a mental disorder who reside in a specific geographic area and are seen in one or more of a defined set of local psychiatric facilities, and (b) maintenance of cumulative statistical records on both the psychiatric care these individuals receive and certain related items.

Case registers have proved their usefulness in the investigation of chronic disease from both administrative and epidemiological aspects. In mental disorder, as in most chronic disorders, the recurrent nature of the illness, the multiplicity of contacts with medical services, and the increasing number and variety of available resources make any investigation complex and particularly susceptible to duplication in counting. With a case register, however, we not only can obtain data from all treatment settings, but also can identify the same individual as he enters the system of psychiatric facilities, progresses through it, leaves, and perhaps re-enters the system later.[2] Case registers can be of particular value as we attempt to coordinate a variety of services in the planning and operation of a mental health center program and to view the latter's impact on the already existing network of psychiatric services in a community.

Dr. Stanley Yolles has noted that "In the attack on mental illness as a serious national problem of public health, we have for years desired to have data which can trace the services provided to a citizen when he becomes mentally ill . . . This is the kind of information we need in planning the new community mental health services that will be part of every community's health protection within the next few years."

In discussing the potential uses of the Maryland psychiatric register, Bahn *et al.* stated that "The State planner, as well as the local leader, cannot properly plan a coordinated program if his facts relate only to services under his jurisdiction or to fragmentary information that cannot be integrated. The problems of mental illness and mental deficiency are multiple and interrelated. They are partly medical, partly social, partly educational. They involve both public and private responsibilities and require the cooperation of all professions and services. The register will aid the State planner by providing information on the flow of patients from one facility to another and the role each plays in serving the mentally ill."[3]

In Maryland, the tricounty area of North Carolina, and in Monroe County, New York, psychiatric case registers have been in existence for several years, providing the knowledge of existing resources and the basic data indispensable to the planning of future services under Public Law 88-164.[4] This paper represents an exercise in the use of data from the Monroe County psychiatric register to illustrate the manner in which each of these case registers may be utilized for planning and evaluation of comprehensive mental health programs.

As described in previous papers, Monroe County is a community with a well developed network of traditional psychiatric services. Until the present time (1967), the inpatient, clinic, and emergency department services of the University Medical Center have acted as a community mental health center for the entire county. In 1967, psychiatric services will be established under Public Law 88-164 in a second general hospital unit, Rochester General Hospital. This center will contain thirty beds, ten of which will be used for day or night hospital care. It will have the full range of clinic, emergency, and consultative services, but it may have a limited psychiatric staff available during the first year for providing much outpatient treatment. Thus, its clinic initially may be devoted largely to aftercare. The present Alcoholism Clinic for Monroe County and the Rochester Child Guidance Clinic also will be housed at the new mental health center. The preparation for this expansion of the psychiatric network occasions a number of questions.

How many persons will be served annually by the new mental health center and which areas of the county will be served primarily? Will the demographic and diagnostic characteristics of the caseload be similar to the patient characteristics of other facilities, or will they be unique? What proportion of its caseload will consist of individuals already revolving through the psychiatric network in contrast to those who might otherwise not have had any psychiatric contact? We must estimate the number of persons in the community who have had no psychiatric care but may now require it and those who have had an episode of service but may now return for a new episode of care. Even with the data from a case register, however, only the grossest of estimates can be made.

Obviously, the total caseload of the new center will depend on a variety of variables such as the number of beds and the amount of staff time available for patient care. In addition, financial arrangements, administrative policies, and staff attitudes will affect the size of the caseload by their influence on the kinds of patients seen, the proportion of patients maintained in treatment, and the duration of treatment. Finally, the number of individuals requiring psychiatric care and the acceptance of such care by the community are factors that will determine the amount of pressure exerted upon the facility by the community; this pressure may well influence the admission rate to the facility and the duration of patient care.

Estimates of the amount and type of service that the new mental health center will provide can be made from data provided by existing mental health centers and from knowledge about the number of beds, the amount of staff time, and the proposed policies in the new mental health center. A case register would not be necessary for these predictions, but as noted above, it may be helpful in providing readily accessible data regarding existing services. A case register can increase the accuracy of these estimates by demonstrating gaps in the current network of services created by areas of the community or sub-groups of the population receiving a disproportionate amount of service. While the register is not indispensable for enumerating those patients admitted for their first psychiatric contact, beginning a new episode of service, or simply continuing within the network of psychiatric services, this data is readily available in the register and can supplement the histories obtained from the patients.

A case register is indispensable, however, in evaluating the impact of a mental health center on the psychiatric network. We can observe the number and geographic distribution of persons admitted to psychiatric care for the year and compare it with an extrapolation from previous years. The register is also indispensable if we wish to study the movement of patients between services and how this will be affected by the addition of a new facility. We may particularly want to examine the pattern of movement between the community services and the public mental hospital, with particular reference to such factors as diagnosis, age, sex, area of residency, private versus public care, facility of first contact, and number of contacts. We may then judge the effect of the new mental health center on the caseload of the public mental hospital. If the Rochester General Hospital center wished to retain all of its patients in a community-based program, and thereby attempt to prevent long-term hospitalization, in what manner must its operation differ from that of the University Medical Center?

To estimate the impact of the new mental health center at Rochester General Hospital on the network of psychiatric services, we have used the University Medical Center as a model of a mental health center.[5] In predicting the operation of any system, whether it be in industry or the health field, one first establishes a model of the system based upon the best available information. To then estimate the reaction of the system to various additions or modifications, a number of assumptions must always be made. Often, these assumptions force us to establish "reasonable limits" for our estimates in contrast to exact projections. In establishing a model for the psychiatric network of Monroe County, and in estimating the future trends of psychiatric service, we have made a number of such assumptions:

(1) The population ages, 15 and over, in Monroe County will continue to increase at the same rate in the period 1964 to 1967, as it did in the years 1961 to 1964 (Table I).

TABLE I. MONROE COUNTY POPULATION, AGES 15 AND OVER

| | By catchment area | | | | |
	1961	1962	1963	1964	1967*
Monroe County Catchment Area	418,158	432,740	429,396	435,127	452,785
Southern Catchment Area	200,871	203,563	206,291	209,055	217,572
Northern Catchment Area	217,287	220,177	223,105	226,072	235,213

* Estimated by linear extrapolation of 1960 and 1964 U.S. Census figures.

(2) The number of persons, ages 15 and over, admitted to all psychiatric services will also continue to increase at the same rate in 1964 to 1967 as in the period 1961 to 1964.

(3) The average bed occupancy rate and the duration of patient stay will be the same at Rochester General Hospital as it has been in the University Medical Center. Although we do not expect the bed occupancy rate to vary significantly, we might expect a considerable differ-

ence in the average duration of patient stay. Depending upon a number of factors, reasonable limits can be established for the duration of inpatient care.

(4) The ratio of readmissions to total admissions will be the same at Rochester General Hospital as it has been at the University Medical Center.

(5) The diagnostic distribution of the patients entering the new

MONROE COUNTY

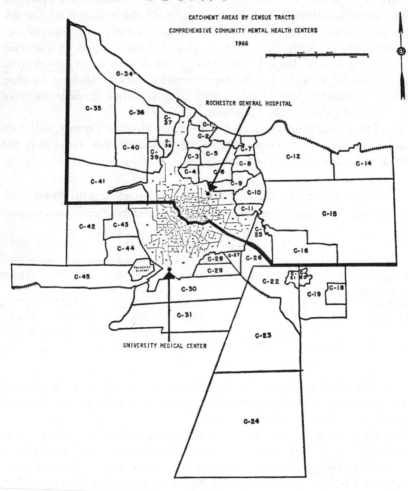

FIGURE 1.

mental health center will be similar to that of the University Medical Center, depending on such factors as the ratio of private to division patients, the area of the community served by the mental health center, and the activity of the emergency department service. The latter tends to draw individuals from the lower socioeconomic districts of the city and may thus alter the diagnostic distribution of admissions. Again, consideration of the varying contingencies may yield different estimates.

(6) The proportion of patients discharged to the community, followed in the clinic, or transferred to the state mental hospital will be comparable to the University Medical Center.

Rochester General Hospital: Estimates of Psychiatric Service in 1967

We can best obtain an estimate of the total caseload of the new mental health center by first estimating the caseload of each of its component services. Using the University Medical Center as a model, we may expect the new mental health center to have a daily percentage bed occupancy of 90 per cent, to have an average patient stay of 16 to 25 days and to have about 10 per cent of the patients readmitted once or more during the year. With an inpatient service of 30 beds, the new center may expect approximately 400 to 650 hospital admissions during its first year of operation. With 10 per cent readmissions, this would mean that between 360 and 585 individuals would be admitted to the inpatient service during the year. Using the mid-point of this range, we might expect 525 admissions or 475 persons to be admitted during 1967.

We know, however, that the average stay in the University Medical Center has decreased from 28 days in 1962 to 21 days in 1965 with no indication of leveling off at this point. If we look at the geographic distribution of persons admitted to the psychiatric services and the trend of admissions to the University Medical Center, we find some other indications that the pressure for admissions to the new mental health center may be relatively great and that the average patient stay on the inpatient service may be closer to 15 days than to 25 days. In 1964 the rate of admissions to all psychiatric services was 18 per 1,000 population from the southern half of the county and 14 per 1,000 population from the northern catchment area (Table II). Projecting to 1967, the discrepancy will become even greater with rates of 21 and 16 from the two catchment areas, respectively. This difference in admission rates of 5 per 1,000 population represents 1,210 persons

TABLE II. MONROE COUNTY RESIDENTS, AGES 15 AND OVER,
ADMITTED TO ALL PSYCHIATRIC SERVICES

| | By catchment area Rates Per 1,000 Population | | | | |
	1961	1962	1963	1964	1967*
Monroe County	13.35	14.38	14.98	16.01	18.58
N=	5581	6148	6432	6966	8415
Catchment Areas					
Southern Catchment Area	14.83	16.36	17.05	18.19	21.26
Northern Catchment Area	11.97	12.80	13.06	14.00	16.11

*Estimated by linear extrapolation of 1961 to 1964 rates.

based on the projected 1967 population for the northern catchment area. Although the psychiatric services are located in the southern catchment area, the similar population characteristics of the two areas (Table III) would lead us to expect equal admission rates with the opening of the new mental health center. In fact, if we examine the admission rates to the University Medical Center inpatient service, we find quite similar rates for the two catchment areas (Table IV). It appears that those persons most urgently needing psychiatric care receive this care regardless of the distance to psychiatric services. The distance seems to become a more significant factor when the service is less urgent and hence, more a voluntary decision. Thus, with the opening of the new mental health center, there may be pressure for hospitalization but not as great as the pressure for outpatient care.

Other data indicating that there may be less pressure on the inpatient service than its outpatient counterpart comes from a study of patients who were seen in the Emergency Department of the University Medical Center and placed on the waiting list for admission. Three-quarters of those patients placed on the waiting list in the year July 1964 to July 1965 were subsequently admitted to the University Medical Center. A few of the others were admitted to another hospital during this period, and only 25 patients were not admitted to any hospital during this particular year.

If we examine the non-psychiatric admissions to the University Medical Center and to the Rochester General Hospital, we find, as may be expected, that there is a greater admission rate from the area surrounding each hospital than from the more distant areas (Table V). Approximately two-thirds of the non-psychiatric admissions to the Univer-

TABLE III. SOCIOECONOMIC CHARACTERISTICS OF MONROE COUNTY
CATCHMENT AREAS, 1960 U.S. CENSUS

EDUCATION: Persons 25 Years of Age and Over	SOUTHERN CATCHMENT AREA		NORTHERN CATCHMENT AREA	
	No.	%	No.	%
Number of Years				
None	2,589	1.6	4,688	2.6
1-7	22,875	14.0	29,189	16.2
8-11	62,957	38.5	72,010	39.8
13 or more	34,775	21.2	28,996	16.1
TOTAL	163,568	100.0	180,526	100.0
Median Number of Years	9.5		10.1	
AGE				
Under 15	77,367	28.1	96,366	31.0
15-24	34,505	12.5	33,891	11.0
25-44	70,487	25.6	86,000	27.7
45-64	59,853	21.7	64,810	20.8
65 and over	33,371	12.1	29,737	9.5
TOTAL	275,583	100.0	310,804	100.0
RACE				
White	261,339	94.8	299,981	96.5
Non-white	14,244	5.2	10,823	3.5
TOTAL	275,583	100.0	310,804	100.0
%DETERIORATING AND DILAPIDATED HOUSING	11.8%		9.8%	
MEDIAN INCOME	$6,369.00		$6,590.00	

TABLE IV. MONROE COUNTY RESIDENTS, AGES 15 AND OVER, ADMITTED TO THE PSYCHIATRIC SERVICES OF THE UNIVERSITY MEDICAL CENTER

By catchment area
Rates Per 1,000 Population

	Inpatient Services*			Clinic-No Inpatient Admission			Emergency Dept. No Clinic or Inpatient		
	1961	1964	1967**	1961	1964	1967**	1961	1964	1967**
Southern Catchment Area	1.92	2.32	2.70	2.25	2.43	3.26	1.94	2.99	4.14
Northern Catchment Area	1.71	2.18	2.53	1.72	2.09	2.50	1.50	2.44	3.23
Total County	1.85	2.25	2.61	1.98	2.25	2.87	1.71	2.71	3.67
N=	722	979	1182	826	981	1298	717	1178	1660

*Approximately 25 percent of the patients admitted to the inpatient services of the University Medical Center are out-of-county residents and are excluded from these tabulations.
**Estimated by linear extrapolation of 1961 to 1964 rates.

TABLE V. NON-PSYCHIATRIC ADMISSIONS, AGES 15 AND OVER,
TO UNIVERSITY MEDICAL CENTER AND
ROCHESTER GENERAL HOSPITAL, 1964, MONROE COUNTY RESIDENTS

| | By catchment area Rates Per 1,000 Population | | | | | |
| | University Medical Center | | Rochester General Hospital | | All Hospitals | |
	No.	Rate Per 1,000	No.	Rate Per 1,000	No.	Rate Per 1,000
Southern Catchment Area	8,630	41.28	4,095	19.59	28,793	137.73
Northern Catchment Area	5,055	22.36	7,110	31.45	24,500	108.37
Total County	13,685	31.45	11,205	25.75	53,293	122.48

sity Medical Center come from the southern catchment area, whereas
the northern catchment area provides about two-thirds of the non-psychiatric admissions to the Rochester General Hospital. Thus, we may
expect some shift in the distribution of inpatient admissions from
the catchment areas when the new mental health center is opened. It
is likely that the shift will not be marked since this center will have
fewer beds than the University Medical Center and most of the psychiatrists will have their offices in the southern catchment area. It is
conceivable, though, that referral from the non-psychiatric physicians
practicing in the northern catchment area may create some pressure
for admission to the new mental health center.

In looking at the diagnostic distribution of the patients admitted to
the University Medical Center inpatient service, we find that a little
more than one-third were schizophrenic, a few less than one-third had
a diagnosis other than psychosis or organic brain syndrome, about one-
fifth were diagnosed as affective psychosis, and the remainder as chronic
brain syndrome or alcoholism. In general, the schizophrenic patients
tend to remain in the hospital longer than the other diagnostic groups,
and those with a diagnosis of chronic brain syndrome have the shortest
hospital stay. Even with a somewhat different diagnostic distribution,
it is doubtful that this would significantly alter the average duration
of patient stay, and thus the admission rate.

Given all of these factors, we are still left with the unknown factors
of administrative policies and staff attitudes at the new mental health
center. Since there is nothing to point more strongly in one direction

than the other, the most reasonable estimate at this point would seem to be an average patient stay of about 20 days in the inpatient service of the new mental health center, allowing a rate of 490 admissions annually. There then would be about 440 different individuals admitted to the inpatient services and, using the University Medical Center as a model, we would expect that approximately 330 of these individuals would have had no psychiatric care for at least one year prior to their admission.

The prediction of the outpatient caseload for the new mental health center provides even more difficulty and is subject to more error than the estimation of the inpatient admission rate. We know from the experience of the University Medical Center that approximately 40 per cent of all persons admitted to the inpatient services are followed subsequently in the outpatient department. Approximately 25 per cent are followed in private practice; another 10 per cent are transferred directly to the State Hospital. Thus, we might expect approximately 175, or 40 per cent, of the 440 persons admitted to the inpatient service of the new mental health center to be followed in their clinic. We might expect one-half of these persons to be followed for less than a three month period and the other half to be followed for more than three months.

If all patients were to receive aftercare and no one were to be transferred to the state mental hospital, then approximately 330 patients (75 per cent) would require clinic care after a hospital admission. (The others would be seen in private practice.) We note from the admission trends to the University Medical Center Outpatient Department that approximately 1,300 individuals would be admitted to the University Center clinic in 1967, with no preceding hospital admission (Table IV). (Approximately 600 of these patients would come from the northern catchment area.) If all 600 were to seek their psychiatric service in the clinic of the new mental health center, then this clinic would serve either 775 persons (600 plus the 175, or 40 per cent, receiving aftercare), or a maximum of approximately 930 patients (using the 75 per cent aftercare figure). If the same number of patients were to seek care directly in the clinic of the new mental health center as estimated for the clinic of the University Medical Center (1,300 in 1967), then we would expect a range of 1,475 to 1,630 patients (1,300 plus 175 to 330 for aftercare) to be seen in the clinic. Thus, we have a minimum of approximately 775 and a maximum of 1,630 patients who might be seen in the clinic during 1967. The mid-point of this range gives us a figure of 1,200 patients, and considering the limited staff that would be available, we might reasonably estimate that 1,000 patients would be seen in the clinic of the new mental health center. Approximately three-quarters of these patients, or about 750, would have had no preceding hospital care. Of these 750 patients, about 85 per cent, or approximately 640, would have had no psychiatric contact for at least one year prior to their contact with the clinic of the new mental health center. Again, these figures are based upon the statistics from the University Medical Center services.

Finally, if we examine the admission rates for the Emergency Department service of the University Medical Center, we find that 1,660 individuals with no prior clinic or hospital contact in 1967 may receive Emergency Department care during that year (Table IV). Of these patients, 760 would come from the northern catchment area. If the new mental health center has at least one staff member available for emergency service on a 24 hour basis, then we may expect this emergency facility to serve a range (from the northern area) of 760 to 1,660 persons in 1967, representing only those patients having no clinic or hospital contact during that year. However, about one-half of the patients seen in the emergency service of the University Medical Center during any year are persons who have had a clinic and/or hospital contact during the same year. If we were to use the 1,660 admission figure for the new mental health center, we might expect a total of 3,320 persons to be seen by the emergency service during 1967. About one-quarter of all the people seen in the emergency service have more than one contact during the course of a year. Thus, we may predict a total of 4,430 visits. If we use the lower estimate of 760 persons with no clinic or hospital contact, this would give a figure of 2,030 visits or 1,520 different individuals. Considering the staff limitations, a more reasonable estimate would be somewhat above the mid-point. We may estimate that about 3,000 individuals would make approximately 4,000 visits to the emergency service and approximately 1,500 of these 3,000 patients would have had no clinic or hospital contact during the year. Of these 1,500 patients, about 1,075 would have had no psychiatric contact for at least one year prior to their Emergency Department contact in 1967.

From this we can, therefore, estimate that approximately 2,690 different individuals (440 inpatient, 750 clinic, and 1,500 emergency department) would be seen in some kind of psychiatric contact at the new mental health center during 1967. Of this group, 2,045 persons (330 inpatient, 640 clinic, and 1,075 emergency department) would have had no psychiatric contact for at least one year prior to their contact with the mental health center in 1967. This latter figure might be used as a very rough approximation of the increase in the caseload for the entire psychiatric network with the opening of the new mental health center.

An exercise such as this serves to demonstrate that, even with a case register, the number of unknown or unpredictable factors permits, at best, only an educated guess of a mental health center case load when it is added to an already existing network of services. Similarly, it is extremely difficult to predict the impact of such a program on the same network. Using the case register, however, we can observe the annual volume and distribution of admissions to all psychiatric services before and after the initiation of the new mental health center. The unduplicated count of patient admissions to all services in Monroe County increased steadily from 1961 to 1964. If it continued to increase at the same rate in subsequent years, we could expect an admission rate of 17.8 per thousand population in 1966 and 18.7 per thousand population in 1967. Any marked deviation from this trend in 1967 could reasonably be interpreted to represent the impact of the new mental health center on the psychiatric network (Figure 2). The same observations can be made for the geographical distribution of the psychiatric admissions.

We also noted that the case register can be used to study the movement of patients between services. Figures 3 through 9 are flow charts showing patient movement between the community services and the public mental hospital. Because we were interested particularly in viewing the impact of a new mental health center on the caseload of the public mental hospital, we have initially used this simple model of the psychiatric network in which all services are categorized under either community facilities or the public mental hospital system. Monroe County residents, age 15 and over, who were admitted to psychiatric service during 1961, were selected for this study and then followed for a minimum of one and one-half, and a maximum of two and one-half, years or until July 1, 1963. While the pattern of movement did not vary significantly by sex or area of residency, the flow charts do show a variance by major diagnostic category, type of service, private versus public care, and by whether a person was beginning a new episode of service (no psychiatric contact for at least one year) or another in a series of psychiatric contacts.

Sixteen per cent of the cohort had their first contact at the State Hospital (Figure 3). In contrast, only five and one-half per cent of the patients beginning a new episode of care were seen initially at

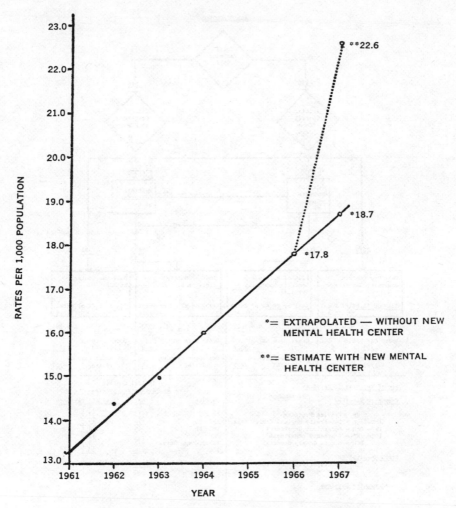

FIGURE 2. MONROE COUNTY RESIDENTS, AGE 15
AND OVER, ADMITTED TO ALL PSYCHIATRIC SERVICES.
RATES PER 1,000 POPULATION.

the State Hospital (Figure 4), but about one-fifth of this latter group did have a state hospital contact by July, 1963. A distribution by diagnosis indicates that approximately one-third of those persons diagnosed as psychotic eventually entered the State Hospital system (Figure 5) and that most frequently these patients, in contrast to all other patients, had first contacted the Emergency Department of the

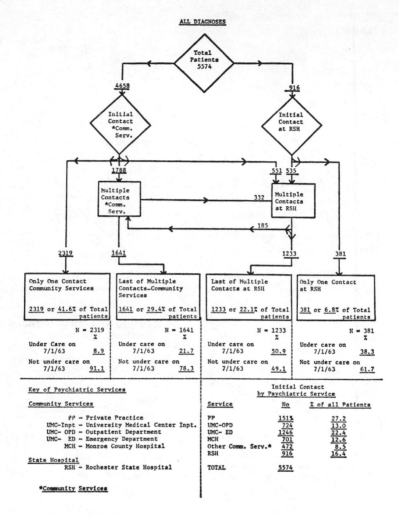

FIGURE 3. RESIDENTS OF MONROE COUNTY, AGE 15
AND OVER, ADMITTED TO PSYCHIATRIC SERVICE DURING 1961,
FOLLOWED IN PSYCHIATRIC REGISTER UNTIL JULY 1, 1963.

University Medical Center. Patients with a diagnosis of chronic brain
syndrome (Figure 6) were admitted directly to the State Hospital
much more often than all other patients, and almost two-thirds of
this group were admitted to the State Hospital by July, 1963. Those
who received a diagnosis of character disorder or neuroses (Figures
7 and 8) seldom entered the State Hospital system and were frequently

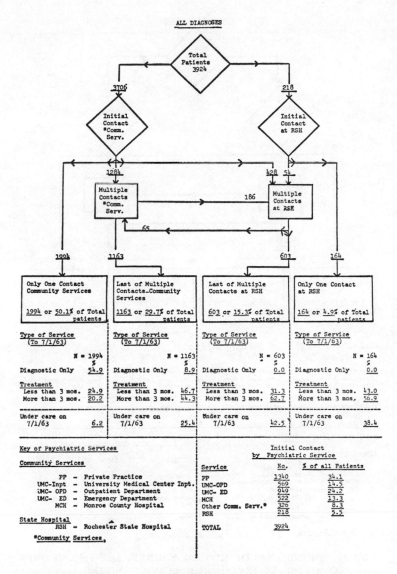

FIGURE 4. RESIDENTS OF MONROE COUNTY, AGE 15 AND OVER,
ADMITTED TO PSYCHIATRIC SERVICE DURING 1961,
NO PSYCHIATRIC CONTACT IN 1960, FOLLOWED IN
PSYCHIATRIC CASE REGISTER UNTIL JULY 1, 1963.

seen first in private practice. A large percentage of these people, as well as all those with a private practice contact (Figure 9), experienced only the one psychiatric contact during the entire follow-up

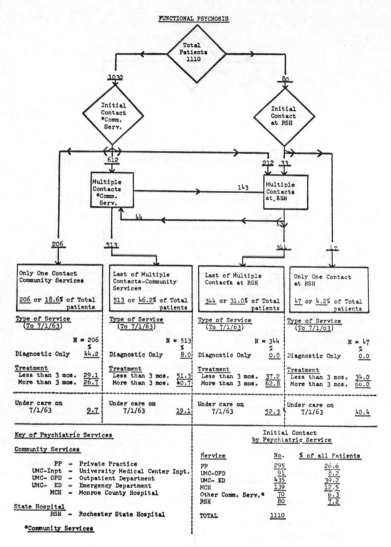

FIGURE 5. RESIDENTS OF MONROE COUNTY, AGE 15 AND OVER,
ADMITTED TO PSYCHIATRIC SERVICE DURING 1961,
NO PSYCHIATRIC CONTACT IN 1960, FOLLOWED IN
PSYCHIATRIC CASE REGISTER UNTIL JULY 1, 1963.

period. Approximately one-half of the patients seen solely in private practice had one diagnostic contact only.

We might expect the caseload of the psychiatric network to be considerably larger by 1967 even without the addition of a new facility,

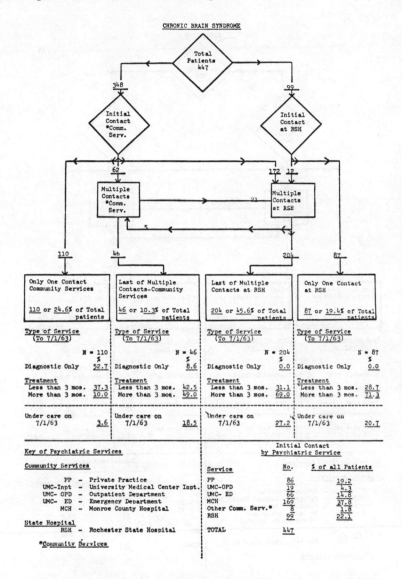

FIGURE 6. RESIDENTS OF MONROE COUNTY, AGE 15 AND OVER,
ADMITTED TO PSYCHIATRIC SERVICE DURING 1961,
NO PSYCHIATRIC CONTACT IN 1960, FOLLOWED IN
PSYCHIATRIC CASE REGISTER UNTIL JULY 1, 1963.

and the pattern of movement among services to be essentially the
same (Figure 10). If a new mental health center is developed, how-

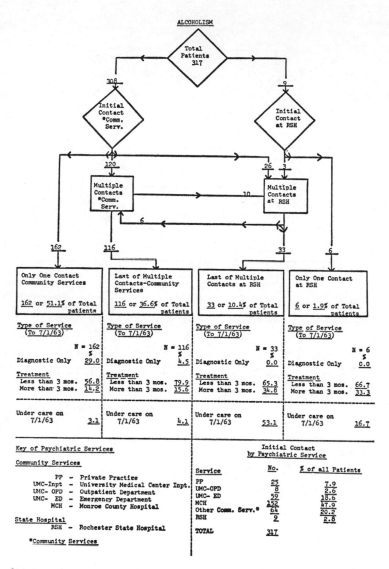

FIGURE 7. RESIDENTS OF MONROE COUNTY, AGE 15 AND OVER,
ADMITTED TO PSYCHIATRIC SERVICE DURING 1961,
NO PSYCHIATRIC CONTACT IN 1960, FOLLOWED IN
PSYCHIATRIC CASE REGISTER UNTIL JULY 1, 1963.

ever, we may predict an additional 2,045 persons to have psychiatric
contact and, hence, the caseload to increase from 8,415 to 10,460 (Figure 11). Again, using the University Medical Center as a model, the

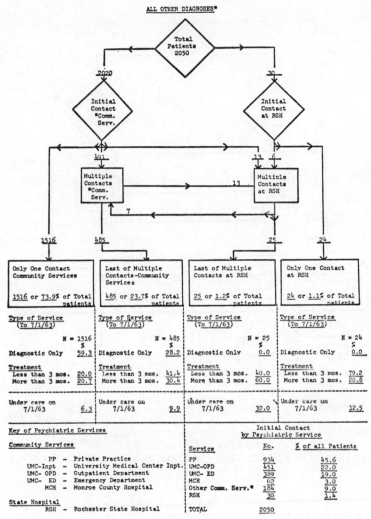

FIGURE 8. RESIDENTS OF MONROE COUNTY, AGE 15 AND OVER,
ADMITTED TO PSYCHIATRIC SERVICE DURING 1961,
NO PSYCHIATRIC CONTACT IN 1960, FOLLOWED IN
PSYCHIATRIC CASE REGISTER UNTIL JULY 1, 1963.

patient flow between services would be comparable to that shown in
Figure 11. An additional 300 patients from a one year cohort would

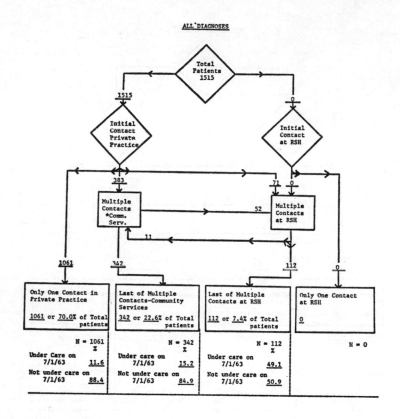

FIGURE 9. RESIDENTS OF MONROE COUNTY, AGE 15 AND OVER,
ADMITTED TO PRIVATE PRACTICE DURING 1961,
FOLLOWED IN PSYCHIATRIC CASE REGISTER UNTIL JULY 1, 1963.

have contact with the State Hospital system by the end of the second
year, increasing its caseload by 12 per cent. Of the 2,690 individuals
seen at the new mental health center during 1967, we might expect
that approximately 250 patients, mostly with a diagnosis of schizophrenia or affective psychosis would have had contact with the State
Hospital system during that year. If the new mental health center
wished to reduce the flow of patients to the State Hospital, or at least
not to increase it, it would have to provide outpatient care for these
patients. The majority of these 250 patients would have had only an
emergency department or inpatient contact at the mental health cen-

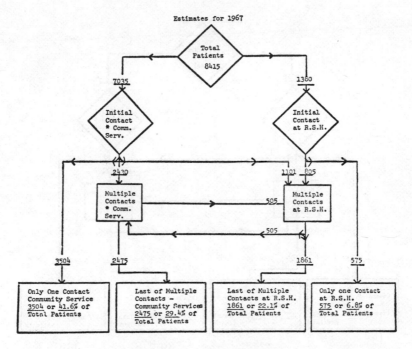

FIGURE 10. RESIDENTS OF MONROE COUNTY, AGE 15 AND OVER,
ADMITTED TO ALL PSYCHIATRIC SERVICES,
EXCLUDING NEW MENTAL HEALTH CENTER.

ter. If, on the other hand, they were to be retained in clinic care, the caseload of that service would be increased by almost 25 per cent.

Again, the many unknown factors preclude any reasonable estimate at this time of the pattern of movement occasioned by the addition of this new facility. The case register can be used, however, to observe any changes in patient flow subsequent to the opening of the mental health center and to guide the necessary operational modifications for a more appropriate movement of patients among services.

Summary

This paper has demonstrated the potential utility of a psychiatric case register in the development and evaluation of a community mental health center program. The register may be used to observe the existing pattern of service in a community and to estimate roughly the changes that might occur with the initiation of a new mental health center. Further, annual trends for the caseload of the entire psychiatric

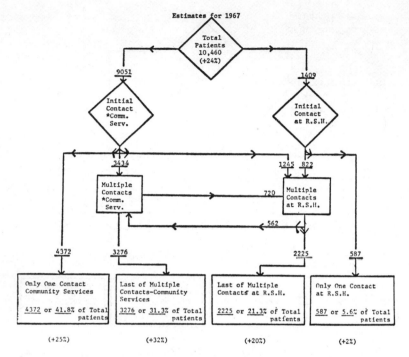

Estimates for 1967

FIGURE 11. RESIDENTS OF MONROE COUNTY, AGE 15 AND OVER,
ADMITTED TO ALL PSYCHIATRIC SERVICES,
INCLUDING NEW MENTAL HEALTH CENTER.

network, the geographic distribution of all patients admitted to psychiatric services, and the movement of patients among services can
be observed in the years prior to, and subsequent to, the opening of
the mental health center. In this manner, the impact of such a new
facility on the entire network may be observed, and subsequently,
operational decisions made which are both informed and documented.

NOTES AND REFERENCES

1. Gardner, E. A., Miles, H. C., Bahn, A. K., and Romano, J. All Psychiatric Experience in a Community. Archives of General Psychiatry, 9: 369-378, 1963.
2. Gardner, E. A., Miles, H. C., Bahn, A. K., and Romano, J. Psychiatric Case
   Register Conference. Publ. Hlth Rep. 77, 12: 1071-1076, 1962.
3. Gorwitz, K., Bahn, A. K., Chandler, C. A., and Martin, W. A. Planned Uses of a

Statewide Psychiatric Register for Aiding Mental Health in the Community. Am. J. Orthopsychiat. 33, 3: 494-500, 1963.

4. Bahn, A. K., Gardner, E. A., Alltop, L., Knatterud, G., and Solomon, M. Admission and Prevalence Rates for Psychiatric Facilities in Four Register Areas. Am. J. of Publ. Hlth. 56, 12: 2033-2051, 1966.

5. In the present paper we have limited ourselves to the adult psychiatric population (ages 15 and over). For this paper, the county has been divided by census tract grouping into two catchment areas, Northern and Southern (see Figure 1).

35

Program Evaluation Models and the Implementation of Research Findings

HERBERT C. SCHULBERG and FRANK BAKER

A SOURCE of great dismay to both the researcher and the clinician is the difficulty encountered in trying to apply the findings of a research project. This consternation is particularly acute in the research specialty of program evaluation, since both the program administrator and program evaluator undertake studies with the fullest and sincerest intention of utilizing the resulting data. The reasons for the gap between research and implementation are varied and considerable attention has been devoted in recent years to analysis of personal and organizational resistances to change. This paper restricts its focus to the issues specifically relevant to program evaluation and program modification and then describes implications of different evaluation research models for the implementation of research findings.

A common approach among those concerned with the utilization of research findings has been the study of the processes through which information flows among scientists. In his review of this broad field, Menzel[1] was able to identify and classify many different types of information-receiving behavior on the part of scientists and to suggest numerous leads for further research. For the past six years the American Psychological Association has been engaged in a wide-ranging study of scientific information exchange and the entire November, 1966, issue of the "American Psychologist" is devoted to a report on this project.

In one of the papers, Menzel[2] discusses five interrelated themes about scientific communication which he considers central to the understanding of this process. Perhaps most relevant to the topic of program evaluation and modification is Menzel's notion that acts of communication constitute a system. He conceives of the flow of scientific information as a set of interaction processes in a social system. As the information-receiving actions of any one individual often involve several of his roles, Menzel urges a systemic view of the problem. The changes and innovations introduced in any one component of the system will have their consequences on the utilization and efficacy of other components.

In considering the processes which intervene between the completion of research and its ultimate application, Halpert[3] identified several barriers to useful communication. The obstacles originate with both the researcher and the clinician. In a perhaps overly stereotyped fashion, we may describe the researcher as suspecting malicious surreptitiousness among those charged with the implementation of his findings and inappropriate defensiveness in striving to maintain the status quo. Conversely, the administrator alleges that the researcher's findings have been presented in an unnecessarily frustrating, abstract manner and that the findings have precious little application to the complex reality of his program. If we are to accept Halpert's contention that "a test of the efficacy of communication is its ability to translate research into altered behavior of key individuals,"[4] we then must sadly conclude that much program evaluation has been unsuccessful.

Proceeding from this conclusion, one should then ask a series of questions whose answers may contain guide lines for future developments. The most basic question is whether the research and clinical enterprises are so antithetical in their nature that they inevitably will be in conflict, particularly when the researcher contends that his findings necessitate modifications in clinical practice. Although we are all familiar with practitioners to whom professional autonomy is so sacrosanct that it even prevents the intrusion of research findings, over the years there have been sufficient examples of research and evaluation directly affecting clinical practice to conclude that under appropriate conditions evaluation and practice can be harmonious. Many of the recent program developments in the field of community mental health stem from demonstrations that alternative patterns of care, e.g., day hospitalization, are preferable to ones used previously and that increased flexibility is possible.

It becomes important then to determine what the appropriate conditions are for bringing program evaluation and clinical practice closer together and to develop them in such a way that they have greater applicability. We will consider now the purposes of program evaluation and the alternative approaches for enhancing the implementation of findings.

Purposes of Evaluation

Even though it is impossible to identify all of the factors associated with the administrator's decision to evaluate an activity, it is essential to identify as many of them as possible. Many aspects of the evaluation procedure itself, and certainly its later utility, hinge upon the administrator's or the organization's motivation in initiating the evaluation. Earlier papers by Greenberg and Mattison[5] and Knutson[6] highlight the complexity of this matter. Knutson thought that the implicit and explicit reasons for program evaluation fall into two categories: (a) reasons that are organization oriented, and (b) reasons that are personally oriented. In both categories values of an unspecified nature exert powerful influences upon decision-making in ways unrecognized by those participating in the process.

The relationship of evaluation purpose to subsequent utilization of findings is indicated in many ways. If the administrator is concerned with achieving status and impressing his peers, he will select for evaluation a program of widespread interest. The evaluation of a relatively obscure service will attract little of the administrator's energy initially and even less if the implementation of findings requires the overcoming of staff resistance.

The purpose of evaluation similarly will affect the depth of investigation to be undertaken and the level of critical analysis to be completed. Knutson suggests that the administrator's orientation will determine the selection of evaluation criteria, since what is valid evidence to one person will not be accepted as such by others. Controversy frequently arises between those subscribing to a "cost analysis" criterion and those advocating a criterion of "human suffering alleviated." In a period of increasing competition for the limited funds in governmental budgets, legislators and economists often reject a program which entails a higher cost per unit of service even when it has been evaluated as successful. The many instances of "successful" demonstration programs which cease operation after the initial funding period demonstrate how the evaluation criteria satisfactory to the professional may leave the legislator unimpressed.

Evaluation Models

In seeking to conceptualize the various approaches to evaluation, two research models stand out: (a) the goal-attainment model, and (b) the system model. The characteristics and limitations of each will be described as they affect the implementation of research findings.

Goal-Attainment Model

There is popular agreement among those concerned with program evaluation that one of the most critical and also difficult phases in this process is clarification of a program's objectives. This emphasis stems from a conception of evaluation as measurement of the degree of success or failure encountered by the program in reaching predetermined objectives. Related to this conception of evaluation is the assumption that if specific program objectives can be defined, then the appropriate methodology and criteria for assessing the program will be selected correctly. The specification of objectives and goals in the evaluation process is considered by some to be so essential that Freeman and Sherwood[7] suggest that if the evaluation researcher is to act responsibly as an agent of social change, then he should actively participate in developing the program's goals. Having failed to do this, he may find himself in the position of either evaluating incorrect objectives or of never even being told what objectives are to be studied.

Accepting the significance of goal clarification as an integral component in the evaluation process, one can proceed then with well-defined methodologies for determining the degree of success achieved in attaining the goal. This *"goal-attainment* model" of evaluation has been widely described in the literature (e.g., Herzog[8] and Knutson[9]) and it has many of the characteristics of classical research. Freeman and Sherwood maintain that evaluation research seeks to approximate the experimental model as much as possible and, when this cannot be achieved, then quasi-experimental designs should be employed. Knutson distinguishes between evaluation of progress, which is conducted during the course of the program, and evaluation of achievement, which measures change between the base line period and some ultimate point in time when the program is expected to have produced results. The data and criteria selected for evaluating progress toward intermediate goals are different from those used in evaluating achievement of final objectives.

In spite of the methodological rigor evident in the "goal-attainment" model of evaluation, a relative lack of concern is found within this approach for technics of implementing findings. Although evaluation research usually is distinguished from other research by virtue of its closely knit relationship to program planning, only rarely has this interweaving been evident in fact. An exception can be found in James's[10] description of the goal-attainment evaluation process as a circular one. It starts with initial goal-setting, proceeds to determine measures of the goal, collects data and appraises the effect of the goal, and then modifies the initial goal on the basis of the collected data.

Nowhere is any indication found, however, of the manner in which the evaluator can insure closing the circle of the evaluation process in the goal-attainment model. More often than not, the previously linked series of cooperative processes between evaluator and administrator break down at the point of goal modification. What had been a reciprocal relationship of mutual benefit suddenly becomes an antagonistic arrangement marked by the stereotyped interpersonal perceptions described earlier in this paper.

What are the characteristics of the goal-attainment model of evaluation that render it relatively ineffective at the point of implementing findings? First, we must consider that one of the supposedly major assets of this model may be mythical in nature. The researcher, attempting to avoid the bias of imposing his own objectives as criteria of the organization's effectiveness, turns instead to the administrator for a statement of the goals to be used as criteria. However, in gaining this "objectivity" and utilizing an unbiased evaluation model, the researcher potentially has sacrificed much of the significance of his work. Etzioni[11] forcefully notes that organizational goals, particularly public ones, have an illusory quality in that they may never have been intended to be realized. When this is the case, the program administrator will be troubled very little by the researcher's finding that his previously enumerated organizational goals are not being achieved. Never having meant to attain the goals studied by the researcher, the administrator sees no need to alter his program to accommodate the findings of the researcher. The program evaluation has little impact upon the organization since the researcher had little understanding of the administrator's purpose in participating in the study.

A second limitation in implementing the findings of the goal-attainment model of evaluation is the relatively circumscribed perspective with which this evaluation model views an organization. Since the model assumes that specific goals can be evaluated and modified in isolation from the other goals being sought by the organization, it constitutes an artificial, if not fallacious, approach. A wide body of literature in the field of organizational study (e.g., Rice[12] and Sofer[13]) highlights the interrelated nature of goals and the manner in which modification of any one is constrained by characteristics of the others.

An example of this process of interrelated goals can be found in studies of the ways in which large mental hospitals establish administrative and clinical structures which will permit them to function in an optimal manner. The hospital administrator is faced by the need to deploy limited resources in such a way as to maximally benefit new admissions as well as long-term patients. Achieving the goal of optimal functioning is further complicated by the fact that the mental hospital as an organizational system is faced with many tasks besides its clinical one. The treating and discharging of patients must be considered as just one among several legitimate tasks including training, research, custodial care, and so on, which affect the over-all framework of the institution's administrative and clinical structure.

A recent study by Schulberg, Notman, and Bookin[14] of the treatment program at Boston State Hospital found that although the total number of inpatients not involved in any specific form of therapy had been reduced by 50 per cent between 1963 and 1965, geriatric patients have received little additional treatment in this period. The implication of this finding is clear-cut in the sense that one aspect of the hospital's treatment program is not functioning up to par and modification of this clinical service's structure seems warranted. What are the obstacles, then, to immediate implementation of the findings in this evaluation of goal attainment, i.e., treatment for all patients?

It becomes immediately evident that alteration of the geriatric unit's treatment program must have reverberations in many other facets of the hospital's total operation. Change in the technological component of the system, therefore, cannot be accomplished without equal attention to the implications of change for social aspects of the system. The goal-attainment model of evaluation often has restricted itself to recommendations about either altered forms of technology or administrative structure, without adequately considering the constraints imposed by other competing factors.

Returning to the services of a geriatric unit, the hospital superintendent might accept the findings of the previously cited treatment survey as a matter requiring his immediate attention and decide to increase the level of care on this unit by assigning additional psychiatric residents to it. In doing so, however, the superintendent must, first, overcome the widespread resistance of many residents to working with this aged population; second, operate within the constraint of his training program's guide lines regarding length of time that residents will spend on any one service; and third, consider the imbalance that will be created in other parts of the hospital by transferring additional residents to this unit. Realizing the complexity of these constraints, the superintendent may possibly decide that although the findings of the evaluation were certainly illuminating, they provide him with little guidance on the merits of altering the present situation in the face of the difficulties that change would create.

It is suggested that this brief example of the fate befalling an evaluation of goal attainment is representative of the process through which many studies have passed at the point when administrators considered implementing their findings.

System Model

In view of the implementation limitations inherent in the goal-attainment model of evaluation, what alternative is available to the researcher concerned with the utility of his findings? An approach which warrants more attention than it has received in the program evaluation literature is the system model. It is described by Etzioni[15] who points out that the starting point in this approach to evaluation is not the program's goal, as it is in the goal-attainment model of evaluation. Instead the system model of evaluation is concerned with establishing a working model of a social unit which is capable of achieving a goal. Unlike the study of a single goal, or even a set of goal activities, the system model is that of a multifunctional unit. It recognizes that an organization must fulfill at least four important functions for survival. In addition to the achievement of goals and subgoals, the system model is concerned with: the effective coordination of organizational subunits; the acquisition and maintenance of necessary resources; and the adaptation of the organization to the environment and to its own internal demands. The system model assumes that some of the organization's means must be devoted to such nonobvious functions as custodial activities, including means employed for maintenance of the organization itself. From the viewpoint of the system model, such activities are functional and actually increase organizational effectiveness.

In contrast to the goal-attainment model of evaluation which is concerned with degree of success in reaching a specific objective, the system model establishes the degree to which an organization realizes its goals under a given set of conditions. Etzioni indicates that the key question is: "Under the given conditions, how close does the organizational allocation of resources approach an optimum distribution?"[16] Optimum is the key word and what counts is a balanced distribution of resources among all organizational objectives, not maximal satisfaction of any one goal. From this perspective, just as a lack of resources for any one goal may be dysfunctional, so may an excess of resources for the goal be equally dysfunctional. In the latter instance, superfluous attention to one goal leads to depressed concern for the others and problems of coordination and competition will arise.

It should be noted that this model of evaluation is a more demanding and expensive one for the researcher. Instead of simply identifying the goals of the organization and proceeding to study whether they are attained, the system model requires that the analyst determine what he considers a highly effective allocation of means. This often requires considerable knowledge of the way in which an organization functions but it carries with it the advantage of being able to include in the analysis much more of the collected data than is possible in classical research design.

Another system model concept deserving consideration in regard to program evaluation is feedback mechanisms, i.e., the processes through which the effects of organizational actions are reported back to the organization and compared with desired performance. Inadequate utilization of research findings is an indication of blocked feedback and thus represents an organizational problem legitimately subject to scrutiny. The system model, therefore, provides not only a more adequate model for determining the types of data to be collected but it also has utility for determining the factors associated with effective or ineffective integration of the findings.

Turning now to the problem of utilizing the system model in producing change, several studies will be cited as examples of how this approach can be applied. An almost classic instance of the greater ability of the system model than the goal-attainment model to offer the program director sufficient guidance for implementing change can be found in the work of the Cummings[17] relative to mental health education. They started out to study to what extent and in what directions attitudes toward mental illness could be changed through an intensive educational program. After completing the six-month program, the Cummings found virtually no change in the population's general orientation, either toward the social problem of mental illness or toward the mentally ill themselves. If the goal-attainment model had been pursued, the researchers might simply have concluded that mental health education is ineffective and that the program should be dropped. Instead the Cummings shifted to a system model of evaluation and considered their data within the context of the functions, both manifest and latent, that traditional attitudes toward mental health play for the community as a social system. From this perspective, the researchers were able to formulate several hypotheses explaining the failure of their mental health education effort and to suggest possible concrete avenues for bringing about future change.

Another example of the use of the system model in evaluating program change can be found in studies[18,19] of the changing mental hospital. Baker[20] contends that viewing the hospital as an open system exchanging inputs and outputs with its environment promises to permit improved evaluation and program modification as the organization moves toward provision of comprehensive services. Three categories were identified by Baker for focus and intensive study: (1) the intraorganizational processes of the hospital; (2) the exchanges and transactions between the hospital and its environment; and (3) the processes and structures through which parts of the environment are related to one another. When attempting to implement the findings from one category, it becomes immediately evident that change may potentially affect the others as well. In a community mental health program the linked interdependence of all components in the system is of particular concern since modification of any one element can only occur within the framework of change for the entire system.

The system model suggests a variety of linkages and feedback mechanisms which can be used to bridge the gap between research findings and program modification. Individuals who have contact with the organization's environment as part of their regular work are considered in the system model to occupy "boundary roles." These people are particularly crucial for research implementation since they often are the first to receive information from external sources about the effectiveness of programs.

Boundary roles may occur at all levels of the organization but they usually are found at the top and bottom of the administrative structure. The program administrator at the top of the structure acts as a filter of research results because of his strong commitment and participation in the implementation of new programs. Negative evaluation of the program's effectiveness, however, may reflect adversely on his decision to back the program and in such a situation research findings may not be utilized properly. On the other hand, those occupying boundary roles lower in the organizational hierarchy often cannot make effective use of evaluation results because they do not have the formal authority to influence individuals at levels higher than themselves. A lower-level boundary role incumbent may pass on only that information which he thinks his superiors want to hear.

Since most health organizations lack a unit or individual specifically concerned with the translation of research into practice, it is suggested that planning divisions be established as one way to fill this void. The planner, being in a relatively objective and highly placed position for analyzing the total organization, can be sensitive to both the data emerging from program evaluation as well as to the unique characteristics of his facility. He, thus, can gauge the flexibility and constraints of his system in accepting the changes suggested by the results of evaluation.

To assist the feedback of research findings to the program administrator, increasing attention is being given to scientific communication. Professional information experts, librarians, abstractors, editors, and others, are employing a variety of hardware-oriented technics for making information more readily available to those who engage in even minimal information-seeking behavior. Examples include computer search programs, abstracting services, review papers, and various types of professional and interdisciplinary conferences. Perhaps these modern technics will partially solve the problem of researchers reporting their findings in forums and language which are foreign to program developers. These devices may be of particular importance when the research conducted in the focal organization is reported elsewhere by the researcher who is without a clear contract to feed back his findings to the organization under study.

A last problem to be considered in the development of feedback mechanisms is the time discrepancy that often occurs between administrators and evaluators. The time dimension of those closest to program implementation is often shorter and more variable than that of the evaluator who focuses upon a more distant horizon. It is suggested that feedback can be enhanced by the design of evaluation procedures which more appropriately fit the scheduled decision-making needs of an organization, and which have data available at a time when they can be used for planning.

Summary

In seeking to conceptualize possible approaches to program evaluation, two research models stand out: (a) the goal-attainment model, and (b) the system model. The characteristics and limitations of each were described as they affect the implementation of research findings. It is contended that the system model, by focusing upon the various factors determining research design and interpretation of the data, offers more promise for programmatic utilization of the evaluation findings. The system model also has utility for determining the factors associated with effective integration of the findings. It is suggested that organizations establish planning divisions because of the problems of blocked feedback to the organization of information on its performance and in order to insure translation of research.

REFERENCES

1. Menzel, H. Review of Studies in the Flow of Information Among Scientists. Bureau of Applied Social Research, Columbia Univ., January 1960. (Mimeo.)

2. Menzel, H. Scientific Communication: Five Themes from Social Science Research. Amer. Psychologist, 21: 999-1004, 1966. Reprinted as chapter 30 of this book.

3. Halpert, H. H. Communications as a Basic Tool in Promoting Utilization of Research Findings. Comm. Ment. Health J. 2: 231-236, 1966. Reprinted as chapter 31 of this book.

4. Ibid, p. 231.

5. Greenberg, B. G., and Mattison, B. F. The Whys and Wherefores of Program Evaluation. Canad. J. Pub. Health, 46: 293-299, 1955.

6. Knutson, A. L. Evaluation For What? Proceedings of the Regional Institute on Neurologically Handicapped Conditions in Children, held at the University of California, Berkeley, June 18-23, 1961. Reprinted as chapter 3 of this book.

7. Freeman, H. E., and Sherwood, C. C. Research in Large Scale Intervention Programs. J. Soc. Issues, 21: 11-28, 1965. Reprinted as chapter 6 of this book.

8. Herzog, Elizabeth. Some Guide Lines for Evaluative Research. Washington: Government Printing Office, 1959.

9. Knutson, op. cit.

10. James, G. Evaluation in Public Health Practice. Am. J. of Pub. Hlth. 52: 1145-1154, 1962. Reprinted as Chapter 2 of this book.

11. Etzioni, A. Two Approaches to Organizational Analysis: A Critique and a Suggestion. Adm. Sci. Quart. 5: 257-278, 1960. Reprinted as chapter 8 of this book.

12. Rice, A. K. The Enterprise and Its Environment. London: Tavistock Publications, 1963.

13. Sofer, C. The Organization From Within. London: Tavistock Publications, 1961.

14. Schulberg, H. C., Notman, R., and Bookin, E. Treatment Services at a Mental Hospital in Transition. Amer. J. Psychiat. 124: 506-513, 1967.

15. Etzioni, op. cit.

16. Ibid, p. 262.

17. Cumming, Elaine, and Cumming, J. Closed Ranks: An Experiment in Mental Health Education. Cambridge: Harvard University Press, 1957.

18. Schulberg, H. C., Caplan, G., and Greenblatt, M. Evaluating the Changing Mental Hospital: A Suggested Research Strategy. Ment. Hyg. 52: 218-225, 1968.

19. Baker, F. An Open-Systems Approach to the Study of Mental Hospitals in Transition. Comm. Men. Health J. 5: 403, 1969.

20. Ibid.

Index